PRAISE FOR

Wired to Eat

"*Wired to Eat* goes way beyond looking at food from a nutritional perspective. Robb Wolf reveals how food serves as information, actually influencing the expression of our DNA. . . . An incredibly user-friendly program that's in line with the most leading-edge research available. A landmark guide for regaining and maintaining health."

—David Perlmutter, M.D., author of the
#1 *New York Times* bestseller *Grain Brain,* and
The Grain Brain Whole Life Plan

"*Wired to Eat* is a scientifically sound and very easy-to-understand road map to optimal health. Robb Wolf presents clear, concise tools and strategies you can use to lose weight, control blood sugar and inflammation, and customize your diet. I highly recommend this groundbreaking program for anyone who has struggled with weight or health issues or who simply wants to get to the next level of well-being."

—Mark Sisson, author of *The Keto Reset Diet*
and publisher of MarksDailyApple.com

"*Wired to Eat* offers a cutting-edge view that goes way beyond Paleo and proves that resetting your metabolism is not about which foods you eat, it's about how your body responds to those foods. Robb Wolf offers readers an easy-to-follow, personal solution of how they can work with their bodies to finally find the foods that are right for them in order to achieve the optimal health they desire."

—Amy Myers, M.D., *New York Times* bestselling
author of *The Thyroid Connection* and *The
Autoimmune Solution*

Wired to Eat

Turn Off Cravings, Rewire Your Appetite for Weight Loss, and Determine the Foods That Work for You

ROBB WOLF

HARMONY BOOKS
NEW YORK

All rights reserved.
Published in the United States by Harmony Books, an imprint of Random House, a division of Penguin Random House LLC, New York.
harmonybooks.com

Harmony Books is a registered trademark, and the Circle colophon is a trademark of Penguin Random House LLC.

Originally published in hardcover in the United States by Harmony Books, an imprint of Random House, a division of Penguin Random House LLC, New York, in 2017.

Library of Congress Cataloging-in-Publication Data is available upon request.

ISBN 978-1-9848-2479-0
Ebook ISBN 978-0-451-49857-1

Printed in the United States of America

Book design by Jennifer K. Beal Davis
Illustrations by Mapping Specialists
Cover design by Jennifer Carrow

10 9 8 7 6 5 4 3 2 1

First Paperback Edition

For Sagan and Zoe

Contents

Beyond Paleo

I'm a forty-four-year-old father of two and husband to one (she is Italian and kind of territorial). I'm in pretty good shape and fiddle with Brazilian jujitsu and "old guy" gymnastics. Twenty years ago, I was a biochemist working in the areas of cancer and autoimmunity research. And I was sick. So sick, due to ulcerative colitis and a number of other niggling problems, that I was facing a bowel resection, statins, blood pressure medications, and antidepressants. That was the good part. The darker portion of the story went like this: I thought I was going to die, and the idea was pretty appealing, considering how much my life and health sucked.

I was a mess.

Through an interesting set of circumstances, which you'll hear about later in the book, the idea of a Paleo or ancestral diet made its way onto my radar, and out of abject desperation, I tried this seemingly wacky way of eating. This decision saved my life. All my health problems resolved in a matter of months. I shared this transformation with my doctors, including my gastroenterologist, rheumatologist, general practitioner, and therapist, all of whom said, "It's great that you're doing better, but it has nothing to do with your dietary changes."

Some people in the medical and academic world play an interesting game—if you say to them, "I hit my hand with a hammer and it hurt," their response is "Well, naturally!" But if you tell these same people that changing your nutrition had a profound impact on your health, their response is, "Well, that's nice, but it's just anecdotal." There is a common saying in Scienceland: "A million anecdotes do not one shred of evidence make." This is true, but if you see a million of the same anecdotes, perhaps it's time to apply some scientific rigor to the question, yes?

Whether my experience of profound health improvement by modifying what I ate was scientific or quasimystical, it convinced me that working through the mainstream outlets was not where I wanted to spend my time. I'd been on a path to attend medical school but the prospect of becoming like my medical providers and professors effectively euthanized my desire to be a doctor. I wondered how I could best help people with their health and fitness, and spending eight years learning about disease and disease management seemed like a circuitous route at best. So I made a serious career shift and opened a gym. Well, actually, two gyms. And they happened to be the first and fourth CrossFit affiliate gyms in the world. I incorporated the Paleo diet philosophy and tenets into my business, which included education about sleep, nutrition, and smart movement. I combined these elements to create a supportive, challenging group health and exercise model that folks loved. Our clients achieved remarkable success, ranging from profound weight loss to dramatically improved health. Our results were so impressive that my little 4,000-square-foot gym in Chico, California, was picked as one of *Men's Health* magazine's "Top 30 Gyms in America."

Word got out that what we were doing was different than the standard approach to health and fitness, and people wanted to know how to do this for themselves, their patients, and clients. I started blogging so I could reach an audience outside our local community and spent a lot of time traveling, not just in the US but also internationally, to speak in front of tens of thousands of people on this topic. The more people who tried something like a Paleo diet, the more remarkable stories I heard. The concept seemed to be spreading faster than a venereal disease on a college campus. I started a podcast that climbed to the top of the iTunes charts and wrote my first book, *The Paleo Solution*, which became a *New York Times* bestseller. I was as surprised as anyone by this success. Soon enough, the "just anecdotal" reports on how this way of eating was changing lives (now in the millions) shifted to some interesting scientific studies. There might be something to this "fad diet" after all.

Still, there were some problems brewing. Both academics and the media loved to portray the Paleo diet as some kind of historical reenactment, poking fun at the "caveman" motif, which became inseparable from the Paleo diet idea. For many people, the whole caveman schtick was a nonstarter. So although many millions were benefiting from the information people like myself were sharing with the world, far more people would not give Paleo eating more than a glance due to an emotional response to the idea. My goal has always been to help as many people as possible, so this "marketing and image problem" was a significant hurdle.

Perhaps even more frustrating, however, was the tendency for folks who actually followed the Paleo diet to turn the general concepts into quasi-religious doctrine. Folks newly converted to Paleo tended to be quite dogmatic in the insistence that this was "the one true way" to eat. Often, these devotees had reversed serious health problems with this way of eating, so their enthusiasm was understandable, but not many people enjoy the company of or the message from someone who comes across as a holier-than-thou diet zealot.

The reality is, some of these folks might have had success on a low-carb version of Paleo and never considered that other people, and even they themselves, might benefit from a higher-carb version. A remarkable number of people are insulin resistant for reasons I will detail later. If these people restore their blood sugar levels through a low-carb diet, better sleep, and exercise (thereby reversing that insulin resistance), they often find they can tolerate eating more carbs and still lose weight. In *Wired to Eat*, I'll explain why this is and detail the latest research surrounding this idea. With my new program, you will discover where you are in this story and learn the amounts and types of carbs you can eat while staying lean and healthy. And that's just the beginning.

The Ancestral Health or Paleo diet model I talked about in my first book is incredibly powerful, but these concepts are tools and starting points, not final destinations. As you'll soon learn, one size does not fit all, and that has never been more evident than now with the newest research on Personalized Nutrition. As you will discover in *Wired to Eat*, you now have the opportunity to go beyond general guidelines and find which foods, including which carbs, work best for you, regardless of your age, weight, or health status. And that's what makes the plan in this book so unique. By the end of your journey, you will understand the genetic and epigenetic factors that govern how you are wired to eat, but perhaps more important, you will finally have a plan customized to your body to help you lose weight, regain your health, and live the life you want to live. No more guessing which foods are right for you. In a little more than thirty days, your life and health could be radically transformed for the better as you heal your gut and refine your personal eating plan.

PART 1

Know Thyself: How You Are Wired to Eat

One Size Does Not Fit All

I f I have learned anything over the years, it's that we all tend to benefit from general guidelines, but our individual needs may be profoundly different than those of our neighbor. This can create a bias that makes us think what worked for us or someone we know will work for everyone. So although we'd like to keep things as simple as possible, when we gear things for an individual's needs, things can get complex in a hurry.

Understanding how and why we need to change our eating and lifestyle to be healthy or lose weight can be relatively easy in practice ("Hey, buddy, just do *this*!"), but if folks need convincing, if they need to understand the whys and the details, well, that takes some work. So which is better: simplicity or complexity? Well, it depends. Both approaches have pitfalls. An overly simplistic view of the Paleo diet led to a mindless process of asking, "Is this food Paleo?" versus the more appropriate question, "Is this food a good option for *me*?" On the other hand, if the details on how the diet works start to look like Advanced Chemistry, a typical reader would rather roll around naked in broken glass. I will aim to strike a balance between the two extremes, giving you sufficient information in a simple way so you understand how these choices will help you live a healthier life.

There is a (likely) fictional account of the famous artist and inventor Michelangelo that describes how he produced his masterwork sculpture

David. He was asked what his process was for creating such detailed and lifelike work, and he responded with something to the effect of, "I cut away everything that did not look like David." Sculptors, woodworkers, engineers, and artisans of all types use a variety of tools and strategies to produce their work. The tools used in the beginning are for the "rough work," while other tools are used to produce the refined, finished product. As powerful as the Paleo diet or Ancestral Health perspective is, in this book, that strategy is used as a "rough" tool. Ultimately, I will help you find your own customized eating plan that will help you achieve your goals.

Recent research has shed light on the need to go beyond doctrine in order to find what works for us individually. In *Wired to Eat*, I will show you how to use this information to create your own effective, customized eating plan that can change your life and your health. How's this possible? In recent studies, hundreds of people were fed a variety of foods and their individual blood glucose responses were tracked over time. To everyone's surprise, there was not a one-size-fits-all "best diet," but rather massive variation, from person to person and in the types of foods each individual reacted favorably or negatively to. This is groundbreaking because it indicates some foods create a healthy response in some people while creating a negative response in others. It shows that we can find the foods that work with our physiology instead of against it. We have never had an opportunity like this, as our previous efforts, although well intentioned, have lacked the precision we now have with this new approach to eating called Personalized Nutrition. Personalized Nutrition, in practical terms, means that you will be able to test specific foods in order to determine which work for your weight loss and health journey. Personalized Nutrition allows us to use big-picture concepts like the Paleo diet to get going in a good direction, but then we can "map" exactly which foods are best (or worst) for us. You'll discover that there may be "bad" foods you've been avoiding for years, like rice or potatoes, that your body can actually tolerate. On the flip side, you may also discover that there are "healthy" foods you've been eating that are causing more harm than good on your weight loss and health journey.

PERSONALIZED NUTRITION FOR PERSONAL SUCCESS

With *Wired to Eat*, I attempt to reach people with two key concepts: one, an understanding of the genetic and environmental factors, such as sleep, stress, hyperpalatable foods, and community, that make it easy for us to overeat; and two, the powerful tool of Personalized Nutrition. Understanding how we are wired to eat will remove the morality and guilt often associated with attempting dietary changes. This is a plan that allows you to refine all the food rules you've been taught while discovering what works best for *you*. The program laid out in these pages will help you rewire your brain and appetite, allowing you to better control your blood sugar, and determine the foods that are right for *your* health and weight loss. Using the science of epigenetics, we will understand that our genes are not our destiny.

By altering our sleep, food, exercise, and social connections, we will shift all the factors governing our metabolism in a way that makes success easy. Additionally, we will lean heavily on the latest behavior change insights, which support the idea that we are not all the same. Some people will find success by abstaining from certain trigger foods. Others will be able to moderate their intake of (rather than avoid completely) certain foods. After reading this book, and doing a little self-experimentation, you will know which strategy will work best for you. Once appetite and blood sugar are in check, you will find it easier to lose weight and prevent or reverse a number of health problems, ranging from obesity and diabetes to heart disease and neurodegenerative diseases like Parkinson's and Alzheimer's.

How will we do all this? Glad you asked. In Phase One, we will determine what your primary needs and goals are (who you are and where you want to go), and from this we will use a simple but powerful 30-Day Reset (a much more detailed program than appeared in my first book) to rewire your appetite and get you moving in the right direction. With it, you will discover if you are insulin resistant (or not), and based on this finding, we will adjust your carb intake to reflect your relative metabolic health. I have teased people in the past for believing they are "unique snowflakes," but the joke has been on me in that regard. We *are* all unique—we are all outliers to some degree. To address the nearly infinite variety of individuals, I have developed Phase Two, a unique 7-Day Carb Test plan based on the latest science concerning Personalized Nutrition. Using easy-to-understand subjective measures, like how you feel after a meal, as well as a blood glucose monitor that will set you back $5 to $20, we can precisely determine what amounts and types of carbohydrates and other foods allow you to keep your blood sugar within healthy ranges.

Let's take a look at what I hope to accomplish in the book and give you a sense of where we are going and how the program will change the way you eat and live for the better.

THE PATH TO PERMANENT WEIGHT LOSS

Millions of people start a diet each year, but the vast majority fail to achieve the results they desire. Why is that? Is it a moral failing on our part, or is there more to the story than a "weak will"? Instead of moralizing eating, perhaps we should consider that we live in a world that is ill suited to our genetics, that our food, sleep, movement, and social connections (the Four Pillars of Health, as I call them) have changed in ways that our bodies find difficult to adapt to. If we understand how our world has changed, how our genetics are wired for a different world, we can free ourselves of the shame and misplaced morality associated with the inherent difficulties of change. We can finally stop blaming ourselves for our inability to lose weight and get healthy. We'll start the book with an understanding of why your weight-loss challenges are not your fault and help you understand how and why the plan in the book will change your life.

Humans are the most adaptable organism on the planet, but our food and environment have changed so rapidly that we are now ill equipped to deal with the modern world. Our genetic tendency to overeat is the root cause of everything from diabetes to neurodegenerative disease. You'll learn about these concepts as well as our tendency to indulge in nearly limitless flavor and palate options. We now eat like professionals. And yes, that's as bad as it sounds.

Before we get to the program and the how-to, I'll help you understand the importance of digestion. It is far more significant to your health than simply understanding how many calories we eat. We will learn that, yes, calories do matter, but so do the amounts and types of food we eat, as the different macronutrients (protein, carbs, and fat) have very different effects on our hormones, which dramatically alter our sense of satiety and fullness.

You will learn that thousands of scientific studies suggest that many of the degenerative diseases we face—from diabetes to obesity to autoimmunity—are tied to a breakdown in our digestive process, specifically in the gut. We will learn how refined carbohydrates alter our gut in ways that predispose us to insulin resistance and a host of conditions, ranging from heart disease to Alzheimer's and Parkinson's. We will also learn how certain foods (such as those containing gluten) may be involved in the development of autoimmune disease and systemic inflammation. Armed with this information we now have a tool to take the general principles of the Ancestral Health approach and create a program customized to your individual needs.

The Paleo diet is more misunderstood than a Goth kid living in Arkansas. As such, we will consider the common misconceptions around the Paleo diet and do something totally wacky: look at the scientific evidence. The Paleo diet approach is a powerful tool, but it is merely a starting place. Human evolution did not stop in the Paleolithic era, and although many conditions may greatly benefit from this basic approach, we can now customize our eating and lifestyle in a way that optimizes weight loss, health, and enjoyment.

GETTING STARTED

Once you've learned why it's hard to avoid the temptations of modern processed food, it'll be time to start doing. With my 30-Day Reset, you'll figure out what your goals are and what eating plan is right for you. Central to this story, we will discover if you are insulin resistant and, if so, to what degree. This information will help us determine which path you take as the insulin-resistant individual and it will have you eating on the lower-carb end of the spectrum (possibly exploring the use of nutritional ketosis and fasting), at least until you reset your system by losing weight and reversing your insulin resistance. We will look at the strategies of prepping your home and outside life to stay on track and make lasting progress.

We'll then move on to the 7-Day Carb Test plan, which will change your life by helping you determine the foods that are right for *your* body and for *your* weight loss. Modern technology like wearable blood glucose monitors allow us to discover which foods and what amounts produce the blood glucose response that is best for us. We will look at some of your commonly consumed carb sources and map how you respond to them. This information is critical if you're going to create the health and weight loss plan that is most effective for *you*. It is a truly groundbreaking feature of *Wired to Eat*, because it's key to understanding how to normalize your appetite, reduce inflammation, lose weight, and get healthy.

And no eating plan is complete without a quick word on cheating. In my twenty years of working with people, I have seen how they undermine their success with regard to food and lifestyle changes. Perhaps the most injurious is the misguided notion of "cheating" on our eating. We don't "cheat" on our food. We do not need a "healthy relationship" with our food. We simply need to understand that there are consequences to our food choices. The mind-set surrounding the "cheating" mentality is almost a guarantee of failure and puts the focus in the wrong place, when the real problem is most likely a lack of love and connection. Now is the opportunity to change our minds and our lives.

Beyond the eating plan, which is crucial for ultimate well-being and health, we also need to rebalance the other three important pillars in our lives: sleep, community, and movement. Our food choices are important, but chow is only part of the story when we consider our health and our waistline. We will first look at sleep and photoperiod, as inadequate sleep and altered circadian rhythm dramatically influence our metabolism and food choices. We will then look at exercise (movement) from an ancestral perspective and understand that the most important activity we can do is the one we love and will stick with. In looking at stress, we will learn that there are important things we can do to minimize stress, but ironically, it may be far more important to change our perception of stress than to try to become a monk on a mountaintop. Finally, we will look at the forgotten feature of health and happiness: community. Humans are social beings, and without adequate social connection our health and longevity can be as negatively impacted as if we had a pack-a-day smoking habit.

The *Wired to Eat* program will make change as simple and effective as possible. You will find easy-to-fix meals that will help you succeed on your weight-loss and health journey. All have been developed by Charles and Julie Mayfield, authors of the bestselling *Paleo Comfort Foods* books. These are delicious, time-efficient meals that will make it easy to maximize your weight loss and stick with the program over the long haul.

For some of you, the basic plan I've outlined may not be enough, so I've also provided a chapter on the ketogenic diet and fasting that might be the answer for your needs, particularly if you are type 2 diabetic or suffering from (or at high risk for) neurodegenerative disease. Ketogenic diets have been used for nearly a hundred years to treat conditions such as epilepsy, while fasting may have been used for several thousand years to remedy a host of ailments. Fasting and ketosis offer profound options for conditions ranging from obesity to neurodegenerative disease, yet most of the medical community considers them to be dangerous, despite the fact research demonstrates them to be both safer and more efficacious than most of the conventional therapies. You will learn if you are appropriate for fasting or ketosis, how to do it, and what to monitor to know if this is indeed the right tool for your needs.

Similar to my first book, I'll offer some latitude as to how you tackle this material. If you are a hair-on-fire self-starter and are ready to jump in and get going, you can skip to the prescriptive chapters in Part Two. I counsel against this, however. If you understand the mechanisms of why change can be hard, many of your questions and possible confusion will be addressed. You do not need to understand this material for the program to work any more than you need to understand the physics of an internal combustion engine to drive a car. *But.* There is a massive amount of conflicting information available at your fingertips. Your family, friends, and coworkers are likely to try to scuttle your progress for both well- and ill-intentioned reasons. You will be deluged with material from the media, which is confusing and contradictory. I explain all these details so you know how your body works, how the world has changed, and why that makes for a difficult set of circumstances with regard to weight and health. This book is not *7 Easy Steps to Jaw-Dropping Abs*. It is a story that builds a chapter at a time, and as that story unfolds, you will understand both how you are wired to eat and how to take advantage of the latest research to work with your genetics instead of against them. All of this cerebral/logical stuff is likely not what will get you to try or stick with the program, but it is the strategy many people use to avoid change, so yes, I do recommend you take each chapter in its due course. How I can help guarantee your success, however, is if I can help you *feel*, not just understand, but *feel* that the difficulty you may have faced your whole life is not your fault, merely a set of circumstances that you and I need to work through. This is the culmination of nearly twenty years of working with people to help them improve their health, lose weight, and live the life they want. This is an amazing time we live in, as we now have the knowledge and tools to make change (almost) easy. I am fully committed to helping you and I hope you are ready to experience life-changing benefits of the plan in *Wired to Eat*.

CHAPTER 2

It's Not Your Fault

Y ou hold in your hands what is commonly referred to as "A Diet Book." If you have good sense—meaning you do not play the lottery, gamble, or worry overmuch about shark attacks—you should likely put this book down and back away slowly. Or perhaps fling it as far as you can and scream, "Kill it! Kill it with fire!" Why? Because . . . well, diets generally fail.

Abysmally.

The only process that fails folks more often than diets is starting a campfire by vigorously rubbing snow cones against wet toilet paper.

You may be wondering, *What the heck is this guy doing? Am I supposed to be inspired by this?* Well, I *am* trying to sell you on the idea of both reading and implementing the contents of this book. But a relationship should be built on honesty. That considered, you need to know there are no tricks, potions, or gimmicks that will make this change easy. Based on my nearly twenty years of experience in and around things like weight loss and elite human performance, cancer, and autoimmunity research, I know the ideas expressed herein can dramatically improve how you look, feel, and perform. I also *know* without a doubt that for some folks, effecting the changes I recommend here will be tough. Critically important, but potentially tough. Slick ad-copy mavens would have me write that this process will entail "effortless weight loss that will leave you feeling satisfied and energized!" That *will* happen for some people. For others, the lifeline I'm throwing you via this book is going to look more like a bag of rocks. But that very toughness, the difficulty most people experience in trying to change diet and lifestyle habits, is completely normal. In fact, it would be silly (or at least uninformed) to expect diet and lifestyle changes to be easy.

If you have struggled with diets in the past, you are not the exception—you are the rule. Conservative estimates are that more than 45 million Americans start a diet each year, many trying four or five times per year to affect long-standing, meaningful weight and health changes. The vast majority fail. A recent piece by NPR made the point that most Americans better understand how to do their taxes than how to eat well. The government and media pummel us with trite bits of advice like "Eat Less, Move More" or, my longtime favorite, "Everything in Moderation." In a world where soda is cheaper than bottled water, what does *moderation* even mean? We are told it's all about "calories in, calories out," so "just eat less." If you can't get with the program, you are a weak-willed glutton, right?

Wrong.

If we look at the epidemic rates of obesity, diabetes, and cardiovascular disease, conditions that are well known to be caused by not "eating less, moving more," it is clear that this simple advice is either too simple or just plain wrong. And the first part of this book will explain why this and many other weight loss theories are, if not wrong then massively ill informed.

I want you to understand that the difficulties you face, be they health or weight related, are not your fault. Thus, we will begin the story of how you are wired to eat by first looking at why the modern world may be working against the fundamental genetic programming we all carry within every cell of our bodies. Once you understand this concept, in the next chapter, I'll begin to explain how and why we are wired to eat and what we can ultimately do about it.

I know we are just getting to know each other, but let me tell you something that you might find preposterous. If you live in a modern Westernized society of relative leisure and abundance but are *not* fat, sick, and diabetic, you are, from a biological perspective, "screwing up." Really. Our species is here today because our genes are wired to eat damn near everything that is not nailed down. Related to this is an expectation, again woven into our genes, that the process of finding food requires that we are active. In unambiguous terms, we are genetically wired to eat simple, unprocessed foods, and to expend a fair amount of energy in that process (walk, run, lift, carry, *dance*!). But modern life affords us the opportunity to move hardly at all, while finding ourselves surrounded by the most varied assortment of delectable food imaginable. It is now possible to order food to your door, work from home, and count the number of steps we take in the dozens, when our not-distant ancestors routinely walked 5 to 10 miles *per day*. This is our conundrum.

IT'S NOT YOU, IT'S THEM

The scientific proposition I will draw from throughout the book is called the Discordance Hypothesis. An oblique-sounding term, but actually quite simple: Organisms, be they sequoias, sand flies, or people, tend to have a set of genes that are reasonably well suited to their environment. Your environment is everything from your food to the weather to how much sleep and sunlight you get. Changes in that environment can be positive, negative, or neutral for the critter in question. I, and many other scientists, make the case that although there have been undeniable benefits from easy access to food, indoor plumbing, and reality TV, this ease and entertainment has come at a price—namely, an explosion in what we call Western degenerative diseases: obesity, diabetes (types 1 and 2), Parkinson's, Alzheimer's, and a host of other conditions.

So it comes down to this: The tendency to "eat all the food," bail on the latest ineffective diet trend, and look at the gym as being just north of a prison sentence, is *normal*. It ain't crazy. But eating a modern diet and sitting on our keister for an endless number of hours is not good for how we look or how we feel.

Overhauling your environment—that is, your approach to food, sleep, and movement—may all seem a bit daunting, but you can make some amazing improvements and obtain life-changing results. The solutions I put forward in this book focus on understanding how changes in our sleep, food, activity, exposure to sunlight, gut microorganisms, and lack of community are causing health problems. By extension, this understanding will provide a road map (which leans heavily on the tool of Personalized Nutrition) for how to fix what ails us. The change is doable, but you need to commit to the process. So it's not your fault you find yourself here, but if you want a different outcome, you will need to do some things differently.

CHANGE IS AFOOT (AND A GENE)!

Change comes in many forms and is most often good: it keeps us growing and engaged and makes life interesting. But we reasonably have only so much capacity to adapt. Sometimes change looks like a slow-moving bulldozer you can see coming from a mile away. Avoiding danger is easy, as long as you are not lying unconscious in front of it. At other times, it happens like a meteor impact wiping out most of life on earth. We need to understand how changes in our food and environment are testing the ability of our genetics to cope with a world that they (and we) may be ill suited to thrive in. Our world in which generations of our ancestors lived has changed in remarkable ways, and although much good has come of this, there are some downsides, too, which need to be managed lest we end up at the hurting end of the change bulldozer.

IT'S NOT ABOUT THE ~~NAIL~~ (FOOD)

Although we will spend significant time exploring the first pillar of health (food) we will also consider how changes to our sleep, exercise, and social connections (community) have worked in a synergistic fashion to undermine our health. I do not use the term *pillar* arbitrarily here: these concepts are all critically important to our success. You will learn how good sleep, healthy movement, and loving relationships all play into our health and appearance.

THE FOUR PILLARS GONE AWRY

Things have really changed for human beings, and some of this change has come at a high price. More than ten thousand years ago, our ancestors lived as hunter-gatherers. They ate largely whole, unprocessed foods that changed with location and the seasons. The work involved with finding food, shelter, and the necessities of life was not easy. Folks were not lifting weights and jogging on treadmills, but they did a lot of hard physical activity. And this hard work was followed by significant amounts of rest; our ancestors generally kept the hours the seasons dictated. Although not an idyllic paradise, people ate nutritious foods, slept a lot, and got significant amounts of exercise during their daily activities. Another important feature of the ancestral life-way was the remarkable amount of social support. People lived in extended family groups that offered literally cradle-to-grave social connections.

With the advent of agriculture, most people shifted from a foraging or hunter-gatherer life-way to a settled, agricultural approach. This transition *generally* meant a reduced variety of foods and a host of well-documented ailments. Living in close proximity to larger numbers of people as well as animals appears to have posed a significant immune challenge for our early agricultural ancestors. Reliance on starchy, low-nutrient foods such as grains also appears to have posed a significant challenge with regard to growth and nutrient deficiencies. From the perspective of sleep and circadian rhythm, we still tended to go to bed not long after the sun went down and got up when the sun came up. And although work on farms required significant amounts of physical labor, we got a lot of downtime.

Fast-forward to about two hundred years ago: Folks left the farm for factory work and urban life. Gas lighting was limited to the large urban centers, so the amount of additional "daytime" people could experience via artificial light was not remarkably different than it had been ten thousand years earlier. Social networks and extended families continued to be relatively strong. Though increased mobility allowed people to follow work opportunities, entire families tended to move together.

And then the lightbulb was invented. The long-lasting, electrically powered, incandescent lightbulb became relatively cheap and ubiquitous, and it democratized a number of things like learning and entertainment. Where previously only the wealthy could afford significant amounts of artificial light, now almost everyone could partake of this miracle. This opened up whole new ways of doing business and dramatically changed industry. Factories could run all night, the concept of shift work was born, and human innovation exploded. As good as all this was for most of humanity, we began sleeping less in general and started our first experiments with shift work. Antibiotics were only a few decades in the future, and although these wonder drugs would save millions of lives, the unintended impact on our gut microbes (and overall health) would not be well appreciated until the beginning of the twenty-first century.

LIFE TODAY: OUR BODIES HAVEN'T CAUGHT UP

About thirty years ago, the explosion of microprocessors and technology innovation ushered in the Internet, 24/7 commerce, and dozens, then hundreds, then thousands of cable TV channels. If we wanted entertainment, education, or distraction, it was only a dial-up phone connection away (and now just a dip into your pocket for your smartphone). We work much more and sleep much less than we did even in the 1980s, about 2.5 hours less per day on average for most Americans. This change in not only sleep but also our constant exposure to artificial light (which affects every body system you care to consider) is perhaps the most profound change humanity has experienced.

As we will see in subsequent chapters, our food system began to rapidly change, shifting us away from largely traditional home-cooked meals to grab-'n'-go options, as well as an avalanche of processed, hyperpalatable foods. *Palatability* refers to how tasty something is. Grass is generally "not that tasty," i.e., it's a low-palatability item (unless you are a horse, in which case it's pretty damn tasty). Chocolate ice cream with toffee chunks and salted almond sprinkles . . . well, that's extremely palatable!

Our gut microbiota likely underwent a profound change due to antibiotic use, modern medical procedures, and an increasing focus on products like hand sanitizers and antimicrobial soaps. It's worth noting that changes in the gut correlate strongly with increasing rates of obesity, cardiovascular disease, and neurodegeneration. In a later chapter, we will explore how alterations in the gut can play into these conditions.

In terms of exercise, until quite recently humans moved to survive. We had to gather food, firewood, and water while shifting encampments based on weather and the season. Anthropologists have estimated that hunter-gatherers walked 5 to 10 miles most days. Today, many of us walk less than a half mile every day as we shuffle from house to car to office and back again.

On a social level, the past thirty years have seen the most profound changes in all of human history. Our highly mobile, information-based society has been a boon for work opportunities, but an unintended consequence has been a profound increase in social isolation, particularly for the elderly. Humans are social animals. We evolved in small groups, and this process has literally altered our genetics to "expect" certain amounts and types of interaction with not just other people, but the natural world around us. Social isolation is recognized as a huge stressor and appears to be a key piece of addictive behavior, including overeating. Although epidemiological in nature, studies have indicated that inadequate social connectivity increases early death potential as much as a pack-a-day smoking habit.

Inadequate sleep, constant stress, and bad food have become the norm. So if everyone is doing it, if we wear our sleep deprivation, hard work, and ability to eat like a garbage disposal as a badge of honor, what could be wrong with that? It's simple: our bodies haven't caught up to these changes. Ten thousand years might seem like a very long time, but in the context of our genes, it's more like a meteoric environmental change than that slow-moving bulldozer.

In the chapters that follow, I'll go into more detail about the health and weight loss benefits of orienting our sleep, food, movement, and community along lines informed by the knowledge of our ancestors. For now, recognizing these changes within the context of how our genetics are wired (a world of more sleep, ample sunlight, whole food, loving relationships, and significant physical activity) makes the bars of an invisible cage suddenly spring into view. We are then faced with the choice of opening that cage and leaving, or clinging to our current condition. I wish we could all keep doing the same things and expect different results, but that does not seem to be the way the rules of this game have been written. If we want a different result, we need to do something different. Shocker, right? You'd be surprised how many people I've worked with who faced potentially life-threatening conditions put a heroic effort into figuring out how to keep doing what they were doing while expecting a different outcome.

IT'S NOT YOUR FAULT, BUT . . .

My main tool to help you is information, which effectively motivates only a small percentage of people. Most of the processes governing eating and movement happen at a deep level in the brain, the level dedicated to sex, survival, and good feelings. So although the information presented here is my best effort to accurately describe the challenges we all face in this modern world of hyperpalatable foods, sedentariness, and abnormal light exposure, I realize that information alone is not enough for most of you.

In my first book I laid out a great "Arthur Murray Dance School" process of "just put your right foot here, your left foot there," and it has helped a lot of people. But as many people as that book has helped, many more need a bit more than to be told to "do this." They need systems, accountability, and tools that bring synergy between the impulsive and logical portions of the brain. To that end, this book will provide detailed plans on how to discover your individual reaction to food so we can get the right "air fuel mixture" (food) to help you look and feel your best. I will also help you understand your psychology and impulses around food, exercise, and relationships so you can leverage your strengths and firewall your weaknesses. I have worked with many high-level mixed martial arts (MMA) competitors, and one of my jobs as a coach is to help the athlete prepare mentally and physically to fight the fight on *their* terms, not their opponent's terms. Helping you understand your wiring and tendencies will put you in a similarly advantaged state.

You hold in your hands what is commonly referred to as a "diet book." For some unknown reason, you have read this far. Now all I ask is that you keep going, give the material honest consideration, and, most important, devote a small portion of what will hopefully be a long, enjoyable life to testing the ideas I've developed here. At worst, in a little more than thirty days, you will decide I'm another idiot who wrote a diet book. At best, you may look at your life as the time before and the time after you understood how you are wired to eat.

CHAPTER 3

Mosquitos, Appetite, and Hyperpalatable Food

I f you take in much in the way of media—be that TV, print, or even the interwebz—you have likely seen ads or offers for seemingly foolproof fat-loss plans. "Try this one weird trick to lose 50 pounds!" The scientist in me says, "Well, maybe it will work." My slightly toned-down public persona might say, "This seems a bit farfetched." But if you catch me in private, after I've had a drink or two, you'll likely hear, "This is a bunch of overly simplistic bullshit."

The lifestyle too many of us find ourselves in—besieged by hyperpalatable foods, poor sleep, and too much stress—is not amenable to a simple solution. Many people try altering their diet and lifestyles each year and the vast majority fail. Again and again. This failure, however, is context specific. In our not-so-distant past, lazing about whenever possible and eating everything in sight was how we survived. Yet in our modern world of plenty, inactivity and overeating are disastrous. This mismatch between our genetics and our modern world is at best complex: our sleep, food, activity levels, gut health, and social connections (or lack thereof) all conspire to make health and a stable weight difficult to maintain.

If there is one "simple" trick that will make better eating easy, it is fixing the neuroregulation of appetite. This is the natural process of our brain literally telling us if we are hungry or not. If the neuroregulation of appetite is functioning properly, we will eat enough to have great energy, but remain lean and healthy. The challenge is that our food, sleep, activity, gut microbiome, stress levels, and emotional connection to food all affect the neuroregulation of appetite in potentially unfavorable ways. So although our sound bite is "just fix your appetite," there are a number of moving parts that go into that. Which is why this is a book and not a bumper sticker.

CALORIES COUNT, BUT ARE THEY THE *SAME*?

You'd be hard-pressed to find someone in this day and age who is not familiar with the concept of a "calorie"—that it is the amount of energy a given food contains. We've all heard that the secret to weight loss and good health is to eat foods with fewer calories or just fewer calories overall. So, we read labels (a problem right from the start, since labels usually mean processed food) and try to keep our total caloric intake under some limit based on our size and activity level. This all seems reasonably scientific and straightforward but this veneer of "science" is actually a problem.

Although our physiology does track our net energy balance via body fat and blood glucose levels, people often reduce this story to the overly simplistic idea of "calories in, calories out." Hormones and neurotransmitters like insulin, leptin, and ghrelin are equally important and inseparable elements of how much we eat (the neuroregulation of appetite) and influence if we are lean or overweight. Calories do count, but not all foods produce the same hormonal and metabolic effects. The strict calories in, calories out folks would have us believe that 2,000 calories of sugar are metabolically equivalent to 2,000 calories of pork loin, broccoli, and sweet potato. Intuitively, this should smell as bad as products from Fukushima Fish Farms, Inc., but we do not need to rely on intuition—science shows this overly simplistic view, that "it's just about calories" is simply not true.

NEUROREGULATION OF APPETITE, OR, HOW DO WE KNOW WHEN "ENOUGH IS ENOUGH"?

You likely have a better social life than I do, so you have probably never asked yourself, *How do I know how much food to eat?* It's a simple yet important question when we think about the process of overeating. We've all eaten meals that have made us feel happy, satisfied, and energized mentally and physically. We do not get hungry again for several hours, and when we do, the hunger is mild, just enough to get our attention and remind us, "Hey, it's time to eat!" We have all also consumed meals that have left us feeling bloated and generally miserable. Our energy was poor, our minds were foggy, and, ironically, we were *hungry* again not too long after eating, often while our stomach was still uncomfortably full. How can this be?

When most people think about hunger or fullness, they largely focus on their stomach and how "full" it has become. There is certainly something to this, but the story is much more complex. Most of what we perceive to be hunger or fullness occurs in the brain.* Stomach distension is an important part of the satiety signal cascade, but it can be overridden by the brain. You could be ravenous, drink a large cup of water (which is often a recommended technique of failed weight-loss programs), and still be ravenous. Our bodies need energy in the form of food—not too much, not too little. We have complex systems that monitor how much food we have taken in versus how much energy we have expended. Additionally, our body-fat level is monitored. These variables, which consider both our short-term and long-term energy status, determine our neuroregulation of appetite. I'm going to go into a bit of detail with regard to the hormones and neurotransmitters that govern appetite, and when you understand how this process works you will appreciate how and why the 30-Day Reset will be so effective in rewiring your appetite, which will help you to lose weight and get healthy. Before we get to that, let me use a simple analogy we are all familiar with to provide some context.

FUEL UP!

It's likely that most everyone reading this has at some point filled a car's gas tank with gasoline. Typically, when the gauge gets close to empty, we hastily make our way to the closest refueling option in order to avoid the amazing exercise of pushing our car to a gas station. If the pump is working properly, the nozzle can sense when our tank is nearly full and will automatically stop the filling process. Occasionally, however, that sensing mechanism is broken and our gas tank can overfill, spilling gas to the ground below. We could also, foolishly, bypass the off function by holding the pump open. That last part is an important point to keep in mind.

---

* Well, if you get right down to it, *all* of our experience occurs in the brain. My point in talking about the neuroregulation of appetite is that our sense of full or empty has much more to do with communication of various hormones and neurotransmitters than it does with precisely how full our bellies are.

The gas tank of our car is analogous to not just our bellies' contents, but also our blood sugar and body fat levels. It is a sense of how much stored energy we have available to us, not just within our digestive tract but our whole body. The fuel pump at the service station is analogous to our brain in that it can sense when we are empty, but, more important, *should* tell us when we are full. However, depending upon the food we eat, the flavor combinations, our sleep status, our stress levels, and our gut biome, we can bypass the off switch in our brain. Conversely, if we are well rested, relatively stress-free, and making good food choices, our brain will alert us damn near perfectly when we've had enough to eat. This is what the second part of the book is all about, fixing the various problems we have with regard to the neuroregulation of appetite.

OPTIMUM FORAGING STRATEGY: HOW WE LEARNED TO EAT ENOUGH, BUT GET BORED OF PLENTY

Every moving critter on the planet, from bacteria to people, unconsciously uses a process called optimum foraging strategy (OFS). OFS is a pattern of movement that tends to maximize the amount of calories and nutrition an individual obtains while minimizing the amount of energy expended to do so. If we think about this like a bank account, it makes perfect sense: you must have more money going into your account than out, or you will have problems. For certain predatory or omnivorous animals, this may mean staking out a choice spot to waylay prey, while grazing animals attempt to find the choicest fodder with the least amount of movement. It's hard out there in the wild when you're a critter both competing for food *and* avoiding becoming someone else's snack! OFS plays into how our genes are wired to experience the world. Our genetics are expecting an environment in which procuring a meal requires a significant amount of energy, but we were pitched a curveball by the changes in not just our food supply but also our sleep and activity patterns. Nature does not exist in a supermarket. We now live in a state of plenty unimaginable a few hundred years ago. It is this mismatch that is at the heart of not just weight gain but also most of the health issues we face.

OFS has another facet that is important when we bring this story back to how and why we overeat in the first place—a concept called palate fatigue. Our palate is our sense of taste (which includes significant input from our sense of smell). In our not-so-distant past, palate fatigue played an important role in keeping us alive. When an organism encountered a new food, there was both opportunity and risk. This new food source *might* prove to be nutritious and calorically dense—a boon for the individual. But what if it contained poisons or toxins? Eating too much of this novel food could mean the end of the line.

Quite literally, palate fatigue means "getting tired of this taste." Palate fatigue sets in for two reasons. The first reason involves minimizing our toxicant load. It may surprise you to know that all plants produce substances that are either poor tasting or outright toxic. This is the natural defense mechanism plants use to avoid being consumed wholesale by insects and animals. Caffeine and nicotine, found in many plants, are substances bitter to our taste and neurotoxic to many insects. Some critters developed an evolutionary strategy to deal with these toxins. Koala bears, for example, are able to eat a diet almost exclusively composed of eucalyptus leaves, which contain substances that are unappealing and toxic to most other animals. Even if a plant tastes good to us, we will become bored of the food at some point because there are still toxins in things as benign as apples, carrots, and blueberries if we overeat them.

The second reason for palate fatigue is somewhat the opposite of avoiding toxins and relates to optimizing nutrient intake in the form of vitamins, minerals, and other food-based nutrients such as polyphenolics (one of the likely health-promoting elements in chocolate and green tea). Human health seems to benefit from getting as much variety as possible, so long as a few guidelines are observed, which we will explore shortly.

The palate fatigue story and its related concept, satiety (a sense of fullness), becomes critically important when we look specifically at the foods we eat, because the macronutrients (protein, carbs, and fat) deliver different degrees of satiety. In broad brushstrokes, lean proteins such as a chicken breast or pork loin are highly satiating. This is likely due to the fact that humans cannot consume more than about 35 percent of their calories from protein before suffering from protein toxicity. We need other nutrients such as fat or carbohydrate to allow us to function properly. Thus, lean proteins send a very strong signal of "Okay, I've had enough." Fiber-rich carbohydrates tend to be the next most satiating, as they effect changes to the stomach's mechanoreceptors, which communicate to the brain that we are filling our stomach.

Most experts consider fat, on a calorie-by-calorie basis, the least satiating of the macronutrients, but there are some important nuances here. It is rare to find a natural food that is all or mostly fat. Most people would find it challenging to guzzle a glass of olive oil. Even butter, which has been a component of traditional diets for ages, has experienced some degree of processing to separate the milk fat from the whole milk. Avocados and coconuts have high levels of fat, but also a decent amount of sugars and carbohydrates.

As we will see, some of these satiety studies look only at the short term (hours) when considering the satiety effects of various foods. This may be a bit misleading, as the effects of hormonal dysregulation and overeating play out over days, weeks, months, and years. Fat does not cause much stomach distension, but it is calorically dense and triggers the release of hormones that provide satiety over the longer haul.

So, although the academic research on the satiety of these macronutrients orders things out as protein > fiber-rich carbohydrate > fat, my clinical experience has shown some variation in this story. For some, a higher fat intake, particularly with adequate protein, causes a spontaneous reduction in caloric intake due to a profound sense of satiety. Folks who eat this way tend to experience fairly easy fat loss and dramatic improvements in health parameters such as blood sugar and inflammation. Keep in mind, however, that this might have nothing to do with the satiety of fat specifically and everything to do with removing junk carbs from the diet, which can hijack the neuroregulation of appetite and make us feel hungry.

Let's now take a look at how human cultural evolution brought about changes in our food and environment, which helped to forge our genetic evolution. What we will find is that these changes are difficult to categorize as "good" or "bad" but rather as tradeoffs with inherent cost/benefit consideration. In direct terms, this means certain adaptations that have been helpful in the past (eat more, move less), may no longer benefit us, given our modern world.

THE FLAVOR AND TEXTURE OF CULTURE

For most of our development as a species, our ancestors were forced to respond to the changes they faced in the environment, just like every other organism on the planet. At some point, however, humans developed the intelligence, sophistication, and culture necessary to begin actually altering the environment in which they lived, which, interestingly, also altered how we evolved. Controlling fire and making clothing allowed us to move into areas that were previously too cold for extended habitation. Language and complex social structures allowed us to plan ahead for hunting and gathering, share key information, and learn from mistakes.

One of the most profound changes our species faced was the transition from hunting and gathering to a more settled, agricultural life-way. Anthropologist Jared Diamond makes the point that abandoning the hunter-gatherer life-way was perhaps the greatest mistake made in all of humanity. His reasoning is controversial but compelling: These new agriculturalists suffered a number of health problems unique to their new way of living. The accumulation of "stuff" allowed for the development of class structures and large-scale exploitation of people and the environment. Our path out of Eden has brought us to a literal existential crisis in which we now have the technology to destroy not only ourselves but most of life on the planet we call home. These ideas are interesting philosophically, but the changes we will consider have much more immediate impact upon our health and wellness. One example of such a change? How slash-and-burn technology set the stage for the development of one of the greatest killers in all of human history: malaria, a deadly blood-borne parasite that can infect humans.

In order to convert large areas of tropical jungle into relatively open spaces devoted to the production of starchy tubers, our ancestors employed a process called slash-and-burn. The slash-and-burn process also made large areas amenable to the formation of shallow pools of water, the preferred habitat for the *Anopheles* mosquito (the carrier of the malaria parasite) to lay its eggs, which in turn led to an explosion in the mosquito population. Slash-and-burn also cleared the way for a shift toward permanent dwellings made with thatched roofs, which provided a safe haven for adult mosquitoes to live, a rich food source (humans), and a nearly limitless reproductive opportunity in the form of those shallow pools of water.

The impact on people living in these affected areas is difficult to describe, but the death and suffering were staggering. Malaria had likely been a problem for people living in these areas since the beginning of our species, but

the application of culture to our environment unleashed a remarkably efficient killer. Fortunately for us, biology is about adaptation, and it appears
an individual in this malaria-affected area developed a genetic mutation,
which, although it carried its own costs, proved to be a boon for the population at large. This single genetic change altered one amino acid in the
hemoglobin protein found in our red blood cells, resulting in a condition
called sickle cell anemia. The effects are not benign on those affected.

Normally, when our red blood cells move through the tiny capillaries
at the ends of our circulatory system, they must move one at a time and
oftentimes fold and change shape to accommodate the tight spaces through
which they move. In the case of sickle cell anemia, this folding does not
occur properly, which can lead to a host of problems ranging from stroke
to limb loss due to ischemia. That may sound bad, and it is, but there is
an upside: folks who carry the sickle cell trait are less susceptible to the
malaria parasite. It's a bit of a Faustian bargain, but well worth it, as we
will see. Individuals with the sickle cell anemia trait can have two copies
of the mutation (homozygous) or they can have a single copy (heterozygous). Homozygous individuals, those with two copies of the mutation, are
protected from malaria, but they have a high likelihood of dying from their
mutation. The heterozygous individuals have resistance to malaria but with
an increased rate of stroke and ischemic problems, albeit much lower than
the rates affecting homozygous individuals. If two heterozygous parents
have four kids, this is what the sickle cell anemia probabilities look like:

One individual will likely be unprotected from malaria, and thus at a
high risk of death or illness. Similarly, one individual will receive two copies
of the sickle cell gene, and will be at a high risk of death due to complications with that condition. Two children, however, are likely to be resistant
to malaria. As nasty as the complications of sickle cell anemia are, the development of the sickle cell trait was a "net win" for the people in this region.

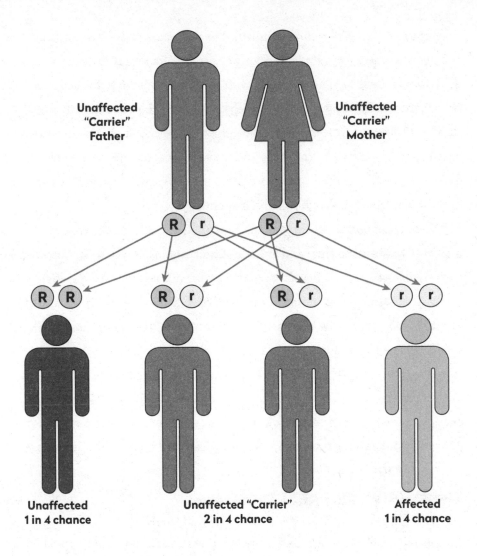

Unaffected "Carrier" Father

Unaffected "Carrier" Mother

R r   R r

R R   R r   R r   r r

**Unaffected
1 in 4 chance**

**Unaffected "Carrier"
2 in 4 chance**

**Affected
1 in 4 chance**

This is evidenced by the rapid spread of this genetic trait within malaria-affected areas. An interesting side note is that the sickle cell trait disappears rapidly (in just a few generations) when folks move to areas unaffected by malaria. The reason is because sickle cell anemia is a net win under the pressure of malaria but a costly, unnecessary adaptation when that disease burden is lifted.

Now, if you are still reading the book and have not lined a birdcage with the pages, you may be asking yourself, *What on earth do sickle cell anemia and malaria have to do with health, weight loss, and food?* Let me ask you a question: Is there any moral failing with people who have sickle cell anemia? No, clearly not, at least not due to the genetics which produce that condition. But the same processes that developed sickle cell anemia were at play in wiring our genetics to eat more and move less. You cannot moralize our desire to "eat all the food" any more than one could make a credible argument to lambast folks with sickle cell anemia.

When faced with a stress, our species can adapt (like in the case of malaria), but it takes time and the adaptation comes at a cost. If, however, the rate of change is sufficiently rapid, we may not be able to cope effectively. This is the salient point of the discordance theory. Our genes are not identical to those of our hunter-gatherer ancestors; there are changes like sickle cell anemia and lactase persistence (the ability to digest the sugar found in milk), but these changes are incomplete in that some novel foods, like refined carbohydrates, still give us problems. Additionally, the rate of change in the factors affecting our health has accelerated with time as evidenced by our rapidly increasing rates of Western degenerative diseases.

THE OMNIVORE'S REAL DILEMMA

The reason we get fat, sick, and broken, the reason it's so hard to affect change in our diet and lifestyle, is simple: our environment has changed, our bodies have not—at least not enough to forestall the development of a host of degenerative diseases. Our genetics are wired for a time when our meals were relatively simple in terms of flavor and texture. We had access to foods that changed with the seasons, and we always had to expend some amount of energy to get the goods. Now, with the magic of food science, convenience stores, and supermarkets, we have access to every flavor combination imaginable, and many that were not imaginable only a few years ago. More than ten thousand new "food" products are created every year in the United States, and the average grocery store stocks tens of thousands of food options. Do you like nachos? French fries? Then you will love chili-cheese nacho-fries, especially with some mole sauce. Given these complex food combinations and our nearly limitless food options, it's no wonder we've broken the neuroregulation of our appetites.

FORGING ELITE EATING

As a kid I was fascinated with eating contests (I know, not much of a social life). Competitors would try to shovel down a mountainous pile of food, ranging from hot dogs to ice cream. My fascination was more akin to watching a train wreck than anything else, but this early interest made me look at some of the modern reality TV offerings differently than most people. I was intrigued by the process and strategy used by these elite eaters, and I found consistencies between how these folks succeed and many of the problems we face today.

The way we construct our meals is remarkably similar to the way professional eaters take home the gold (and the bacon). These folks instinctively understand the underpinnings of the neuroregulation of appetite and how to bypass those signals to eat as much food as possible.

Adam Richman, host of the Travel Channel's popular *Man v. Food*, was tasked with eating an Everest-size ice cream sundae. He tackles the process like the professional he is and digs in. But partway through, he bogs down. Badly. You can see a bit of a green tinge come to his gills and you wonder if he is going to pull this off. What does he do? In a move that would befuddle most people, Adam asks for . . . *more food*, specifically, a plate of crunchy, extra-salty French fries. Adam begins nibbling on the fries, and in a short time he is back in the fight and manages to eat his bucket of ice cream in the allotted time.

What happened here is that Adam hit complete palate fatigue on something most of us would find pretty tasty: ice cream. Even a good thing can become too much and result in palate fatigue, with severe nausea as the result. Adam craftily employs a workaround in the form of a food that is as different from ice cream as one might imagine: the crunchy, salty, savory French fries played perfectly against the cold, sweet ice cream. Prior to the fries, consuming more ice cream might have caused him to become physically ill and vomit, yet *adding more food*, specifically a food that is profoundly different in taste, temperature, and texture, allowed him to not only finish the ice cream, but the fries, too.

Want to see how this goes down? Go to robbwolf.com/icecream to see this disaster.

Inadvertently, we eat like professional eaters. We construct complex meals that in general allow us to eat more than we'd otherwise eat. Add to that the problem of nearly limitless food options, options that have the same effect on us, allowing us to eat *more* food, just like Adam did. This phenomenon has been well documented for decades and is called the dessert effect. Simply put, this is the observation that someone may claim to be full after a meal, commenting, "Oh, I cannot eat another bite!" only to eat much more than a bite once the dessert tray comes out. This is just the short-term effect of hyperpalatable complex foods. The long-term hormonal story is equally important and relates to why we not only can eat more at a given meal, but also why we tend to get hungry more often in response to these types of meals—but we'll get to that story in a bit. Right now, I want to make a solid case for why it is so easy to overeat, why simple, wholesome meals may become unappetizing relative to refined, hyperpalatable foods. And ironically, I'll make this case with porn.

SUPERNORMAL STIMULI
(PORN WITH A SIDE OF NACHOS)

One could make a strong argument that sex and food are the reasons every living thing exists. No food? You die. No sex? No potential for offspring, and the species dies. Sex is a . . . sticky subject in the United States, as we tend to be remarkably puritanical relative to most other Westernized societies. I mention this because the forthcoming section is likely to make many of you uncomfortable, but sex and the related topic of pornography are actually educational from the perspective of how supernormal stimuli can alter our neural architecture and consequently our behavior.

Iterations of the Internet have existed since the 1960s, but it was around the mid-2000s that some researchers and clinicians became aware of a confounding trend among healthy young men who displayed an odd set of symptoms: depression, apathy, lack of motivation, and erectile dysfunction. Men ranging from their teens to their twenties were not only suffering a bad case of the blues—they were literally incapable of achieving any type of sexual performance with mere humans (this process occurs in both homosexual and heterosexual men). The only way these young, seemingly virile men could achieve any type of sexual function was via Internet porn consumed in a particular fashion: these men would open multiple tabs within their Internet browser, each tab housing a different clip of porn. What these young men found via trial and error was that having a broad range of scenes, genres, and actors (variety) would bring them to a remarkable degree of arousal (for a while). A degree that *could not* be replicated or matched by any real-life sexual experience.

In Gary Wilson's book *Your Brain on Porn*, he relates the problems these men face and the stories are startling as well as informative as to how supernormal stimuli (SNS) can break the normal functioning of our brain.

Just like with sex, food is regulated in ancient regions of the brain called the hedonic centers. As the name implies, this is related to the experience of pleasure and, perhaps more important, the behavior of pleasure seeking. Although a bit mechanistic, it should make sense that sex and food carry some kind of reward—in this case, feelings of pleasure and satisfaction. Again, if we do not eat, we die. If we do not have sex (and babies), the species dies. These hedonic centers operate with a host of neurotransmitters but perhaps the most important for this story is the neurotransmitter dopamine.

Serotonin gets a lot of airplay in the media due to its use in antidepressants such as Prozac (which increase the levels of serotonin in the brain), but dopamine is the key player in the hedonic (reward) centers of the brain and in drugs such as caffeine, nicotine, and cocaine. I'm sure it's no surprise to you that the aforementioned drugs are addictive, but you may not know why. Stimulating the dopamine centers of the brain creates a positive feedback loop in which one desires more of the substance or activity that elicited the initial good feelings. All of this would be fine were it not for the opportunity to experience SNS and unleash a cascade in which the "dose" of stimuli that made us feel good last time will not do anything for us the next time. In fact, without that next dose, we can feel depressed, anxious, and compulsive. The only solution is to increase the dose and/or change the stimuli, which in our modern world is all too easy to do.

The ability to open dozens of Internet browser tabs with every form of porn imaginable (and many that defy any thoughts of good taste or common sense) sets up the user for ever-diminishing returns from their "dose." Eventually, nothing on the Internet is kinky enough for normal sexual function. Having six different flavors of ice cream in our freezer in addition to an easy selection of highly processed, hyperpalatable foods (chili-cheese nachos for lunch, Sriracha fries for dinner) is analogous to the dozens of tabs of Internet porn. Simple, healthy meals are so lacking in stimulation *relative* to our nearly limitless options that people will describe these normal meals as being just north of cardboard with regard to flavor. Add to this story the deep social ties (friends, family, coworkers) that often come with our meals, and we not only have food urges that are on par with a cocaine addiction, but we also have the societal pressures to keep doing exactly what we have always done.

I've noticed a fascinating story playing out in churches, workplaces, and family gatherings, which you will likely identify with: most people are unlikely to say anything to a person who eats terribly. Doughnuts and a sugary coffee drink for breakfast, constant snacking on sweets, a lunch that could not be identified as "food" if an FBI forensics squad analyzed it, and dinner from a fast-food joint elicits not a comment from most folks. *But.* If a person is trying to "eat better" and brings a salad to work or forgoes the refined carbs at a family gathering, that person is at the least questioned and at the worst heckled, cajoled, or guilted into capitulation. I'll share some of my thoughts on why this is the case later, but for now I hope you better understand why it's so hard to make meaningful dietary changes stick. We live in a world full of foods that have been engineered for overeating. Remember the Lay's potato chip slogan, "Betcha can't eat just one"?

I'll take that bet all day, so long as the big junk food producers are very good at their job. The problem today is that we have a near infinite variety of foods that completely bypass our neuroregulation of appetite. These foods produce a degree of stimulation in the brain that leaves normal food looking (and tasting) awful. Our main mode of addressing this issue is to tell people to "eat less, move more" (completely at odds with our genetics) while moralizing the "failure" we see. None of this is your fault, but it is a predicament we all face. The way through this is completely doable, as is evidenced by the millions of people who have benefited from my work and the work of others in this Ancestral Health scene. With the 30-Day Reset, we will rewire your neuroregulation of appetite, allowing you to restore your health and trim your waistline.

This is an overview of the "outside" story of why we get fat, sick, and broken. This chapter makes the case that moralizing food choices and shaming people (including ourselves) about difficulties in changing eating behavior are as misplaced as chastising someone for simply wanting to breathe. Would you begrudge someone for grasping at a tree branch while drowning? If not, then you cannot vilify someone for struggling with their eating habits. Both processes deal with survival. Our modern world is so safe, so secure, so rich with food, that we largely forget starvation was a constant companion of our human predecessors. The people who figured out this game, the people who ate more and moved less, are the folks we call ancestors—the ones who didn't die. Their success is the reason we are here today, but that success also presents some challenges. Nothing insurmountable, just things we need to be aware of. It's understandable if you have beaten yourself up in the past about the difficulty of changing your eating, but that time is now done. You are well along your way to understanding how you are wired to eat.

In the next chapter, I'll shift gears and look at what happens "under the hood" when we overconsume food in general and refined carbohydrates and sugars in particular. This story will take us through the digestive process and introduce us to the microorganisms that play a remarkably important role in our health (or disease). We will learn about how specific macronutrients play into the neuroregulation of appetite and also how our metabolism can be broken by chronically overconsuming foods that our genes are ill prepared to handle.

CHAPTER 4

On Digestion and Obesity

Health educators often become known for a specific genre or process that they champion. Some are known for abs, others are known for helping to produce diamond-hard glutes. Me? Well, somehow I became an expert on poo. I know—pretty sexy, right?

Hopefully by now you understand a few of the many factors that play into our tendency to overeat the ubiquitous hyperpalatable food we are exposed to. But overeating is only part of the story. How specific foods are properly or improperly digested, and how those foods communicate with our brains and bodies are also quite important. "Important how?" you ask. Food produces dramatically different hormonal and metabolic consequences depending on whether we are adequately fed or overfed and also based on the amount and types of protein, carbs, and fat in our diet. We will use the 30-Day Reset to get your digestion moving in a good direction and then use the 7-Day Carb Test to determine what amounts and types of carbs you do best with.

Deep knowledge of the digestive process is not usually something that will garner one high social standing, but we need to take a quick trip down our alimentary canal to understand how things can go right or wrong with regard to our waistline. In addition, a remarkable story has emerged over the past ten years linking problems with the digestive process to everything from diabetes to autoimmunity to obesity to neurodegenerative diseases such as Parkinson's and Alzheimer's. In a somewhat Zen-like proposition, in order to talk about digestion, we must first (briefly!) consider what is getting digested.

Digestion is simply the process of making large things smaller. The things in question here are the foods we eat. Starches, proteins, and fats are broken down into their respective building blocks: sugars, amino acids, and fatty acids. There is a dizzying degree of potential detail we could go into with digestion, but I'm just going to hit a few key points relating to protein, carbs, and fat so you will better understand why I make the recommendations I do in the prescriptive portion of the book.

Protein

Most people associate the word *protein* with meat, tofu, and supplements like the whey protein used in shakes. Depending on the structure of a given protein, it can be easier or harder to digest. This is an important point we will consider when we look at food intolerances and food-borne immune responses such as celiac disease.

Carbohydrates

Carbohydrates are built from sugars and, similar to proteins, come in a vast assortment, from rice to bananas to wood! Possibly the two most common sugars in our world are glucose (also called blood sugar, as this is what we use to fuel much of our metabolic machinery) and fructose, found in a number of fruits and vegetables but also a major part of the rightfully vilified high-fructose corn syrup. For our purposes, we just need to be aware that carbs can come in the form of sugar, starch, or fiber and that depending on the makeup of a given food (its relative mix of sugars, starch, or fiber), it can create vastly different blood glucose responses. We will learn much more about this when we look at the science of Personalized Nutrition a bit later in the book. Our knowledge of digestion in general and our unique response to carbs in particular will influence our food choices to affect weight loss and improve our health.

Fat

The most contentious of the three macronutrients, fats are also called lipids in science lingo. Fats fall into one of three categories based on their chemical structure: saturated, monounsaturated, and polyunsaturated. There is a massive amount of confusing information surrounding fats and their role in health and disease, and whole books have been written on the topic of fats alone. This book has a lot of detail, but I want to keep all this as practical as possible, so for our purposes we will just try to get the bulk of the fat in our diet from whole, unprocessed foods. If we stick to this plan it's hard to vilify *any* fats. It's when we start eating refined foods that we see not just problems with the amounts and types of fats, but also the carbs.

Now that you have a sense of what the items are that we digest, we will look at the actual process of digestion.

DIGESTION STARTS IN THE BRAIN, THEN GOES SOUTH

Believe it or not, digestion starts before we have set teeth to grub. Simply seeing and or smelling food begins a process of increasing the release of gastric juices in anticipation of the upcoming meal. We will talk a good bit about the hormones released in the digestive process, but it's worth mentioning that certain hormones can be released in anticipation of a meal. For some folks, simply seeing or smelling a dessert (or a damn tasty meal) can cause the release of insulin, which is a key hormone in health and body fat levels. This is a fully neurological process that can contribute to some of the problems we will consider. If our neuroregulation of appetite is broken, we will tend to respond much more strongly to hyperpalatable foods. I guess you could categorize this as "your brain on food porn."

Digestion involves both mechanical and chemical activity. The digestion that occurs in the mouth is a beautiful illustration of the physical breaking down of food via chewing and the enzymatic activity of amylase (the primary enzyme involved in breaking down starches to sugar). While this physical process is occurring, the act of tasting the food and the mechanical action of chewing primes the stomach to begin releasing hydrochloric acid and enzymes involved in protein digestion. It's perhaps worth mentioning that thoroughly chewing food is an important aspect of proper digestion. Our time-crunched lives tend to make people multitask while eating, and this does our digestion no favors. Some people, like my wife, have developed the "boa constrictor" method of gumming their food a few times, disarticulating their jaw, and gulping the food down largely whole. My wife is tougher than 99 percent of the people I know, so perhaps she can get away with this gustatory option, but I don't recommend it for you.

The stomach is really a marvel of biological engineering, as it is host to an environment so acidic (the pH of the stomach should be around 2 to 2.5) that it can dissolve metals. This highly acidic environment begins the process of protein digestion in earnest, while starch and fat digestion will ramp up once we hit the small intestine. The enzyme pepsin is released in the stomach and begins cleaving large proteins into smaller units. The stomach contents are mixed and given time for the action of acid and digestive enzymes to break down protein. The physical action of the stomach and the (ideally) high acid environment send signals to the small intestine to prepare for its role in digestion.

The small intestines are a "hot spot," as it were, with regard to digestion. A lot happens here if things are working properly, but a lot can also go wrong, as we shall see. The contents of the stomach squirt into the small intestine and a number of processes occur simultaneously, including important roles by the pancreas and the gallbladder. Ideally, at the end of the process, carbohydrates in the form of starch are reduced to sugars (mainly glucose), while proteins are degraded into amino acids. In this stage, the proteins and carbohydrates can be absorbed at the intestinal wall and enter the circulation for a trip to the liver and eventually into the body, where they may be stored or used as energy or building blocks for the growth and repair of our bodies.

Two critically important features of our digestive tract are structures called villi and microvilli. These finger- and hairlike structures increase the surface area of the gut, thereby increasing its ability to absorb nutrients, and play a crucial role in the digestive process. They allow certain molecules to be absorbed into our circulatory system, while screening out the billions of bacteria that live in our gut.

Absorption of nutrients is best accomplished with what is called an intact gut lining. As the term implies, this means the cells making up the gut, villi and microvilli, are not damaged and are functioning properly. If the gut lining is not fully intact, amino acids and sugars can still be absorbed (albeit inefficiently), but fats will not be absorbed. This can be a serious problem, as a remarkable number of nutrients—antioxidants, beta-carotene, etc.—can only be absorbed by the body when eaten with fat (a fact those preaching low-fat diets often overlook).

Undigested fat that makes its way into the large intestine and colon can have . . ."remarkable" consequences. The medical term is *diarrhea*, but around the Wolf household we like to call that "disaster pants." I do not want to go into so much detail that you decide to hang yourself with a computer cord, but there are a few more points we must consider with regard to digestion in the small intestine. In general, we see more absorption occur in later sections of the small intestine. The consumption of highly refined foods can alter this process, causing more nutrients to be absorbed early and effectively starving the gut bacteria later in the GI tract. As we will see in the next section, properly feeding our gut bacteria and the mucosal layer of our gut is critically important, whether our main goal is fitting into a pair of skinny jeans or avoiding a heart attack.

Beyond the small intestine are the large intestine and the colon. When I've lectured on the gut and health in the past and I got to the large intestine and colon, I've mentioned that water and minerals are reabsorbed in this region, and declared, "It's all poop from here!" However, in the past ten years we have witnessed an explosion in our understanding of the role gut bacteria plays in health and disease. Undigested fiber and a wide variety of starches called resistant starch are the primary food source for our gut bacteria. The bacteria ferment these starches and fibers, producing certain vitamins and a not insignificant amount of short-chain fatty acids, which not only feed the cells of the gut but can also make their way into our circulatory system and play a role in our own energy needs. Ideally, most of the protein and fats have been long since absorbed into our circulatory system. Problems in the digestive process (such as low stomach acid) can leave large intact food pieces present in the "southbound" regions of the GI tract, and this can stimulate the growth of bacteria that are not benign to our health. Ulcerative colitis, Crohn's disease, irritable bowel syndrome (IBS), and a host of other GI and non-GI related problems can occur when we get either the wrong types of bacteria growing (as happens when food is poorly digested) or bacteria growing in the wrong places (as happens when we eat large amounts of refined carbs, which stimulates the growth of bacteria inappropriately in some places and starves bacteria in other regions). The plans you will use in this book will help you avoid these problems by improving digestion and avoiding the foods which cause the most problems.

Okay, from this point on it really is "all poop from here." In the gut chapter, we will discuss what good poo versus not-so-good poo looks like. This information will not only impress friends and family, but when properly applied to improve digestion, it can dramatically improve your life, possibly even save it.

WORLD'S SHORTEST ENDOCRINOLOGY COURSE

Most people are familiar, at least at a passing level, with the term *hormone*. Folks have a sense that things like estrogen, testosterone, and insulin are important in regulating our physiology. Hormones are chemical messengers released into the circulatory system by specific glands or tissues. If they come in contact with something called a receptor site, the hormone can effect changes in specific cells, organs, or the body at large. Hormones and receptor sites come in very specific shapes, and we can think about the hormones a bit like a key and receptor sites like a lock. The right key will open certain locks due to the complementary shape of each. When a hormone has bonded to its receptor site, we generally see a change in DNA expression in a given cell, which means we will see changes in how certain proteins are produced within the cell, and *this* is how we change our physiology. This is a very superficial view of this highly complex process, but it's good enough for government work, er . . . our needs here.

There are at least fifty different hormones that govern human metabolism, but we are going to focus on just a few of the major players tied to digestion, namely insulin, glucagon, adrenaline (epinephrine and norepinephrine), and cortisol.

In broad brushstrokes, insulin helps us regulate blood sugar levels, as it is critical for helping glucose enter the cells of our body. For example, if you eat a banana, you will get an increase in blood glucose levels, and this increase in blood glucose will stimulate the release of insulin to bring glucose levels back down. Under ideal circumstances, we require only a small amount of insulin to deal with a given amount of carbohydrate, and thus our blood sugar does not go too high or too low.

When our cells do not respond properly to insulin (insulin resistance) our blood sugars tend to rise too high after a meal.* The unfortunate side effect is that blood sugars tend to then crash to abnormally low levels, leaving us shaky, hungry, and irritated, what I and others have taken to calling "hangry" (hungry + angry = hangry). In general, carbohydrate releases the largest amount of insulin on a calorie-by-calorie basis, with protein releasing (generally) less insulin and fat releasing a relatively small amount. There are some exceptions to this, as certain proteins and amino acids do stimulate the release of large amounts of insulin.

Glucagon is insulin's counter hormone. Released by hunger and also by protein, it is able to convert proteins in the body to glucose via a process called gluconeogenesis. In short, insulin helps to store nutrients in the body, while glucagon helps to liberate those fuels.

Adrenaline is a hormone produced in the adrenal glands, which sit atop the kidneys. I think most people are familiar with the notion that

---

* Some folks who really buy into the insulin hypothesis of obesity say that with elevated insulin levels, we cannot get fats out of cells. Research indicates we do release fats from adipocytes in the overfed state, but this is not really doing us any favors, as we already have a situation of nutrient excess in the body. Elevated insulin levels certainly play into the ease of liberating fat from adipocytes; this is why insulin-sensitive people can lose body fat on relatively high-carb, low-fat diet. Conversely, however, folks with insulin resistance will find the high-carb, low-fat approach almost impossible to lose weight on, but may thrive on a lower-carb, higher-protein/fat mix. Once the underlying insulin resistance has been addressed, these same people may find they tolerate more carbs and can shift their diet accordingly but this is a highly individual thing. The fervor and acrimony around this topic only have parallels with religion and politics . . . people have their pet theory and no amount of information counter to their pet theory will sway most folks. I wish this story was a simple black/white dichotomy, but life is a bit more complex than that.

adrenaline is a stimulatory hormone long associated with thrill-seeking activities. It is also a handy way to restart the heart during a heroin overdose, as evidenced by John Travolta's quick thinking in the movie *Pulp Fiction*, when he plunged a syringe full of adrenaline into the unbeating heart of Uma Thurman, who had inadvertently gotten her cocaine and heroin mixed up. Silly kids! Adrenaline is released under a number of circumstances: physical (or psychological) threat, physical activity, and hunger. Adrenaline has a number of actions, including dilating pupils and constricting blood vessels, but our main focus is that adrenaline increases blood glucose levels by stimulating the liver.

Cortisol is generally considered a stress hormone, and you may have even heard of the contentious medical condition adrenal fatigue, which indicates low or altered adrenal function. Cortisol has a number of functions, including aiding in blood sugar control and modulating inflammation and immune response. If you or someone you know has received a prednisone shot for a cranky back, knee, or shoulder, this person has received a dose of synthetic cortisol in the hopes of decreasing inflammation in a particular area.

It's important to note the sensitivity hormones have for their receptors, as many of the pathologic conditions we will consider have, at their core, a state of resistance on the part of the hormone's desired action. In general, the more receptors there are for a given hormone, the higher the likelihood its respective hormone may bond to it. An insulin-sensitive individual usually has a relatively large number of insulin receptors. When insulin is released, the body tends to begin reducing the number of receptors in the never-ending counter-regulatory dance. When insulin goes up after a meal, it begins effecting metabolic changes, and one of those changes is a decrease in the number of insulin receptors. This is a normal process unless insulin becomes chronically elevated and the individual's body greatly reduces the number of insulin receptors and thus becomes insulin resistant.

This process of down regulation or resistance can happen with any hormone and is again part of the feedback loops that keep our physiology working effectively. As you might suspect, this process (and others) is not exactly straightforward, and the action of glucagon on insulin sensitivity is an interesting case in point: glucagon tends to increase insulin sensitivity. This makes sense from the perspective of fasting, as we are in a "low food" state and we'd certainly like our body to be ready to receive any nutrients we throw its way. You simply need to know that in the insulin-resistant state in which glucose levels are elevated, increased glucagon levels do play a part in attempting to improve insulin sensitivity. The problem, as we shall see, is that our bodies are ill equipped to deal with uninterrupted, chronic overfeeding.

You likely need a smoke, a cup of coffee, and a hug by this point! I know this is a lot of dense material, especially if you do not have a biology background. Hang in there. I would not take the time to cover all this if it were not important. Whether your goal is improving evergy levels, losing body fat, or avoiding a nasty condition like a heart attack or Alzheimer's disease, digestion and gut health are quite important. I'd love for folks to have a 100 percent understanding of this material, but if you have a general understanding of digestion and gut health and how problems in these areas can affect your wellness and waistline, you will be much more likely to not only give my recommendations a shot, but to stick with them.

We will now take a look at the specific neurotransmitters and hormones which regulate our appetite. Ideally, when we finish this next section you will understand what is occurring mechanistically when we either overeat or eat foods that may pose problems to our digestion and gut health.

LAYERS UPON LAYERS

The scientific process is a bit like peeling an onion, in that today we have what is our best cataloging and understanding of how a process works, but tomorrow or a few years down the road we will likely discover another layer to the story. The hormones and chemical messengers that govern our physiology are a great example of this "onion peeling" process, as we have had a comprehensive understanding from which to describe how the human body works for more than a hundred years, but with the advent of modern genetics, biochemistry, and information processing, the degree of detail and nuance has become nothing short of staggering.

For many decades, there was a rough understanding that digestion and appetite had some connection to the brain and nervous system. The simple association between the brain and digestion has taken on a remarkable degree of complexity over the past few years, with dozens of hormones and neurotransmitters acting on the appetite-control centers of the brain. We will look at all this just deeply enough to appreciate how things like our food, body fat stores, and hormonal status can influence hunger, and therefore how much (and what) we eat.

There are a number of hormones that govern the neuroregulation of appetite, including leptin, ghrelin, peptide YY, and more, but beyond their specific functions and names are a few important points I want you to understand:

1. Appetite is controlled on a short-term basis by hormones such as insulin and ghrelin largely in response to immediate food intake (or lack thereof).
2. Appetite is controlled on longer time frames by our level of body fat (leptin is the big player here). Under normal circumstances, a relatively

high level of body fat should suppress our appetite, while low levels increase appetite. Intuitively, this should make perfect sense. Though our physiology is quite adaptable, hyperpalatable foods, disordered sleep, stress, and GI problems can damage normal functions, making it easier to overeat.

3. As complex as this story is at the detail level, simple steps (good sleep, exercise, quality food, and community) can fix what ails us.

TO THE LIVER, AND BEYOND!

Many of our decisions in life have an optimum in which things work best. Too much savings with inadequate spending can make one's life a bit dull and uneventful. Too much food can score us a host of problems ranging from obesity to diabetes while too little food will bring on the Big Nap a lot earlier than any of us would like. Ideally we'd like to get our food intake "just right" but do it in a way that does not necessitate putting every meal into measuring cups. Fortunately, eating real, whole food (as we do with the 30-Day Reset and the 7-Day Carb Test) makes this process pretty easy, but we still need to learn a bit about how overconsumption of food negatively affects us. In essence, we still need to understand what happens on a metabolic level when we overeat. To do this we need to understand how and where nutrients are stored in our bodies as well as what happens when we consume too little, too much, or just the right amount of food.

UNDERFEEDING

Underfeeding can mean a few different things: inadequate calories, inadequate nutrients (essential amino acids, fats, vitamins, and minerals), or outright fasting. When in this state, we are generally using more calories than we are taking in,* and this has some very specific metabolic consequences: low insulin levels juxtaposed with elevated levels of cortisol, adrenaline, and glucagon. Glucose is released from the liver, and fats are released from the liver and fat cells. Proteins take on an interesting life, as our bodies become quite thrifty with protein when we are chronically calorie deprived. We tend to see damaged cells and tissues getting broken down in order to be recycled and used in other purposes. Calorie restriction or fasting appears to be quite beneficial, as some of our cells can sustain damage over time that induces a state called senescence. In this condition, cells are technically alive, but they are not behaving as they should. Under ideal conditions a cell that becomes damaged will undergo a process called apoptosis and do us the favor of dying and being recycled. In certain circumstances, however, these senescent cells can become cancerous and/or produce large amounts of inflammation, which increases our likelihood of a host of diseases, including cancer, cardiovascular disease, and neurodegeneration.

If calorie restriction and/or fasting are of sufficient magnitude and duration, we enter a state called starvation ketosis, whereby our metabolism shifts from a primarily glucose-based fuel to being fueled by free fatty acids and ketones. Ketones have received a bad rap by the medical community, as most practitioners are unfamiliar with the difference between ketosis (induced by calorie restriction, fasting, or a low-carb, moderate-protein, high-fat diet) and ketoacidosis, which is a state of significantly elevated ketones generally seen in poorly controlled diabetics. I go into much more detail on ketosis and fasting later in the book, but it's important for you

---

* Dr. Jason Fung has published research indicating a prolonged fast can completely reverse the effects of type 2 diabetes. Dr. Fung is also a fan of ketogenic or low-carb diets for his diabetic patients, as the ketogenic state mimics many of the features of fasting. These ideas are far outside the mainstream and need significant validation, but if Dr. Fung's theories prove to be correct, we have at our fingertips simple interventions that can halt, possibly reverse, one of the greatest problems facing Westernized societies.

to understand that this is a normal physiological state, and it's likely that humans have gone in and out of ketosis throughout our history.

Understanding that the underfed state involves hormonal signals that release stored nutrients will be important in understanding the pathology of the overfed state. As we will see, when we break our neuroregulation of appetite and chronically overeat, we actually produce a state in which the brain and liver "think" we are starving, despite being awash in energy in the form of excess food.

THE OVERFED STATE

Overfeeding, as the term implies, is the process of taking in more calories than we use. You could think about overeating as a bit like filling up rooms of a house. Once one room or storage location is filled up, we move on to the next—until things start spilling out in the street! When too much food is consumed, we fill up liver and muscle glycogen with excess carbs and protein (once it has been converted to glucose), and excess fat is stored in fat cells and to some degree within the muscles. This is all fine, as long as the process does not go on too long, but once these locations are topped off, the body must get a bit creative in how to handle additional food. Blood sugar and blood lipids creep up, as the body has nowhere else to put these substances. The why behind this is simple: our genetics are not wired for this type of novel stress. Although we are meant to store some fat as a hedge against starvation, we are not meant to carry significant amounts of extra weight.

Excess fat increases the inflammatory signaling in our body, which, unfortunately, accelerates the cascade of problems related to elevated blood glucose. This is particularly true when fat is deposited in two key locations: the liver and around the visceral organs.

Our physiology is designed to keep blood glucose levels within tight ranges. The brain does not do well if glucose levels get too high or too low, or if they change rapidly in a short period of time. In the chronically overfed state, we can see blood glucose levels rising as our liver and muscle glycogen stores are full. Elevated blood glucose can be toxic to the brain, kidneys, and capillaries. So in a fascinating adaptive response, our bodies convert the highly reactive molecule glucose into fat. Although excess body fat can have problems of its own, elevated blood glucose can kill us quite rapidly.

Under ideal circumstances, when we consume a large amount of food, we will receive strong satiety signals that put the brakes on further eating (the plans in this book do exactly this). If our body fat levels are rising, we *should* have strong feedback signals telling us "stop!" But hyperpalatable foods, poor sleep, altered gut bacteria, and systemic inflammation can all undermine this process and allow us to continue to overeat. There is a fair amount of controversy surrounding exactly how this process rolls out, but here are a few things we know with reasonable certainty:

The brain becomes leptin resistant and the muscles become insulin resistant. This fools the brain and the liver into believing we are starving. So despite being awash in excess calories, the body releases glucagon, cortisol, and adrenaline, behaving as it would if we were in an underfed or starvation state.

The release of these catabolic hormones leads to a host of problems, not the least of which is muscle and bone wasting. This occurs in anyone with insulin resistance (estimates range as high as 50 percent of the US population) and particularly for diabetics. What's worse, when you lose muscle mass, you have even *fewer places to store glucose*, which further exacerbates the problem of excess glucose storage.

High insulin levels down regulate insulin receptors, which increases insulin resistance and puts more and more stress on the pancreas. This is the race toward uncontrolled type 2 diabetes, accelerated aging, increased rates of cancer, neurodegenerative disease, cardiovascular disease, and kidney failure.

In addition to hormonal dysregulation and increased inflammation due to overeating, one's mitochondria can be badly damaged by overeating. Mitochondria are tiny organelles found in most cells and are responsible for the process of converting the basic molecular constituents of food—amino acids, lipids, and carbohydrates—into energy. Similar to a coal-fired power plant, this process produces waste products—in this case, free radicals, which can be harmful if not well controlled. We ideally want some of this oxidative stress *sometimes*. But we do not want this process running all day, every day.

Under normal circumstances, the mitochondria, and by extension our metabolism, should be very flexible in shifting between fat and carbohydrate as a fuel. Unfortunately, the damage created by the overfed state can impair our ability to use fat as a fuel source, which makes us all the more dependent on carbohydrates. As we get a little broken, we metabolize fat less well, which forces us to rely on carbohydrates, often the readily accessible, highly refined carbohydrates, which adds to overeating, which drives this process another step forward. Assuming you are still alive (if you are reading this from the afterlife, let me know, as I do not think I have royalties set up there) and you are in this downward spiral, all is not lost. We will explore strategies to help restore your mitochondria (and metabolism) and get you moving toward health. As the guy said in *Monty Python and the Holy Grail*, "I'm not dead yet!"

THE NORMAL FED STATE

You may want to roll me in honey and bury me in an anthill for what I'm about to say, but here goes: What constitutes the "normal" or optimal feeding state for any given person varies. It depends on their genetics, stress levels, sleep status, exercise, gut health and, of course, the amount and type of food they eat. This need for customization is why we will use the 30-Day Reset to heal our metabolism and normalize our neuroregulation of appetite. Then we will use the 7-Day Carb Test plan to discover what carbs we do best (and worst) with.

In the normal feed state, we take in sufficient calories and essential nutrients (including protein, fats, vitamins, and minerals) to support our activity, growth, and repair. How do we do this?

We eat whole, largely unprocessed foods, sleep well, get a little exercise, and do the best to keep our gut bacteria happy. This should not be earth-shaking stuff, but when the message from the government and media is "everything in moderation" and when "moderation" includes remarkable amounts of foods that hijack our neuroregulation of appetite, we have a serious problem. But the normal or optimally fed state, when it is built around whole, largely unprocessed foods, is not a balancing act like walking a tightrope over Niagara Falls. Nor is it akin to doing a calculus problem.

Our physiology seems to be wired with an expectation of variable food intake, not an absolutely solid, steady state. This fact is quite liberating once we get a sense of what foods work for us; we do not need to stress about how much or when we eat. We eat when hungry, eat to satiety, and then do something amazing: we live our lives. Food fixation and the health consequences of overeating negatively impact the quality of life of tens of millions of people. It does not need to be this way. In the prescriptive chapter, we will look at how you can find the plan that works for you, including how to map what foods you respond well to and developing an eating schedule that maximizes energy and gets you to an optimal—for you—body fat level. As I've mentioned previously, we will use the 30-Day Reset to get your neuroregulation of appetite back on track and then we will use the 7-Day Carb Test to precisely dial in the amounts and types of carbs that work best for you.

CHAPTER 5

Glucose, Guts, and Genes

GUT PROBLEMS: ALL IN YOUR HEAD, RIGHT?

I'm a fan of etymology (the study of word origins) as the context of how words come into usage is pretty fascinating. Many years ago in a medical terminology class, I was working on a number of Latin-derived words and perhaps one of the most commonly used words in all of medicine really caught my eye and my imagination: *hypochondria*.

The word refers to a condition in which a person thinks he is always sick, often presenting a constant rotation of ailments ranging from severe to vague and diffuse. Despite the litany of problems the person presents, standard medical screening provides no answers as to the cause of the phantom ailments. The blood work and tests check out. Everything is normal. This is the malingerer, the problem patient. The person the medical staff roll their collective eyes about when they see the name on the schedule. Digging into the term *hypochondria* provides some interesting insights. *Hypo* means "beneath or below." *Chondria* literally means "cartilage" but also refers to the ribs, which are largely composed of cartilage. Literally, *hypochondria* means "conditions below the ribs." That, my friend, is what we generally refer to as the gut.

There's a quote from Hippocrates, who is generally regarded as the father of Western medicine, that I love: "All disease begins in the gut." Most non-Western medical traditions also consider the gut to be the genesis of a remarkable number of diseases, but this was lost within our medical systems until fairly recently. It would be funny, were it not so tragic, that instead of Western reductionist medicine recognizing that a myriad of nonspecific conditions have a potentially common origin (the gut), it has labeled these people, these "hypochondriacs," as mentally unstable. If you enter the terms "gut health mental illness" into a search engine, you will find thousands of peer-reviewed research papers detailing the emerging connections between gut health and mental illness. One article you are likely to find, "The Gut-Brain Connection, Mental Illness, and Disease: Psychobiotics, Immunology, and the Theory of All Chronic Disease," was written by my good friend Emily Deans, MD. In this fantastic piece, Dr. Deans makes the point that in order to understand mental illness and most of our Western degenerative diseases, we must understand our hormones, the evolutionary biology of our fight-or-flight response, the bacteria we share this life with, and, perhaps most important, the overall health of our gut.

The truth is that the gut may be the genesis for most of what ails us. It is the heretofore "invisible" common denominator for diseases as seemingly unrelated as diabetes, Alzheimer's, and cardiovascular disease. We will learn more in the next five years about the role of the gut as it relates to our health than we discovered in the past fifty years. It's exciting times, even if you are *not* a geek! In this chapter, I'll review what we know about the role the gut plays in health so you will better understand why the programs recommended in this book hold such promise for your health and waistline. Fixing the gut may be the key to addressing everything from cardiovascular disease to neurodegenerative diseases such as Parkinson's and Alzheimer's. One could rightfully call gut health "a pretty big deal."

We have covered a lot of ground on our journey to understand how our wiring has gone awry. This understanding puts into context the programs we will use to rewire your appetite and find what is optimum for you. For instance, we explored how our genetics are wired for novelty yet tempered with palate fatigue; how hyperpalatable foods make it easy to overeat, breaking our metabolism. This chapter, which looks at the gut, represents a possible unified model for most of the diseases that plague us.

If you recall from the digestion chapter, our GI tract has an important job of breaking down food into base molecules that are easily transported into the body. This is a balancing act. We need nutrients to enter our body, but we do not want the billions of bacteria residing in our GI tract to enter as well. The bacteria that live in our digestive system have co-evolved with all life on earth, and when all systems are in order, they have a mutually beneficial relationship with our gut. All we need to do is eat the right foods and our bacterial co-conspirators are more than happy to do their part to keep the whole system working smoothly. This process can run aground, however, if the gut lining is damaged by certain gut irritants and/or if we feed or "trim" the bacteria in a way that shifts the bacterial population from one that is beneficial to potentially harmful.

QUASI-SCIENTIFIC/PHILOSOPHICAL/GEE-WHIZ DIGRESSION OF A POSSIBLY HELPFUL NATURE (QSPGWDPHN) #1

In this mortal shell, we face many deep philosophical questions: What is the sound of one hand clapping? What is the meaning of life? Did my wife eat all the guacamole? Again?? Deep stuff, clearly, and I'm just scratching the surface of ponderables, but a question of equal merit that you have likely never heard of or contemplated is, Is what we eat inside or outside of our body? Seriously! Have you ever thought about this?! The answer to this question may seem obvious. Of course what I've eaten is inside my body. But the truth is that we have a tunnel from our mouth directly to our PEP (Posterior Exit Port), so the contents of that tunnel are in fact outside the body. Why the heck does this matter? Well, the most basic unit of life, the cell, is really alive only so long as it has a barrier between itself and the environment. If that barrier (the cell membrane) should be damaged or disappear, that cell has "become one with the infinite" (i.e., died). This does not mean the cell is impervious and does not let anything in or out. But the cell, ideally, lets only certain things in and out, and this happens in a very specific way. Our digestive tract is somewhat like the cell membrane in that it allows certain things both in and out of our bodies in a very specific way. (I'm not sure if you've noticed, but poo is pretty nasty stuff. I have two young kids, and I've learned the horrors of poo migrating to locales to which it was never intended to go.) I mention all this because our modern diet and lifestyle tend to damage the gut in a way that allows the contents of our gut to enter our bodies, and the results are disastrous. Conversely, the approaches we will use in the book will ensure we keep our poo where it belongs.

HOW THINGS CAN GO WRONG: THE HYGIENE HYPOTHESIS

Until recent human history, infectious disease was one of the primary causes—if not *the* primary cause—of early death and was responsible for untold suffering. Infectious agents ranged from viruses like smallpox to the bacteria responsible for scarlet fever, ooogly-googly parasites like tapeworms, and the always cocktail-party-worthy liver flukes. A primary goal of modern medicine has been to eradicate infectious disease and between public health initiatives, sanitation, and antibiotics, we have accomplished much in this regard. Where once children were crippled for life by polio, the disease has been nearly eradicated. Infections, which are now routinely treated with a course of antibiotics, once proved fatal to millions of people worldwide. It's difficult to describe how much good has come from these efforts. But like most things in biology, the gains we have made in certain areas may have provided challenges in others.

The Hygiene Hypothesis posits that many of the problems we face today such as asthma, allergies, and autoimmunity may be an outgrowth of *too little* interaction between our immune system and infectious agents. Our genetics are "expecting" a certain degree of infection to help fine-tune the process of recognizing self from nonself. However, antibiotics, hyperclean environments, and hand sanitizers may be overly limiting the amount and types of infectious opportunities our immune systems face. Without this tuning, we may overreact to dietary or environmental agents, or perhaps even our own body in the case of autoimmunity. Here are some key observations that support the Hygiene Hypothesis:

1. The gut bacteria of non-Westernized populations appears to be quite different from that of most Westernized populations. Western populations have much less bacterial diversity in general and appear to be lacking a significant number of species common to non-Westernized populations.
2. Children in Westernized societies who are raised around animals and on farms appear to have a gut bacterial profile far more diverse than those who are not. Their microbiome may not be as varied as the one seen in non-Westernized populations, but is significantly different from that of individuals born and raised in urban settings.
3. The likelihood of the two aforementioned groups to develop allergies, autoimmunity, and inflammatory bowel issues is much lower than that of the folks with what we'd call "Western guts." We do not know exactly why this is, but it is reasonable to conclude that the increased microbial diversity in their guts provides immune tuning and possibly unique

metabolic products that are beneficial to their health. These "novel" bacteria may help to break down otherwise problematic foods, preventing allergies and food intolerances.

For us to understand how alterations in the gut can lead to conditions as seemingly unrelated as autoimmunity and type 2 diabetes, we need to understand two important ways the gut environment may be altered. The first situation involves an overgrowth and/or change in gut bacteria, while the second consideration will actually involve damage to the gut lining. These are important distinctions, but it's worth mentioning that the problems we will look at often have elements of both bacterial changes and damage to the gut lining.

BACTERIAL OVERGROWTH AND REFINED CARBOHYDRATES

There have been an equal number of nutritional darlings and demons over the past sixty years of nutritional research. As we have seen, dietary fat has been in and out of the proverbial frying pan many times. Although never demonized like fat, dietary fiber has been alternately in and out of favor within the scientific community as well. Sometimes a study will show that fiber is beneficial for health, other times the connection is weak or nonexistent. This is not dissimilar to the story of the Macronutrient Wars themselves, in which researchers appeared to be circling around a problem using the same techniques and methodologies and expecting a new insight or result. Are carbohydrates good? One study says yes, another no. A recent paper* cut through

---

* Titled "Comparison with ancestral diets suggests dense acellular carbohydrates promote an inflammatory microbiota, and may be the primary dietary cause of leptin resistance and obesity."

this confusion in a remarkable way by not starting the conversation from a reductionist perspective (which parts and pieces may be important) but rather in looking at our ancestral environment to ascertain if changes in our modern diet might be at play in modern disease.

If you recall from the digestion chapter, under ideal conditions, digestion and absorption of nutrients should occur at specific points in the digestive tract. Ancestral diets that are rich in a wide variety of fibers appear to provide a form of carbohydrate that is not broken down by the action of our digestive enzymes, but instead feeds the bacteria in our large intestine and colon. Bacteria convert certain types of fiber to short-chain fatty acids, which appear to play an important role in feeding the intestinal cells while also decreasing inflammation throughout the body. Additionally, and really to the point of the paper, cellular carbohydrate, like that found in fruits, vegetables, roots, beans, and *whole* grains are packaged in such a way that their digestion is slow, and this appears to "save" the carbohydrate for digestion later in the digestive tract. By contrast, refined carbohydrate alters the digestive system by encouraging the abnormal growth of bacteria in the small intestine (SIBO), while also encouraging the growth of pathogenic bacteria in the large intestine and colon. You might wonder, *Okay, bacteria are growing in the wrong places, and the types of bacteria may have shifted from benign to nasty, so what?* That's a great question, and the answer involves one of the most ancient processes in all of biology: What happens when a complex organism is infected with certain types of bacteria?

SEPSIS: IT'S NOT WHAT'S FOR DINNER

If you are a fan of medical shows or if one of your loved ones has had the unfortunate luck to develop a condition called sepsis, your ears may have perked up at this point. Sepsis is a condition in which an organism (let's say you or me) is infected with bacteria, like the often heard about *E. coli*. Sepsis is a dire, life-threatening situation, and it looks eerily similar to, in fact nearly indistinguishable from, poorly controlled type 2 diabetes. Blood glucose is dramatically elevated, free fatty acids are released into circulation, and inflammation is rampant. This process of insulin resistance and altered metabolism appears to be in response to a substance produced by bacteria called lipopolysaccharide (LPS). LPS is a molecule that can be fatal in humans (and virtually all animals) at elevated levels. Certain types of bacterial infections can be incredibly dangerous for an individual, and although a significant response is needed to wall off the infection, the septic response is so powerful that individuals often die, not specifically from the infection, but rather from the body's inflammatory response to the infection.

Although less severe (at least initially) the development of SIBO and changes in our microbiota allow for abnormally large amounts of LPS to make its way into our circulation. While these levels are not as high as those seen in life-threatening sepsis, it establishes a chronic inflammatory state that increases risk for cardiovascular disease, neurodegeneration, and a host of other conditions. This pathogenic shift in gut bacteria is largely independent of the total amount of calories consumed (although overeating makes things worse) but is most certainly initiated by eating pro-inflammatory carbohydrates typical of those found in the modern junk food diet.

Studies of Western versus non-Westernized populations show striking differences in not only disease rates and risks, but also levels of inflammatory markers and the hormones governing the neuroregulation of appetite. Ancestral diets show a remarkable spread in macronutrient profiles. Some are rather low carb, while others may be as high as 70 percent carbohydrate. This spread in macronutrients appears to have little if any impact on health so long as the foods are largely unprocessed and the carbohydrates come mainly from fruits, vegetables, and tubers.

I've mentioned whole grains and beans a few times thus far. Although this may wrinkle the Paleo purists, I think these foods may be consumed in moderation without perturbing our gut microbiota, but there are important caveats to this. If your gut is already damaged, if you have SIBO, or if you are reactive to proteins found in these foods (like gluten, in the case of wheat), you should likely avoid these foods altogether. I will dig into all this in much greater detail later.

For now, I'd like you to understand that ancestral diets appear to confer remarkable health benefits to the folks who eat them. People naturally eat to satiety, overconsumption of food is actually difficult due to the satiating quality of these foods, and the gut microbiome is healthy. This means the hormones and neurotransmitters responsible for the neuroregulation of appetite are all functioning properly. Refined modern foods clearly pose a problem for the gut, as they tend to shift bacterial growth in unfavorable ways. Several studies have linked an altered gut profile with type 2 diabetes and insulin resistance, and although suggestive, it's important to note that correlation does not equal causation. With this in mind, researchers have taken the gut biome from obese mice and inoculated lean healthy mice with the altered gut profile. The result? The healthy mice gained weight and became insulin and leptin resistant. The opposite experiment was also done: obese mice were reverted to health after receiving a poo-cocktail from healthy mice. It's worth mentioning, however, that it appears much easier to shift from healthy to unhealthy. It's not impossible to undo this damage, but it's not easy. This research helps us understand that as long as the carbohydrates we eat are unrefined (and our guts are generally healthy), the amounts of macronutrients we consume may not matter. Conversely, if our guts are damaged and we are suffering from SIBO or related problems, a low-carbohydrate diet (which prunes back the microbiome) may be a smart treatment option, at least until we can fix the gut. Some people (like myself) seem to do better long term by keeping carbs on the low side (100 to 150g/day), while other people may find they tolerate larger amounts of unrefined carbs. We will talk about what factors may be driving these differences in just a bit, and I'll help you figure all this out by using the 30-Day Reset to get your gut healthy, then using the 7-Day Carb Test to optimize your hormones and gut flora based on your individual needs.

As if altering our gut bacteria were not enough, certain "Neolithic" foods also appear to damage the GI tract directly. Let's look at that.

FOOD AND THE GUT: FRIENDS OR FOES?

Everything in nature has thorns, horns, teeth, claws, shells, or some kind of poison. If a given critter does not have a solid system of defense, said critter will end up being a snack for another critter. People generally do not think about this in terms of our food, particularly plants, but I'm telling you *everything* has some kind of defense mechanism or antipredation technique. Don't believe me? Next time you go out to eat, find the most authentic Thai food place available, wander into the establishment, and ask for a curry that is "Thai hot." The proprietor will nod in agreement, and likely roll out some video equipment to document for posterity the disaster about to unfold. As you bring the first steaming mouthful of curry to your face (assuming your metal spoon has not melted), you can actually smell the heat. Chomp, chew, swallow. Your face is on fire, your nose is running, and your eyes are watering like you have been watching dog rescue shows on Animal Planet. You have just consumed a food with hot peppers that contain an irritant called capsaicin. This irritant evolved as a means of dissuading most critters from eating hot peppers. Humans have found that the right dose of hot peppers can make food pretty damn tasty. Traditional cultures have attributed medicinal qualities to many spices such as ginger, turmeric, and hot peppers, and science has borne this observation out. All these spices contain potent antioxidants as well as antimicrobial compounds. These herbs and spices provide a number of health and medicinal benefits, as long as the dose is appropriate. Thai-hot curry is generally not an "appropriate" dose for most people! That mouthful will burn all the way through the GI tract, and the individual who regularly ventures down that path would be wise to invest in toilet paper futures.

Similarly, the bitterness most people find appealing in coffee is caused by alkaloids, which dissuade critters from eating coffee beans. Most of the selective breeding and genetic tinkering humans have done to our food over the past ten thousand years has focused on making certain types of plants larger, sweeter, and milder in flavor. Mellowing flavor typically involves decreasing the amount of bitter or irritating chemicals the plant makes. With these natural deterrents removed, our modern fruits and vegetables are, not surprisingly, an easy target for pests.

I'm taking the time to mention all this because I'm about to implicate a number of staple foods as being highly problematic for our digestion and therefore our health. When I mention to people that grains like wheat, rye, oats, barley, pseudo-grains like quinoa and amaranth, and legumes like black beans and pinto beans all contain chemical defense substances that may be irritating to the gut as well as to our immune system, people . . . well, they freak out. Anger, denial, I get it all. Let's consider for a moment that these foods I've mentioned follow trends that we see in nature, and one of those trends involves the need for some kind of chemical or physical defense system to dissuade critters from eating what is essentially the reproductive structures of these plants.

If we eat an apple or a watermelon, we generally discard the seeds. If we eat the seeds, they pass through our digestion unchanged, and if we deposit this payload somewhere other than in the municipal sewage system, those seeds get a nice start wrapped in a warm, nutrient-dense blanket of poo. Grains and legumes *are* the reproductive structures of their respective plants, and they have a host of defense mechanisms including enzyme inhibitors, which limit the breakdown of the seed. A grazing animal that consumes some ripe grain may in fact pass most of the seeds intact through its digestive system, and this is due in part to the enzyme inhibitors. This can be problematic as these enzyme inhibitors may negatively affect the digestion and absorption of other foods, but the seeds do not stop their defense efforts here. They also have a number of proteins, many of which are classified as lectins, which can raise hell on the GI tract if not properly prepared. Some of these lectins, like those found in beans, can actually cause the cells in the GI tract to rupture. In properly prepared beans, this is rarely, if ever, an issue, but this may be something to consider if one has autoimmune disease or serious gut issues.

Other molecules, like the family of proteins related to gluten, cause an inflammatory response in the gut. We will look closely at gluten in a moment, as it appears to be particularly problematic for many people. Before I get to that, however, I'd like to make the point that there are many methods of preparation that can reduce the activity of these toxic substances. Many traditional cultures have soaked, sprouted, and fermented grains and legumes as a means of reducing the deleterious effects of consuming these foods. If you are going to eat these foods, I think employing these methods is a wise decision. But in my nearly twenty years of working with people, I've found that the vast majority of folks do well to keep consumption of these foods relatively infrequent, at least until we have built a strong healthy gut and the individual is willing to monitor how he or she responds to these foods. More on that in Part Two of the book.

AUTOIMMUNITY BEGINS IN THE GUT

We now understand that certain foods can directly irritate the gut. This is typically not welcome news to most people and is received with the warmth one might confer on an old diaper that has been left in the car for a few weeks. Why? Because this information paints many of the foods we love to eat in a pretty poor light. Perhaps at the top of that list is wheat, which is the main ingredient in most cakes, cookies, cereals, and other cocainelike "food" items.

Most people are aware that celiac disease is a condition in which certain individuals cannot eat wheat (and usually some related grains like rye, millet, and oats) without suffering serious health consequences. Celiac is an autoimmune disease triggered by the protein gluten (really it's a subfraction of gluten called gliadin, but we'll stick with calling it gluten for now), but it also happens to be a model for autoimmune diseases such as rheumatoid arthritis, multiple sclerosis, and lupus (to name but a few). Gluten is a tough protein for humans to digest. Its chemical structure makes the protein resistant to the action of protein-degrading enzymes. This tends to leave the gluten protein intact, which makes it available to interact with the epithelial cells of the intestines, which leads to a process that allows for intestinal permeability and ultimately to undigested food particles entering our bodies. This may be a factor in the cause of allergies, autoimmunity, and multiple chemical sensitivities. As if that were not bad enough, this process also releases a cascade of inflammatory cytokines that brings the immune system in that area into high alert.

The suggestion that intestinal permeability (commonly called leaky gut) is a major factor in autoimmune diseases such as multiple sclerosis, lupus, and rheumatoid arthritis strengthens daily. There is not yet an airtight case of causation, but the evidence is compelling: of the autoimmune diseases studied, all appear to present with intestinal permeability. This is "just" correlation, but it's interesting enough to warrant a closer look at this problem.

Using celiac disease as a model, we have a solid mechanism for how the intestinal barrier may be breached, allowing our immune system to inadvertently produce antibodies against either our tissues or food particles that have protein structures that look like proteins in our bodies. The net effect is the same: our immune system attacking our organs, cells, and tissues.

Repairing intestinal permeability has halted the autoimmune process in a number of studies. Several years ago, my good friend Dr. Terry Wahls started experiencing profound fatigue accompanied by loss of strength and fine motor control in her arms and legs. Eventually, her worst fears were confirmed with a diagnosis of multiple sclerosis (MS). Although her situation seemed dire, she did not give up. She looked at what was then the fringe elements of the autoimmune research community and noticed that intestinal permeability was implicated in her condition. Using a special variant of the Paleo diet called the autoimmune protocol (of which there is a meal plan in the prescriptive chapter), Dr. Wahls was able to reverse her condition and ditch her wheelchair. Dr. Wahls released a TED Talk on her experience, which has been watched nearly 2.5 million times. Fortunately for all of us, Dr. Wahls is in a perfect position to investigate this story in a rigorous fashion in order to provide evidence for the medical community. Her preliminary work indicates significant success for patients with various autoimmune conditions and recommends the adoption of an autoimmune Paleo diet, which appears to improve intestinal permeability, lower blood glucose levels, and reduce inflammation. You can watch Dr. Wahls's amazing TED Talk by searching for "Minding Your Mitochondria."

This brings us full circle in the story of Western degenerative diseases, as it would appear that many autoimmune conditions share an interesting relationship with type 2 diabetes and other conditions in the form of mito-chondrial dysfunction. If you recall, one of the final stages in the "overfed" state is characterized by damage to the mitochondria, which increases inflammation while also limiting energy for the cell. Recent research in a number of conditions such as rheumatoid arthritis, type 1 diabetes, and MS indicates that damaged mitochondria are quite common.

An interesting workaround for this problem involves the use of a keto-genic diet to provide alternate fuel for the mitochondria, bypassing our reli-ance on glucose. Ketosis also appears to help repair damaged mitochondria and select for those mitochondria that are more metabolically flexible. This is why many people find that an autoimmune Paleo program mixed with a smart ketogenic diet can greatly improve their autoimmune and systemic inflammatory symptoms. Some people need to remain on a fairly low-carb diet if they are to remain symptom free, while others find they do well on appropriate levels of unrefined carbohydrate. This is a highly individual story and I'll help you understand how to navigate this process in Part Two. Fortunately for all of us, recent research has provided a simple tool (the blood glucose monitor) and protocol that will help you refine your dietary program to meet your needs. I'll talk about that presently, but I'd like to take a moment and pull all this together. I know this is a lot of thick mate-rial, but we have nearly crested the top of this information mountain. Let's look at all this with just a few key points:

1. Refined (acellular) carbohydrates appear to negatively alter gut bacteria, causing overgrowth in the small intestine (SIBO) while starving the bacteria in the colon and large intestine. This shift causes inflammation and damages the liver, and impairs leptin and insulin sensitivity. This is a state of low-grade sepsis and likely the cause of diabetes and a host of insulin-related conditions.

2. Immunogenic foods such as grains and legumes can damage the gut lining, allowing intact food particles and bacterial products to enter our bodies. This sets the stage for autoimmune disease via a process called molecular mimicry. Additionally, inflammation can damage mitochondrial function, shifting our cells even further toward a proinflammatory state.

3. Whether one develops autoimmunity or insulin resistance, these diseases appear to be largely driven by genetics. But there appears to be similar cause in both cases: increased intestinal permeability, an unhealthy shift in gut bacteria that creates increased inflammatory signaling in the body.

IS THIS REALLY A ONE-WAY STREET?

I'd like to briefly make the point that this whole process is not likely a "one-way street." Yes, our food has a massive impact on our gut health, but so too do stress, sleep, exercise, birth history, antibiotic use, and light exposure. Each of these topics feeds back on gut health in highly complex ways that are outside the scope of this book, but this *is* why I put such emphasis on these topics as part of our overall program.

Let me share some of my personal history as a means of illustrating how all this fits together.

I was born via vaginal delivery, which, in theory, should have imparted a solid microbiome within me. Unfortunately, my mother had a lifetime of GI and health issues, including rheumatoid arthritis and lupus. It's likely that her biome was shifted in an unfavorable way. I was formula-fed due to problems my mother had with breastfeeding. This means whatever microbiome I did receive was not set up as well as it could have been, and I did not take in the immune-enhancing proteins and sugars that make breast milk so beneficial. Additionally, I was exposed to soy, rice, and a number of other foods far too early. The infant gut is naturally permeable, which allows the large, intact proteins found in breast milk to make their way into the infant body, tuning the immune system and setting us up for success. Early exposure to foods other than breast milk dramatically increases the likelihood of allergies and reactivity to foods, as the highly permeable infant gut is ill prepared to deal with these novel foods.

I had an almost constant run of strep throat throughout my childhood. I frequently had sinus and ear infections, and my tonsils would swell to elephantine size. This was likely a consequence of food sensitivities that increased inflammation in my throat and sinuses while also suppressing my immune function. I took a lot of antibiotics as a kid. My adolescent years were not much of an improvement, as puberty, mixed with a strong reaction to cow dairy, produced acne on my face, back, and neck that was volcanic in proportions. I still get acne from cow dairy, despite being closer to "manopause" than puberty. Food reactivity was not remotely on the radar of medicine at this time, so instead of looking at a root cause for my acne, I was put on the antibiotic tetracycline from the age of fourteen to twenty-one. I only discontinued the tetracycline due to severe acid reflux and GI distress that seemed to coincide with taking the medication.

In my mid-twenties, I did what most people do in college: I adopted a vegetarian and then a vegan diet. I was convinced this was a healthy way of eating, but I spent the next three to four years absorbing almost nothing from my food. I went from a lean, muscular 180 pounds to a sick, emaciated 135 pounds, eventually receiving a diagnosis of ulcerative colitis. My condition was so bad that my doctors were recommending a bowel resection at the ripe old age of twenty-seven. Not only was this scary, but the prospect of major surgery and possibly carrying around a colostomy bag did not bode well for my dating life. Neither I nor my doctors could think of anything good to do for me other than immunosuppressant drugs and/ or surgery.

Interestingly, it was my mother's health crisis that provided insight into what I needed to do. My mom had been sick as long as I could remember. She had her gallbladder removed in her thirties and suffered from a myriad of nonspecific health problems for decades. She was often labeled a hypochondriac, which was completely accurate, only not in the way modern medicine would look at that term. My mom had a very sick, terribly damaged gut. She went into the hospital suffering from inflammation around her heart, lungs, and many other tissues. Her doctor eventually gave her the diagnoses of celiac disease, rheumatoid arthritis, lupus, and several other less-known autoimmune conditions. My mom nearly died from this autoimmune flare, but the aggressive use of anti-inflammatory and immunosuppressant drugs saved her life. This was a harrowing experience for my whole family, and I remember talking to my mom on the phone asking her about how she was doing. She described the laundry list of conditions she'd just been diagnosed with and then said something almost offhand that was to completely alter my life and the lives of everyone who has ever read one of my books or blogs, or listened to one of my podcasts. Mom mentioned that her doctor had told her she was remarkably reactive to most grains, legumes, and dairy.

Given that I was vegan at this time, my first thought after getting off the phone with my mom was, *What the hell do you eat if you do not eat grains, legumes, and dairy?* I thought about this and my mind drifted to the following flow: *Have people always eaten these foods? If not, when did consumption start? Agriculture . . . that's when we domesticated animals and plants, dramatically altering our food system. What was this time called? The Neolithic, birth of modern culture. What was the time preceding this? The Paleolithic. What did people eat at that time? What they could hunt and gather . . . not much in the way of grains, legumes, and dairy.*

It may seem crazy, but this flow of consciousness took just seconds; it was like my mind was primed for this discovery and I just needed the right information to push me in the proper direction. This was around 1998, and I used a newfangled search engine called Google to search a term I'd heard of: the Paleolithic Diet. I found work from Dr. Loren Cordain that painted a picture of remarkable health for our hunter-gatherer ancestors. His seminal paper "Cereal Grains, Humanity's Double-Edged Sword" suggested the transition to agriculture as critical for the development of our modern world, but this cultural evolution came at a price in terms of individual health. These Neolithic foods appeared to be potential sources of inflammation in the human gut, possibly setting the stage for autoimmune disease, obesity, and conditions like celiac disease.

I've now eaten what is generally termed a Paleo diet for nearly twenty years, and my health in my mid-forties is far better than it was in my mid-twenties. I've learned how to heal my gut to a remarkable degree and my health has improved tremendously. There are people who have never eaten a Paleo-type diet who are healthy and vibrant, but they do not have my life history. Millions of people *do* have a similar life history as I do, and these folks have greatly benefited by healing their gut with something like a Paleo diet. Unfortunately, many millions of people have never heard of this idea and thus suffer needlessly.

I'm driven to do the work I do because I have information and experience that I'm pretty sure can save lives. I share this information not from a position of religious conviction, but rather a sincere desire to help as many people as I can. Although the ideas about nutrition and wellness I have shared with you are gaining traction, most doctors and health care providers are not aware of the evolutionary medicine model. They do not yet have access to the tools that could dramatically alter the health of their patients. I know that some of the material I have shared with you in this section can be emotionally charged, but I ask you to follow my Greasy Used-Car Sales Pitch: Give this program a shot for thirty days. See how you look, feel, and perform. Do some basic blood work and then evaluate if the effort of following the program is worth the rewards. If you are still with me, you may be wondering, *What the heck am I supposed to do?* Great question, and we will get to the answer soon.

This may feel like a lot of background information (and it is!), but it's been my experience that taking the time to explain the whys will help you relax into the hows. My job is to strike a balance between providing information and practical, easy-to-follow guidelines that fit as many people as possible, while also maintaining the flexibility necessary to address individual needs. The basic 30-Day Reset presented later in the book addresses the needs of most people. As well as the program works, there is still significant individual variation that can make the program both easier to stick with long term and more effective. The next chapter looks at research highlighting the power of Personalized Nutrition. We are on the threshold of a new era in nutrition, one in which clunky one-size-fits-all approaches give way to the elegant solution of tailoring our nutrition to our specific genetic and gut microbiome needs.

CHAPTER 6

Personalized Nutrition

The Future Is Now

There are tens of thousands of medical research papers published every year. The vast majority are not that helpful in providing better insight into our health and in particular what we can do to affect positive change. One could spend billions of dollars on research and not come up with better health recommendations than: eat whole, unprocessed foods, get outside in the sun, move a lot, sleep like you are on vacation, and surround yourself with loving relationships. Pretty common sense, right? The scientific process is amazing in that it is mainly focused on asking "why?" I consider myself a scientist, but I actually think about things more like an engineer than a scientist. I am interested in the why, but if I have a problem to solve, I don't want to wait fifty years for the peer review process to give me actionable steps. The paper "Personalized Nutrition by Prediction of Glycemic Responses," which appeared in the prestigious journal *Cell*, is one of the most important research projects in the past fifty years.

These researchers tackled the problem of "what the hell should I eat" the way an engineer would address the problem. The goal was not specifically to answer another "why," but to find a way of helping people eat and live in a way that would keep them lean and healthy. This is what is called outcome-based medicine. Theory be damned, what actually works? Here is the gist of the research: Eight hundred people were screened for the composition of their gut biome, in addition to basic blood work looking at cholesterol levels, blood glucose, and inflammatory markers. They also had a continuous glucose monitoring device inserted into their skin, which checked blood glucose every 5 seconds! They answered extensive lifestyle questionnaires and were instructed to log their food throughout the course of the study.

Under ideal circumstances, this study would have been done in what are called metabolic ward conditions. This is a step above prison life in that folks are continuously monitored in a hospital while their food intake is fastidiously tracked. It is both invasive and incredibly expensive to put together a study like this. If you make the study experience too difficult, people will opt out of the program. If researchers are overly ambitious in study design, they will never get funding. This is why so much of the published research is not particularly helpful: the studies are small and poorly designed.

This study was fairly unique in that it was incredibly comprehensive while not being so onerous as to cause most of the participants to quit midway through the project. Although this was *not* a metabolic ward setting, the participants were fed one meal per day at the research institute conducting the study, thus providing a solid baseline consistent among all participants. People were also instructed on how to log the contents of their other meals using a simple smartphone app. Knowing what folks actually ate is a difficult process in dietary intervention studies and is notoriously fraught with error. Did folks *really* weigh out the right amount of food for a meal? Did they forget to include everything they ate? The daily baseline meals, composed of an equal amount of carbohydrates from either bread, bread plus butter, glucose, or fructose, provided a massive, consistent source of data that offers many of the advantages of a metabolic ward intervention, but without the cost and complications. Using a subdermal continuous glucose monitoring device, the researchers were able to track the response these people had to all the meals they consumed. The groundbreaking highlight from this research was that a person's glycemic response (how much blood glucose increased for a given meal) appeared to be influenced by genetic factors, exercise, body fat levels, and, perhaps most interesting, the composition of the gut biome. One of the most important findings of the study showed there was massive variation from person to person in how they reacted to various foods. Some foods that we'd normally assume would cause blood glucose problems were not problematic for some people, while foods normally thought of as "good" caused some people to experience significant blood sugar increases. Again, this was interesting data, but it was not yet at a point that anyone could do much with the information. What the researchers needed to do was find the connections between genetics, gut microbiome, and people's responses to the various foods.

To create a predictive model, one that could tell us what or what not to do, the researchers took the genetic, lifestyle, and microbiome information from the initial eight hundred participants and created an algorithm, which they then used to validate (or invalidate) their process. The researchers collected the same metrics as they did previously, but in a fresh group of one hundred participants. This time the researchers used their algorithm to predict what each individual's response to a given meal would be, and their predictions were spot on. The machine-learning algorithm the researchers used could accurately and consistently predict what an individual's glycemic response would be to a given meal. As good as this information already was, the researchers asked another critical question: If we know the genetics, gut biome, blood work, body fat, and activity level of a given individual, can the algorithm recommend a carbohydrate type and amount that will keep the individual within healthy levels? Once again, the algorithm did what only painstaking trial and error has been able to achieve: provide customized nutritional guidelines that resulted in healthy glycemic response. Let me give you a real-world example to provide context: Some people find they do well on a lower-carb diet. They avoid bread, rice, beans, and most other foods that contain significant amounts of carbohydrate. These folks lose weight and are no longer ravenously hungry, but they are often left wondering if they must eat this way forever, or if they have more latitude in their eating, are unsure how to proceed. Instead of blindly experimenting with dozens of foods and waiting for often subtle changes in how one feels, by using Personalized Nutrition one can zero in on problematic foods quickly and easily. In this book, we will start with a 30-Day Reset to get you moving in a good direction, then with the 7-Day Carb Test plan we will use a blood glucose monitor to help find the amounts and types of foods you do best with.

It's perhaps worth noting that the two main variables that determine what foods work best for folks involved eating either more fat and fewer carbs or avoiding problematic foods. We will use this same strategy to dial in your program by finding both the right amounts and types of food to suit your unique situation.

When we look at optimal nutrition from the perspective of Personalized Nutrition, it's no wonder the macronutrient wars have raged for so long! There are people who do far better on lower-carb, higher-fat diets (like me) and other people who excel on higher-carb, lower-fat programs. Similarly, there are foods that seem to elicit a negative blood glucose response in some people but are seemingly benign for others. I mentioned that there was a high degree of variability from person to person with regard to individual glycemic response. Let's look at a few of those examples from the study, as they are both interesting and educational:

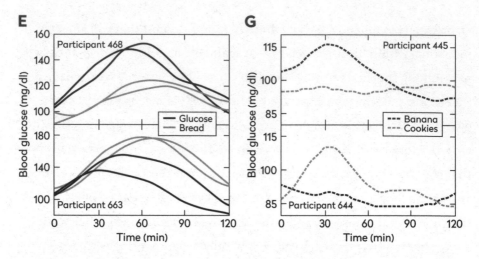

In the graphic labeled "E," we see two different participants, #468 in the upper box and #663 in the lower box. The blood glucose response to both glucose and bread are noted. What is interesting is the participant 663 had a better glycemic response (lower overall blood sugar increase) to pure glucose than to bread! Participant 468 had what we'd expect to be a more typical glycemic response in that glucose drove blood sugar levels higher than bread.

That first example is interesting, but the second example, where equal amounts of carbohydrate from bananas and cookies are compared is frankly stunning. In graphic "G," participant 445 had a pronounced increase in blood sugar from eating a banana, but a good blood glucose response from a cookie, while the opposite occurred in participant 644! Although tempting to label these folks as "cookie or banana" profiles, the story is not that simple. This is just a snapshot of how these two people responded to these specific foods. Although this research was aimed at finding how folks responded to various foods, the results do raise the question of "Why the variability?" In talking with some of the researchers, I discovered it is possible some of this seeming randomness is an outgrowth of food intolerances, like gluten or dairy, for example. This round of research did not address that topic specifically, but it is an area of investigation for the future. The point is that everything you have learned about the immunogenic/gut-irritating nature of certain foods still holds true here; we are just looking at the problem in a different way.

Conventional wisdom would have us believe that "a calorie is a calorie," and equal amounts of carbohydrate should cause the same blood glucose responses. Clearly, this is not the case. More sophisticated models that look at glycemic load, fiber, and cellular versus acellular refined carbohydrate would tell us that we should see a uniformly better blood glucose response from a banana relative to a cookie. However, this was also not the case. What the heck is going on here? It appears most of this variability can be ascribed to differences in the gut microbiome. There are trends to this story, with certain species of bacteria being more strongly associated with favorable glycemic responses, but there was still significant variation. The next bit of information I'll share with you cements the need to use big-picture nutrition models, even the Paleo diet, with a bit of caution, as even the most benign of foods can prove problematic for some people. Participants were fed either "good" or "bad" foods, and this was tracked over the course of one week.

A few foods were almost universally good or bad, but others, like hummus (a mix of garbanzo beans and sesame seed paste), were mixed. Some people did well when eating these foods, but others did not. If you talked to most doctors or dietitians, they would likely say beef is bad for blood glucose (because of its saturated fat content), while hummus is good. They would be flatly incorrect in the case of beef, and doing little more than a coin toss in the case of hummus. You may be thinking, *Bloody hell! What am I to do with this?* Don't worry—a final piece of this research gives us a great tool to figure out what to do with our own diet.

In the final stage of this study, the researchers put participants on a diet that, based on previous blood glucose response and the insights of their machine learning algorithm, would provide favorable glycemic responses. The results were quite interesting. Although the specific dietary protocols varied from person to person, there was a consistent shift toward a gut biome that is more associated with leanness, low inflammation, and favorable glycemic control. Eating a diet that did not negatively alter blood glucose levels appeared to "rehabilitate" the gut. The participants were not evaluated for abnormal growth of bacteria in the small intestine (SIBO) or for reactivity to specific foods, but as we now know, both conditions can negatively alter inflammatory state and therefore glycemic response. An individual with SIBO, but with no reactivity to, say, wheat, will likely need a different protocol than an individual with gluten sensitivity but no SIBO. Although gut biome and genetic testing like that done in this study could certainly be informative, we can likely bypass these tests and go directly to simply monitoring our blood glucose responses with an inexpensive glucometer. I'll talk about how to do just that in a later chapter.

This was a lot of ground to cover, but I think you can now better appreciate the influence of the gut on our health and how important it is to recognize that we all have unique nutritional needs. This is exactly why the one-size-fits-all diet approach does not work—and why the plan in this book is so groundbreaking. Whether you are concerned with cardiovascular disease, neurodegeneration, autoimmunity, or cancer, lowering inflammation and controlling blood glucose levels appear to reduce our likelihood of developing all these conditions. It is also clear that the same process that gets us healthy is what will help us to lose weight and keep it off permanently.

In the next chapter, we will look at the science behind the model we will use to get you started on your path to health and skinny jeans: the

Paleo diet. It may seem odd that I've talked at length about the need for Personalized Nutrition, only to shift gears to a specific eating approach, but this is just the launching pad to get you moving in the right direction. My program starts with Phase One: The 30-Day Reset to get your body primed and ready before moving on to Phase Two, where you will begin the 7-Day Carb Test plan to find what specific foods you do best with.

CHAPTER 7

Is There a Case for the Paleo Diet?

I mentioned at the beginning of this book that people are *generally* not swayed to action by information. A few people are driven by information, and those people tend to be geeks, like yours truly. Most people, however, make changes in behavior due to emotion, not facts and figures. This is not a bad thing; our emotions, coupled with our logical intellect, are what make us human. It's an amazing combination that serves us well for most things. But if we have strong emotional connections to a behavior that is unhealthy for us, it can be tough to change.

Given all this, you might wonder why I have devoted so much space to . . . well, facts and figures. Although people often do not find cold, hard facts to be compelling enough to change a behavior, these same people *will* dig up information to defend a particular position. I'm going to recommend some specific diet and lifestyle changes for you; if those suggestions do not sit well with you, the likely course of action is for you to jump on the Internet and find counterpoints to my suggestions. Other folks just ignore any new information out of hand.

Here is a hypothetical situation: You have a friend with the gender-ambiguous name of Charlie who smoked and drank heavily for years. You care about this friend, and want to see him/her live long enough to see his/her kids grow up and go to school, and maybe even see some grandkids. One day, you invite Charlie to lunch and have a heart to heart.

YOU: So Charlie . . . when did you start smoking?

CHARLIE: Oh, about age twelve.

YOU: Holy cats! You've been smoking that long?

CHARLIE: Yeah! It's awesome.

YOU: Ugh . . . yeah. So, how long have you been drinking to a blackout stage each night?

CHARLIE: I got started drinking kinda late. I think around eighteen. And I don't drink to black out. It helps me relax and sleep.

YOU: Listen, Charlie, I don't want to be nosy, but you are one of my best friends, and I care a lot about you. *Also*, you have two young kids. Do you ever think about not being around to see them grow up? Don't you want to see your grandkids one day?

CHARLIE: I will totally be around to see my kids grow up, and I expect to see great-grandkids! What are you talking about?

YOU: Well, you don't exercise, you eat like a cockroach, and you smoked and drank for years like you are in *Leaving Las Vegas*. You must have read or heard about studies that say how bad smoking and drinking in excess are for you!

CHARLIE: Look, I appreciate the concern, but my grandfather and grandmother both smoked and drank the same way, and they lived into their late eighties. If they didn't have that ice-fishing accident, they would have lived to be a hundred. And all the "scientific research" just contradicts itself year to year. This week broccoli is good, next week it's bad . . .

This hypothetical conversation may seem far-fetched, but I know I have played both roles, and I suspect you have, too. Perhaps it was not about smoking. Maybe it was finances or bad driving. But we have all been held accountable at some point and used some specious logic to dismiss well-intended advice or information. The reasons for this avoidance of the truth are manifold. Fear and inertia are clearly factors. Blockheaded stubbornness is also occasionally a player.

The reason for change to finally occur in these situations tends to be a jolting life event. Something that grabs you by the short hairs (so to speak) and makes you wake up, pay attention, and reevaluate how you do things. I've seen this a lot in the work I've done with people over the years. A brush with cancer. A diagnosis of prediabetes. Learning that a parent has Alzheimer's. At critical moments such as these, people make changes they might not have otherwise enacted.

Several things can get in the way of this process. A particularly vexing problem is simply confusion. What the heck should a person do if they discover they have a disease like type 2 diabetes? A few minutes on the Internet will provide enough contradictory information to crush that individual back into business as usual. *Should I go vegan? Drink green smoothies? Do Atkins? Just follow the Standard of Care?* The information is not only contradictory, but the volume is enough to make one curl up in the fetal position or rock back and forth on the floor making mewling noises.

The purpose of this book is to provide you with both the information and the emotional support to make a change. Simplicity is the key to effective change, particularly in the beginning. Getting buried under a million details just makes the process too hard. If you learn a language or work your way through a series of math classes, it's important for you to get small chunks of information you can work on daily. If your instructor dumps a massive amount of information on you, you'll likely get overwhelmed and mentally check out. Knowing this, I will provide you with simple guidelines that help you keep on track so you can see some success and maintain the motivation necessary to make changes around your sleep, food, and activity, forming lifelong habits.

So here's my Greasy Used Car Salesman (GUCS) pitch for getting started with Phase One:

- Try the 30-Day Reset.
- See how you look, feel, and perform.
- Check your blood pressure and waist-to-hip ratio (WHR).
- Do some basic blood work (if you want) before and after.
- Critically evaluate the results.
- Decide if the rewards outweigh the costs.

The 30-Day Reset period is a short enough time that most people feel they can do it, while it's long enough that you can critically assess if the program is working. If it is working, you also have the ability to ask a very reasonable question: Are the results worth the effort?

The 30-Day Reset is based on a Paleo eating plan similar to the one outlined in my previous book, but with some alterations and tweaks I have learned since the book's publication. Most of those tweaks involve a process of better determining where your health is and helping you delineate goals. This builds a map for you to follow, as you know where you are and where you want to go. This 30-Day Reset is incredibly effective at resetting your neuroregulation of appetite, healing your gut, and reducing inflammation. Those are the features; the *benefits* are that you can get healthy, increase your energy, and lose weight easily.

Before we go any further, though, I want to set up some rules of engagement to keep us all honest. Be open-minded, but also critical. I want to empower you to become an expert via your own experience. Give the process a shot and evaluate it based on the results you obtain. Also, ask yourself what *my* motivations are in making the recommendations I do.

I'm a health educator. I serve on the board of directors of a medical clinic in Reno, Nevada. I do speaking gigs around the world on this Ancestral Health topic to entities ranging from Twitter to NASA to Naval Special Warfare. My success is driven, completely, by how effective I am at helping people. Junk food companies, by contrast, make their money by exploiting our evolutionary wiring, which compels us to seek out new foods and flavors while expending as little time and effort as possible (the optimum foraging strategy, or OFS). My job is to help you understand the rules of this game so you, your family, and our society as a whole can be winners instead of unwitting victims of our modern junk food catastrophe. *That* is my motivation—and if you're successful, I'm successful.

I hope this resonates with you on both intuitive and cognitive levels. Some of you may think all this reads like a legal disclaimer, and in a way, you are correct. Some folks will launch into this program, give it a go, and let the results speak for themselves. A painful number of people, however, will vigorously pump the brakes at this point, for reasons they are likely unaware of. Based on thousands of conversations I've had with people about why this program is not for them, I can say that the individual has a story that makes him or her fear change. We often tell ourselves stories about why we are a certain way, why we can or cannot change. And the common denominator with most of these stories is fear . . . fear of change, failure, or wasting time. This fear sends the logical mind searching for credible reasons why embarking on a new solution seems like a bad idea. Some people have developed an identity tied to their condition, be that obesity or a specific disease. It's a tough loop to break. If you have reservations about getting into the program, you have to find what the block is and then find a "why" that is compelling enough to get past that point. Your "why" may be personal health concerns, your kids, or any number of other motivators. But as Yoda might say, "Need this, you do."

WHAT IS THE PALEO DIET?

One of the greatest challenges surrounding the Paleo diet, both from a research perspective and implementation, is the tendency to make the recommendations written in stone as if it were religious doctrine. I'll detail where and how this has happened and how this rigidity has created significant drama and confusion. For now, we can look at the Paleo diet in two complementary ways. By inclusion, the plan is generally composed of fruits, vegetables, roots, shoots, tubers, nuts and seeds, meat (including organ varieties), seafood, and fowl. By exclusion, a Paleo diet is one that *generally* avoids grains, legumes, and dairy. If we simply called this way of eating an "anti-inflammatory diet" and then looked at how certain foods cause inflammation, either in the digestive system or the rest of the body, we'd arrive at largely the same place and avoid a lot of the confusion on this topic. Similarly, if this way of eating had been called an evolutionary diet and some specific caveats were applied, we would also likely see less backlash from elements of the research community.

The Paleo diet is the basis of the 30-Day Reset you'll embark on in Phase One of my plan. There are several reasons for using the Paleo diet as a starting point, here are the highlights:

It's effective. The Paleo diet removes many common allergens and foods that may cause an inflammatory response, particularly in the gut. Due to its high nutrient density and low relative caloric load, the Paleo diet is highly satiating. By reducing inflammation and repairing the neuroregulation of appetite, we tend to naturally eat what we need. Most people are concerned about losing weight and overeating, but the powerful satiety effects of the Paleo diet can actually be a problem for some highly active people. Although athletes can and do follow a Paleo diet with good results, it's not uncommon for folks to add rice and dairy to their plan if they find it difficult to eat enough to maintain their activity level and body weight. If you want to be the size of an NFL lineman, you might benefit from adding certain non-Paleo foods, but the inverse is also true: if you want an easy way to eat to satiety that allows you to remain lean, strong, and healthy, the Paleo diet might be the best plan for you.

It's easy. Although the Paleo diet is a departure from the way most people eat, you have already eaten thousands of Paleo meals, whether you knew it or not. Ever had scrambled eggs, fruit, and coffee for breakfast? How about a chicken salad for lunch? Perhaps some grilled fish with a salad and a glass of wine for dinner? That's pretty damn close, and no, we do not need to get wrapped around the axle of whether coffee and wine are "Paleo" or not. In moderate amounts both are healthy, and when taken in the fuller context of our overall eating, they are just fine. My point here is you have already eaten many "Paleo"-type meals, I'm just suggesting you eat more of these than not. The cooking is simple and the meals are delicious. This makes sticking with the program easy and it quickly becomes a habit, not a "diet."

We will use this 30-Day Paleo Reset to get you back on track, losing weight (if you need to) and feeling great. My expectation is not that you try to follow this plan perfectly for the rest of your life. I want you to experiment with foods outside the basic Paleo diet (this is what the 7-Day Carb Test Plan is for) and figure out what foods you can eat that do not cause you problems. This provides for as much variety as possible while maintaining our health, sanity, and waistline. In my own diet I tend to include a fair amount of properly prepared beans and lentils, as well as some goat's- and sheep's-milk-based dairy, mainly cheeses. I am highly reactive to gluten, and cow dairy (of all types, with the possible exception of butter) gives me acne. Being middle-aged is bad enough; I do not want to be over the hill and looking like I'm going through puberty at the same time, so I generally follow Paleo guidelines while adding foods that I feel good with. This is the process I want you to follow. If you have specific health concerns such as autoimmunity or diabetes, I'll recommend some possible modifications to the basic plan. My greatest challenge in helping people has always been just getting them to follow a Paleo diet for thirty days; see how they look, feel, and perform; then evaluate the merits of the process. If I can get folks to just do that, they are sold. This is why I have the lengthy, quasilegal disclaimer at the beginning of this chapter. If you are whipped into a Paleo frenzy, I'll give you an option of skipping to the next chapter to learn how sleep, stress, and community all play into how you are wired to eat. You do not need to know the science behind the Paleo diet for it to work. If you are not sold on this idea, or if you have been confused by the many negative news pieces surrounding this way of eating, read on: I tackle all that in the coming pages. There are many whys answered in this next section, and that can be helpful for folks who may be concerned about ill-informed media pieces on the Paleo diet. This information is valuable, but it pales in contrast to just following the program and evaluating the results. Many of you reading this book may have a medical background, and you may be at best skeptical about this "fad diet." That's fine; check out the research, tinker with the process, then let me know your thoughts at robbwolf.com

HISTORY: IT AIN'T WHAT IT USED TO BE!

Most dietary approaches, from Atkins to The Zone to South Beach, tend to have a person or persons who come up with ideas about what constitutes the best way to eat for health or weight loss. Most of the plans I just mentioned tend to focus on the carbohydrate—and therefore insulin—load of the diet. The Paleo diet, by contrast, was arrived at by the observations of anthropologists and explorers studying contemporary hunter-gatherers and archeologists studying the remains of our human and pre-human ancestors. What anthropologists *observed* was that despite the lack of modern medical practices, hygiene, and sanitation, free-living hunter-gatherers, from the Arctic Circle to the savannas of Africa or the jungles of South America, tended to be remarkably healthy and largely free of what we'd call the diseases of modernity. When I say "observed" I don't want you to dismiss that out of hand as many researchers do. This observation ranged from spending a few days or weeks with certain groups or, like in the case of the Kitavan people of Papua New Guinea, being studied for more than thirty years with blood work, medical evaluations, and even autopsies.

These populations show little if any of our modern afflictions such as type 2 diabetes or heart disease. Now, it might be reasonable to dismiss these findings of good health among hunter-gatherers as nothing more than an aberration. But anthropologists have been able to observe an experiment of sorts in that most of these free-living hunter-gatherer groups' diets and living patterns have been incrementally altered with their exposure to Westernized foods and lifestyles. In simple terms, as these people were exposed to increasing amounts of refined foods, sedentism, alcohol, etc., they developed ever-increasing rates of modern degenerative disease. Some researchers posited that these groups had genetic protection against these diseases, but after only a generation of living in modern housing and eating modern refined foods, these recent hunter-gatherers had rates of degenerative disease similar to and often greater than their counterparts who had lived this way for generations.

This information may come as a surprise to you, and it can be counterintuitive to many people. Life has arguably gotten better with the advent of modern medicine and science. We live in relative abundance and leisure that was unthinkable only a few generations ago. But this very abundance and ease carries with it certain challenges and risks. Civilization is great, and there are many laudable features of modern medicine. *And* there are inescapable downsides to our modern world. I've found a remarkable number of people are incapable of having two seemingly contradictory "truths" in their mind at the same time. This is a great example: civilization is good, but it does confer some downsides that might be remedied by looking at our remote past.

The information about the relative good health of pre-Westernized societies is well known in anthropological circles, yet it was only recently that people asked the question, "Could this discordance story have implications for modern health?" One of the first people to ask this question was Dr. Boyd Eaton of Emory University. In 1985, Dr. Eaton and his research associate Melvin Konner, PhD, wrote the groundbreaking review paper *Paleolithic Nutrition: A Consideration of Its Nature and Current Implications*. In this paper, Eaton and Konner lay out a case similar to the one in this book, citing the impressive anthropological and archeological observations to theorize that changes in our diet and lifestyle may be at play in our epidemic of modern disease. Although this was not primary research and did not include a randomized controlled trial, the paper was important because it laid out the discordance theory of disease as it relates to the rapid change in our diet and lifestyles since the Paleolithic era. It also compelled curious minds to begin the process of considering the Paleo diet in a rigorous, scientific process.

Slowly, research has emerged showing the clinical efficacy of the Paleo program. Though early on, the concept of the Paleo diet was criticized as having no scientific backing, that is no longer the case. There *is* scientific research indicating that the Paleo diet is effective not just for weight loss, but potentially for a host of degenerative diseases from cardiovascular disease to diabetes to autoimmunity. It's worth remembering that although modern degenerative diseases appear to be quite different (they affect different organs and systems), the root causes tend to be the same: poor blood sugar control, elevated insulin levels, systemic inflammation, and intestinal permeability. Given all this, it's reasonable to assume that if we address these underlying problems, we will likely improve not just the conditions mentioned shortly, but also a number of other degenerative diseases. Let's take a look at some of the research.

The first study was performed by Professor Staffan Lindeberg of the University of Lund in Sweden and is entitled "A Palaeolithic diet improves glucose tolerance more than a Mediterranean-like diet in individuals with ischaemic heart disease." In this study, twenty-nine men who were either type 2 diabetic or suffering from elevated glucose and diagnosed heart disease were instructed to eat either a Paleo diet (fruits, vegetables, roots, shoots, tubers, nuts, seeds, meat, and seafood) or a Mediterranean diet (whole grains, legumes, low-fat dairy, lean meats, and seafood). A number of factors were tracked, including weight loss (or gain), waist measurements, and glucose tolerance. After twelve weeks, the Paleo group had lost more weight than the Mediterranean diet group and showed markedly improved glucose tolerance.

The "A" graph is the Paleo group; the "B" graph is the Mediterranean group. The black circles are the pre-diet oral glucose tolerance numbers, while the open circles are the post-diet numbers. The Paleo diet group saw a 36 percent improvement in blood glucose response, and every member of the Paleo diet group saw their blood glucose levels return to "normal" values, while the Mediterranean group saw a barely statistically significant improvement of 7 percent and only half its participants returned to normal.

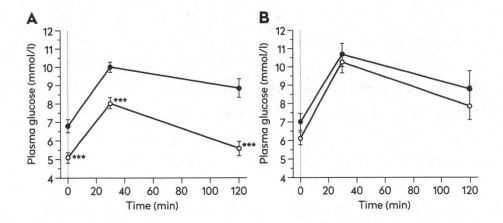

Effectively, the folks in the Paleo group were no longer type 2 diabetic, and their risk factors for cardiovascular disease were dramatically reduced.

It's worth mentioning that this was not a metabolic ward study. These folks were instructed how to eat, and then it was the honor system as to whether they followed the program and accurately recorded their food. Although this is a legitimate concern often raised with regard to this study, it ignores the results. These folks were previously eating a standard Western diet and suffering the ill effects of such a practice. Not only did the Paleo group see impressive results, but the plan was clearly "doable." As of the writing of this book, there are studies planned that will perform essentially this same study, except all meals will be provided to the participants. Check in at my blog for updates on that story.

Also worth mentioning is that there was not a huge difference in weight loss between the two groups, yet the Paleo group saw a much better reduction in visceral fat and clearly also much better blood glucose control. Although this study did not look at what might be driving these changes, our understanding of the pro-inflammatory and gut-irritating nature of grains, legumes, and dairy point us in a likely direction. Calories clearly count, but for far too long the research community has ignored the therapeutic potential of a Paleo-type diet with its low glycemic load and general absence of pro-inflammatory foods.

The next study we will look at is titled "Beneficial effects of a Paleolithic diet on cardiovascular risk factors in type 2 diabetes: a randomized cross-over pilot study." As the title implies, this study involved patients who had been previously diagnosed with type 2 diabetes. Similar to the previous study, these patients were instructed to eat either a Paleo diet or a "Diabetes" diet (which is quite similar to the Mediterranean diet used in the previous study). These people followed one diet for three months and then switched to the other diet. Results were similar to the previous study in that participants generally improved on both diets, but the Paleo group showed better weight loss and blood glucose levels. They had a greater reduction in abdominal fat, improved HDL levels, and reduced triglycerides.

From a scientific perspective, this study has some gaps. It's small in participant number and the people were free-living (we do not *really* know what they ate), but again we see a dramatic difference between the supposedly "healthy" Diabetes diet and the "fad" Paleo diet. That said, I think this is a good moment for a reality check: Does it make sense that diet is a black-and-white story, or might we see many shades (perhaps fifty??!) of gray? What do I mean by this? I think it's reasonable to assume that shifting from highly processed junk food to whole grains, legumes, and low-fat protein is likely going to be a significant improvement. We have just seen that played out in the last two studies.

An interesting feature of the previous two studies is that people consuming the Paleo diet spontaneously reduced calories despite being told to eat until satisfied. The foods were tasty and satiating to a degree that people naturally felt full and were unlikely to overeat. Ironically, this is a common critique of many Paleo diet studies, as the results we see like improved blood glucose response are commonly seen with "simple" weight loss. Do you get that?! "Simple weight loss"! If weight loss were simple, you probably wouldn't be reading this book, we would not have national health crises of obesity and type 2 diabetes, and I would have started farming coconuts in Central America instead of writing this! Experts who have criticized the Paleo diet have gone out of their way to minimize the incredible ability these specific foods have to send the right satiety signals to our brain when we have both adequate nutrition and calories, while standard recommended plans like the Diabetes diet fail when compared head-to-head. What these researchers have said essentially is that there is "nothing special" about the Paleo diet. So long as we can get weight loss, we will get similar results. This is clearly inaccurate, as we have seen weight loss in both of these studies for both the Paleo and Mediterranean/Diabetes groups, yet we have seen metabolic improvements in the Paleo groups that cannot be explained by "simple" weight loss.

In the next study, we will look at a group that was fed a Paleo diet but was instructed to eat at a level that does *not* allow for weight loss. These people had to be tightly monitored by daily weighing and were told to eat well past the point they would otherwise stop eating. In essence, these people were forced to overeat. Sounds like a recipe for disaster, right? Let's see if it was.

This study appeared in the *European Journal of Clinical Nutrition* and is titled "Metabolic and physiologic improvements from consuming a paleolithic, hunter-gatherer type diet." Nine healthy individuals were fed a Paleo diet for ten days, eating one meal (breakfast) each day at the clinic, while subsequent meals and snacks were provided by the research institute brown-bag style. This brown-bag approach brings a much higher level of accuracy to the study. We do not know for sure that the participants ate that food (and only that food), but most people participating in studies like this genuinely want to do the right thing. Another interesting wrinkle in this case was that the participants had a hard time even finishing the food they were given due to the highly satiating nature of the meals. A number of parameters were tested before and after the trial, with the following results:

1. Triglycerides decreased by 35 percent
2. Total cholesterol decreased by 16 percent
3. LDL cholesterol decreased by 22 percent
4. Insulin secretion decreased by 39 percent
5. Blood pressure reduced by 3.4mmHg

Okay, let's unpack this study. As I highlighted above, this intervention involved only "healthy" individuals. Folks with outstanding health problems or who could not pass a basic exercise tolerance test were excluded. We are often lulled into complacency by seeing dramatic changes in folks who are sick, but these changes occurred in young, mainly college-aged participants. One of the most striking features of the study was the duration: The test ran for only ten days! This is a point that is brought up about this study when researchers or keyboard warriors on the Internet are trying to paint this study as insignificant. What this in fact shows is that we can see dramatic metabolic changes in a little over a week (if people follow the damn program). Finally, we have the feature that, when taken with everything else, is really icing on the Paleo cake: *these participants had to force-feed themselves in order to maintain weight*. Read that piece again, please. The Paleo meals they were fed were so satiating that they would normally have stopped eating much earlier were they not instructed to "eat everything provided" so that the participants did not lose weight. *Despite* the fact these participants were not allowed to lose weight, their blood work improved dramatically.

Had these individuals been allowed to eat only to satiety, the results would almost certainly have been more impressive, as all these metabolic parameters like blood sugar, cholesterol, and triglycerides do tend to improve with weight loss, regardless of food composition. But in this case it is clear, the improvements were due to the quality of the food, not the amount eaten nor weight lost (none).

What this means is that if you follow the 30-Day Reset in this book, you will be able to eat to full satiety, you will not be "hangry," you will have great energy, your metabolism is likely to improve dramatically, and losing weight, be that a little or a lot, will be damn near effortless (if you follow the plan!).

I'm not going to bombard you with more studies. If you really want to go down the Paleo rabbit-hole, you can check out my first book, *The Paleo Solution*. I also recommend you do a little research of your own by doing some searches using the terms "Paleo diet + research." That will keep you off the streets for a few months!

This should be a reasonably compelling case for trying the 30-Day Reset to help you get a handle on your weight and your health. I've walked you through where the Paleo diet came from and some of the research highlights that have come to light in the past few years. This next section deals with the common counterpoints to the Paleo diet. If you share some of these concerns, read on. If you read a negative news piece or have a know-it-all coworker who is certain this way of eating will kill you, you can refer back to this material at a later date. I provide this information because although people will literally save their lives with a Paleo diet—and look and feel better than they have in years—the first news piece they encounter will shake their conviction and cause them to question the results of their own experience.

Common Concerns about the Paleo Diet

Almost daily one can find both new research supporting the Paleo diet and news pieces that say the concept is a worthless fad. The critiques follow a very predictable course. Here is a brief accounting of the common misconceptions and negative news pieces you will see on this topic.

THE PALEO DIET IS "UNSCIENTIFIC"

For the past several years, *U.S. News & World Report* has figured out a way to garner enormous site traffic with its yearly ranking of the "best and worst" diets. They consistently rank the Paleo diet dead last as the worst diet one could possibly imagine doing. Yes, they actually deemed the Paleo diet, built around whole, unprocessed foods, as "worse" than the standard American diet of processed junk. In fact, it is also ranked behind a number of diets built around eating protein shakes for most of the meals. Now, why does the Paleo diet (in the eyes of *USNWR*) rank so poorly? One of the main points made by whatever "expert" *USNWR* manages to find cites "lack of scientific research on the Paleo diet." Yeah, really. I just gave you a short list of some well-done Paleo diet studies. Clearly, these are not hard to find if one can perform a simple Internet search. Folks spouting similar nonsense are either not bothering to do *any* research or are ignoring the scientific studies in order to whip people into a lather and get some cheap exposure for their awesome journalism. Something that is also interesting: A number of the plans that ranked better than the Paleo diet—including the SlimFast plan, which focuses on proprietary bars and shakes—have not one scientific study supporting it. Nada. A plan based around fake food, with no scientific research, is consistently ranked ahead of the Paleo diet, yet the main argument against the Paleo diet is that it lacks scientific research. I hope you can appreciate the irony here. I have no idea how many SlimFast ads have appeared in *USNWR* over the years ...

THE PALEO DIET IS "ALL MEAT"

No, no it's not. In Professor Loren Cordain's paper "The nutritional characteristics of a contemporary diet based on Paleolithic food groups," we learn that of the more than two hundred hunter-gatherer groups studied, there was a huge difference in the amounts of fish, meat, and fowl consumed by these groups. Individuals living in the far North consumed relatively little plant material (we don't find a lot of kale and bananas in the Arctic), while equatorial peoples tended to consume significant amounts of plant material. I make the point in future chapters that you may do better on more or fewer carbs, but I'm *not* recommending that you eat only meat, and none of the research on the Paleo diet has ever recommended this.

THE PALEO DIET WILL LEAD TO NUTRIENT DEFICIENCIES

This argument actually sounds pretty good at first, since most people assume bread, pasta, and whole grains are "loaded with nutrients." This argument, however, is also one of the easiest to put to bed as it's essentially the game we all likely played as kids: "You show me yours and I'll show you mine." By inputting either a Paleo diet based on commonly available foods, or whatever other diet you might want to compare, you can see that the Paleo diet wins by a mile. Check out the table from the same paper referenced above from Professor Cordain. This looks at the vitamins and minerals from a 2,200-calorie diet for an average-size twenty-five-year-old female:

TRACE NUTRIENT	TOTAL	% RDA
Vitamin A (RE)	6386	798
Vitamin B_1 (mg)	3.4	309
Vitamin B_2 (mg)	4.2	355
Vitamin B_3 (mg)	60	428
Vitamin B_6 (mg)	6.7	515
Folate (µg)	891	223
Vitamin B_{12} (µg)	17.6	733
Vitamin C (mg)	748	1247
Vitamin E (IU)	19.5	244
Calcium (mg)	691	69
Phosphorus (mg)	2546	364
Magnesium (mg)	643	207
Iron (mg)	24.3	162
Zinc (mg)	27.4	228

What this describes is the total amount of the various nutrients as well as the recommended daily allowance (RDA; now called the recommended daily intake, or RDI). A quick word on the RDA/RDI: These levels are set just above what causes disease. They are *not* set with an idea of optimum health in mind. Virtually all our research is devoted to disease, not health, so when you think about these RDA/RDI numbers, I'd like you to consider the possibility that they are set far too low if you want to do anything besides avoid scurvy. In the example of the Paleo diet cited above, you can see that with the exception of calcium and vitamin D, a Paleo diet (in most cases) has several hundred percent more of these vital nutrients than the RDA. Calcium is an interesting topic, as the main source in the modern diet is dairy products, yet the main sources from a Paleo diet are vegetables, nuts, and seeds. The Paleo diet is much higher in magnesium than the modern diet, which physiologically appears to buffer the need for calcium. Additionally, we have examples of cultures that both do and do not consume much dairy, but all grow tall, strong, and healthy.

In the case of vitamin D, the diet described in Professor Cordain's paper does not contain any organ meats. A weekly serving of liver can take care of that need just fine. Don't like liver? Okay, I'll make this super hard for you: go out in the sun for a few minutes with your shirt sleeves rolled up. It only takes a few minutes of sunlight for most people to hit their vitamin D needs. If you are a Nervous Nelly about being in the sun, I'll defuse that anxiety a bit later in the book. From a scientific perspective, this nutrient-density topic is actually the most credible argument *for* the Paleo diet; it arrives at this position not from anthropological observations, but rather from the best that reductionist science has to offer. My good friend Mat Lalonde, PhD, of Harvard University performed a remarkable analysis by comparing the nutrient profiles of thousands of foods relative to their caloric content. He found that the top ten nutrient-dense foods include organ meats, herbs, spices, cacao, beef, pork, and eggs, all of which are mainstays of the Paleo diet.

THE PALEO DIET IS "JUST ANOTHER LOW-CARB DIET"

This counterpoint is interesting in that it somehow implies that low-carb diets are inherently bad. Just the opposite appears to be true, especially for folks who, for a myriad of reasons, have suffered the poor luck of literally breaking their metabolisms with modern food, sleep habits, and stress. The literature on the Paleo diet shows that it does tend to be a "lower"-carb diet relative to the standard American diet, which is rich in refined carbs, but is generally not formulated as specifically a low-carb diet (less than 100g carbs per day.) All that said, I've made the point for years that the Paleo diet is "macronutrient agnostic." The concept is not concerned so much with specific macronutrient levels but rather food quality. As you will see in Part Two, you will be able to determine the protein, carb, and fat levels that work best for you.

THE PALEO DIET IS NOT SUSTAINABLE ON A GLOBAL LEVEL

It is outside the scope of this book to go deep into this topic, but it is popular with those who are legitimately concerned with the current structure of our food system and rightfully so. However, I'd like to turn this around and ask you a question: is our current food and medical system sustainable? Our artificially cheap, hyperpalatable food, which is government subsidized, has created a population that is so sick that our health-care costs are growing exponentially and represent an existential threat to our financial systems. If you want to talk about a system that is unsustainable, let's start with the sinking ship we are currently on, not a dietary and lifestyle approach that shows promise in addressing diseases ranging from diabetes to neurodegeneration. I know I did the literary equivalent of a hit-and-run by implicating foul play in our financial system with our current health problems. Like I said, it's outside the scope of this book, but I will address these topics on my blog and a subsequent book.

PALEO FOR COPS AND FIREFIGHTERS, OR, HOW TO SAVE YOUR CITY A METRIC TON OF MONEY

I've shared a lot of research with you about the Paleo diet concept, but what about beyond the research and the numbers? How does the Paleo way of eating, sleeping, and moving work in the real world? Once you put it into action, how can it affect your life and the lives of those you love? Let's look at how it's helped some real people on an everyday level.

If you or someone you know is in police, military, or fire service, you know these are remarkably difficult jobs. High stress, high stakes, with an incredible amount of scrutiny. The demands of this work take their toll, as evidenced by the dramatically shortened life-spans we see in these communities. Although controversial, studies indicate the average life-span of a police officer may be as much as twenty years shorter than the rest of the US population. Many factors contribute to this story, but one of the most profound impacts appears to be insulin resistance and systemic inflammation, which is an outgrowth of the generally poor diet, altered sleep patterns, and excessive stress (called "hypervigilance"), which is endemic in these populations. Quite a number of police and fire personnel die or are sidelined due to either a heart attack or stroke.

In Reno, Nevada, a number of local doctors, including my good friend Dr. Jim Greenwald (we call him "Greenie"), wondered if some kind of screening in the police and fire departments might find indications of these problems early, which would then allow for diet and lifestyle modifications designed to change the outcomes to something more favorable than an early death. When the doctors started looking at the blood work obtained from the cops and firefighters on their yearly physicals, they sorted the data in a way that most general practitioners do not consider. They looked for signs of insulin resistance and inflammation, and what they found was stunning. A remarkable number of these public servants were not just a little insulin resistant, but severely so. This tended to get worse with age, but youth was no guarantee of protection. Even young, seemingly fit individuals, folks who lifted weights and did triathlons, were insulin resistant. At first these insulin-resistant individuals were instructed to eat a high-carb, low-fat diet. Almost to a person, this standard of care recommendation made these people worse. Their triglycerides went up, their HDL went down, and total cholesterol increased. Their docs were stumped, but fortunately they were also curious. They continued to ask questions, and when the high-carb diet failed, they flipped the problem on its head: If these people are insulin resistant, and if dense carbohydrate is the primary promoter of insulin release, perhaps recommending a low-carb diet would be better? Money was found for a small pilot study.

For two years, they followed a low-carb diet and received counseling on how to improve sleep and reduce stress. The results were telling. Based on the changes in blood work (which provide a predictive measure for these people developing cardiovascular disease), it was estimated that the pilot program alone saved the city of Reno $22 million with a 33:1 return on investment. I became involved with the Specialty Health clinic four years ago, and in addition to its already successful low-carb program, I helped integrate the Paleo diet principles to address conditions ranging from traumatic brain injury to autoimmune disease.

This part of our journey together is important, as it marks the spot where we go "beyond Paleo." We live in a world of technological marvels. If we can use the type of testing that made the Reno study such a success, coupled with an Ancestral Health template that considers food, sleep, exercise, and community, we can literally change the world. First, however, we need to start with you.

I think about this a bit like the instructions we receive just before an airplane takes off. In addition to how to buckle your seatbelt, the flight attendant tells us that "in the event of an unexpected loss of cabin pressure, oxygen masks will deploy from the bins overhead. Please put on your mask before assisting others . . ." We need to start first with ourselves; then we can think about fixing the health care system and possibly the rest of the world. I'm not sure if it comes across in my writing, but I'm incredibly excited by all this. I feel like my work matters.

As much success as I've had in helping people help themselves, I am haunted by my inability to really help my parents. I could never get my dad to alter his ways and we lost him in 2005 due to a heart attack. We lost my mom in 2013. I managed to get my mom to change a few things, but for whatever reason the prospect of change was just too much for her to deal with. She did get to meet my elder daughter, one time, and talked to her a few times via video chat . . . but even the prospect of seeing her granddaughter grow up was not enough leverage to effect the changes she needed. This is a hard enough story to relate, but there is another layer that brings a decided urgency to my work. My wife's mother, Candy, died in 2003 due to complications from rheumatoid arthritis. Unlike my mother, Candy was highly motivated to find a way to beat her condition. In an ironic twist of fate, the same rheumatologist who helped my mom track down her autoimmune triggers, which is likely the reason I became aware of this Paleo diet concept, was also Candy's rheumatologist. Although anecdotal, we now have thousands of testimonials of people reversing or dramatically reducing their symptoms of not just rheumatoid arthritis but a host of other ailments by adopting the Paleo lifestyle. The painful part in all this is that I met my wife a few months after her mom died. I'm haunted by the notion that if I'd met her sooner, Candy might still be alive and their lives would be dramatically changed. So although I may come across as a hard-ass at times, I feel a profound sense of urgency. This is my "why." This is why

I do what I do. If you still have reservations about this program or if you are struggling at a future point, don't look to the studies or the science I've related to you. Think about how your health and the health of those you love may be affected by your decision to make these important lifestyle and dietary changes.

I've made about as compelling a case as possible to give the 30-Day Reset a shot and follow that up with the 7-Day Carb Test. We've gone from theory to research to real-world application in first responders. In less time than it takes to close escrow when buying a house, you will know if this program is working. It's not a big ask, but it may be a huge reward. Now let's take a look at the other pillars of health: sleep, stress, and community. Armed with this information, you will be ready to start the program.

CHAPTER 8

Rebalancing the Pillars of Sleep, Community, and Movement

We've come a long way together, and if you have absorbed 10 percent of what we've covered you likely know more practical information about human health than most health care providers. We have clearly focused the bulk of our attention on food, but there are a few other pieces to this story that are of similar, if not greater, importance. The final pieces to the puzzle involve sleep, stress, and social connectivity.

Some of what I will present on sleep and stress may be completely at odds with your notions of these subjects. There are a number of fantastic resources on these topics, and they are all valuable, but the media and most researchers tend to look at all of these critical pieces in isolation and forget that we are not parts and pieces—we are a whole, dynamic system. As such, we need a systems-based approach if we are to achieve lifetime changes in not just our health, but in our waistline as well. The Italian saying *Vivi bene, ama molto, ridi spesso* means "Live well, love much, laugh often." If we can apply that advice and add in sound eating, we have the opportunity to live a truly blessed life. Although I'm the "food guy," over the past ten years I have spent more and more time talking about the importance of sleep, stress, and community. These topics are critical elements of health and happiness, but they also dramatically affect our food choices. In short, our sleep, stress, and social connections (if properly managed) can make our dietary changes stick. If these considerations are out of control, they can make lasting dietary change almost impossible.

Before we dig into the topic of sleep I'd like to make an important point: if people "just" slept, we'd likely not need to concern ourselves about diet much at all. I'm not saying you could eat refined junk all day long and not suffer the consequences, but good sleep buys us a lot of latitude in our eating. The opposite is also true, as poor sleep necessitates a fair amount of focus on our food, lest we find ourselves facing some serious health problems. If you want more latitude on your food, you need to sleep better. If you can't sleep well due to work demands, you *really* need to pay attention to your food, particularly carbohydrate amount and type. If you want to get the best health and aesthetics possible, you will make both good sleep and good food your priority more often than not.

SHUT-EYE

Let's start with a topic that should be nearly as exciting as sex: sleep. My good friend Dr. Kirk Parsley is a physician and also a retired US Navy SEAL. Kirk is an amazing guy and he has arguably taken on two of the toughest professions one can imagine (okay, three: he is also a father of three children!), as becoming a doctor or a SEAL are understood to be tough due in part to the dramatic demands placed on sleep. To become a SEAL, one must go through a "weeding-out" program called BUD/S (Basic Underwater Demolition/SEAL). Early in this program, recruits are subjected to what is accurately called Hell Week. Recruits are kept awake for over five days, typically getting two to four hours of sleep per night. They must perform prodigious amounts of physical and mental activity, typically while wet and cold, and clearly sleep deprived. Not many people make it through this process due to extreme mental and physical discomfort that assail them at every moment of the selection process. Medical school, although less physically demanding and offering a bit more temperature control, is no cakewalk. Medical school is a grind necessitating the mastery of anatomy, physiology, biochemistry, and pathology . . . and that's just in the first year. Once one has made it through the four years of medical school, fledgling MDs must spend several years working as residents where *weekly* sleep totals may be around twenty to twenty-five hours.

As I said, Kirk has succeeded in both of these professions, but he is the first one to admit the process has left its mark on his health and vitality. After completing his medical training, Dr. Parsley took on the position of monitoring the health of most of the West Coast SEAL teams based in Coronado, California. On Kirk's first day of work, his first two patients (current SEALs) came into his office with largely the same problems. Both of these formerly athletic but still young SEALs generally felt like hell and had seen their performance and cognitive abilities slide dramatically in the previous six months to a year. Both were attempting to exercise to stay in shape for their work, but also to "get tired enough to sleep." These guys would work themselves to exhaustion, then triple their normal dose of prescription sleep aids. Unfortunately, their heroic efforts appeared to be, if anything, making things worse.

Over the coming months Kirk saw dozens of young SEALs with similar complaints. There was such a consistent pattern that emerged: Kirk called it the "SEAL flu." It took him the better part of a year to piece together what was happening. What Kirk figured out was that the SEALs were suffering from profound circadian rhythm and sleep disturbances. There were many factors for this but one of the most powerful was likely the flipped schedule SEALs endure by doing "night ops." Essentially, they tend to work at night and sleep during the day. The SEALs slept during the day using prescriptions like Ambien, and they woke up using loud music and energy drinks. Despite often being in desert environments, these SEALs tended to have remarkably low vitamin D levels, as they actually spent little time in the sun, and when they were in the sun they usually had on their full gear (they weren't lazing around in a pair of shorts).

You may be wondering why I'm relating all this to you. What does the situation of Navy SEALs have to do with you? The process that was literally breaking these SEALs is essentially the same that is breaking most people in Westernized societies. We are not sleeping enough, and not sleeping at the right times. We do not get outside enough, and as a whole, we tend to have low vitamin D levels due to a lack of adequate sun exposure. I worked for more than six years with Dr. Parsley as part of the Naval Special Warfare Resiliency program, and the lessons we both learned from this hard-charging community have been invaluable in helping everyone from student-athletes to parents to CEOs of Fortune 500 companies. If what I'm going to share with you worked for SEALs, it will likely work for you. The only caveat is that you actually need to do it!

WHAT IS SLEEP?

I've had the good fortune of traveling with Dr. Parsley to a number of different events, and he has a fantastic sleep lecture that he starts with a seemingly simple question: What is sleep? I've seen audiences ranging from doctors to cops to athletes squirm in their seats trying to come up with a good response. Everyone "knows" what sleep is, right? We typically do it every day and have been doing it our whole lives. But getting a technical definition is tricky. After a bit of floundering, Kirk saves the crowd by explaining that no one really knows what sleep is. We can only describe and characterize some elements of sleep like brainwaves and hormone levels.

For something that should be pretty scientific, that seems a bit flimsy, right? It is. Sleep is still largely a mystery, but here is an operational definition of what sleep is, according to Dr. Parsley: Sleep is a barrier between the individual and the environment. During this period, we are not aware of sight, sounds, smells, or feelings. However, we *can* be awakened.

If you drink a bottle of vodka or get hit in the head with a brick, you would most certainly not be aware of sight, sounds, smells, or feelings. But the brainwaves of someone on a vodka bender or who is unconsciousness are not the same as those of someone who is sleeping. This may seem a silly point to make, but think about it this way: prescription sleep aids (as well as the OTC options) and nonprescription sleep aids (such as alcohol) do not cause sleep. They cause unconsciousness. This means that although you are not technically awake, you are not gaining most—or sometimes any—of the benefits of sleep. Just going by basic statistics, a number of you who just read that had either a bout of incredulity or a seriously puckered backside, or both. If you use booze or sleep meds, you are unfortunately only making your situation worse, not better. I can best explain that by looking at what sleep does do for us and what happens when we do not get enough.

At a basic level sleep restores us. Tissues damaged via normal wear and tear heal. Antiaging hormones such as growth hormone and melatonin are released. Our immune systems are rebooted. Systemic inflammation is reduced and our guts are given a break, thus allowing them to heal and recover from the work of digesting food. Whole books have been written on each of these topics, so I want to keep this discussion at a 30,000-foot level. All that you need to take away from this is that when you sleep well, you will feel better and have a more youthful hormonal profile and immune function while minimizing inflammation.

And . . . lack of sleep? Not surprisingly, sleep loss, either in total amount or quality, produces the opposite of these benefits. Let me share with you what a few nights of poor sleep does for us:

1. Impairs insulin sensitivity. Want to become diabetic overnight? Just sleep poorly. A night of poor or missed sleep can make one as insulin resistant as a type 2 diabetic. Luckily, good diet, exercise, and getting caught up on sleep can undo this mess, but the effects of sleep deprivation on insulin sensitivity and thus glucose tolerance are profound and nearly immediate.

2. Increases gut permeability. I know the gut chapter is a long way in the rearview mirror by now, but hopefully you remember that leaky gut is not good. Increased intestinal permeability itself impairs insulin sensitivity while increasing our reactivity to certain foods.

3. Increases systemic inflammation. Even with very little sleep loss we immediately see increases in C-reactive protein and the tendency of platelets to stick together (not great if you're at risk for a stroke or heart attack). If you recall, all modern degenerative diseases have a commonality of increased systemic inflammation. It is not surprising that we tend to see increased rates of Western diseases in lockstep with poor sleep. Internet blowhards will argue about whether this is correlation or causation. I just say, "Go to bed."

4. Impairs immune function. Even short bouts of sleep loss increase our likelihood of infections. This is a hot area of immunology, and we do not yet have a full accounting of what sleep does for the immune system, but it is clear that inadequate sleep is not congruent with a healthy immune system.

5. Alters anabolic hormones. Whether you are male or female, it behooves you to have your hormones within certain optimum ranges and in appropriate ratios. Sleep debt tends to shift us toward a "catabolic" or breakdown state. Want to lose muscle and gain fat? Don't sleep.

6. Causes cravings. Sleep deprivation is a stress, and when a stress becomes chronic, one of the first adaptive mechanisms our bodies shift toward to deal with the stress is to seek out any food, but particularly highly processed foods. We crave and tend to eat "bad" foods. This is a survival mechanism that bites us in the backside in our modern world. Not only do we tend to crave highly processed foods when sleep deprived, but we also tend to have less willpower to resist these foods. This phenomenon is not confined to food: anything that may tempt you is made more appealing with sleep deprivation. Addiction programs routinely counsel the need for adequate, consistent sleep to avoid a relapse.

7. Cognitive impairment. What if I told you that perhaps 50 percent of the drivers on the road are as impaired as someone who is at the blood alcohol limit for drunk driving? Crazy, right? If we look at studies of how much people sleep (or do not sleep, in this case) and our understanding of how even modest amounts of sleep debt impairs us, we can conclude that up to half the drivers on the road, though not literally drunk from alcohol, have reaction times and decision-making ability that is comparably impaired.

THE BRIGHT IDEA

Why we don't sleep is a simple question with a complex answer. There is no one single reason, but we can trace some of the issue back to the invention of the lightbulb and the remarkable transformation it has brought to humanity. Prior to the incandescent bulb, lighting amounted to gas lamps, candles, and fires. Not particularly effective, cheap, or safe. The lightbulb dramatically expanded both our learning and leisure time, and it's hard not to marvel at all the amazing advancements that have come about as a result. But, just like ubiquitous food and little need for physical work, this advancement had its downsides. Historically, we went to bed not long after the sun went down, got up when the sun came up, wash-rinse-repeat. With electrical light our time in the rack decreased dramatically as we had opportunities to read, socialize, and binge on reality TV, as just a short list of sleep-curbing diversions.

The Puritan Work Ethic. Folks in the United States tend to sleep about 2.5 hours per night less than they did in the 1970s. That may not seem like much, but it adds up when we think about all the negative effects of inadequate sleep. It's little wonder we see the increasing rates of degenerative diseases that we do. People work hard everywhere in the world, but there is this "Puritan Work Ethic" that still permeates much of the US psyche. Hard work is not in and of itself a bad thing, but when we sacrifice sleep to do this work, we are striking a Faustian bargain. Dr. Parsley describes this process as "wearing sleep loss as a badge of honor." We all know (or are the person) who brags about how little sleep we get and how much we achieve. There are certainly times when we need to knuckle down to get a project done, but we have a tendency to not step back from that frenetic pace and cultivate downtime, which fosters better sleep. Instead, we pack every moment of every day and make sleep a last priority.

I love the nightlife, I got to boogie. Lots of fun things happen after the sun goes down. Parties, social gatherings, hookups! I've always been a morning person and have been a little jealous that no one wants to get together at six A.M. for social hour. Coffee is fun, but booze and dancing are, admittedly, on a whole different level.

TechCrunch. The rise of the Internet, smartphones, tablets, and five hundred channels of cable TV has given most of us access to a limitless number of titillating options. Want to watch a zombie movie? You can lie in your bed and do it from your smartphone. Curious what your friends from high school are doing now? You can stalk them on social media. Not only does this tend to push back our bedtimes, but we are exposing ourselves to light at a time when we should be in the dark.

I'm not saying a strong work ethic, a thriving social life, or enjoying the Internet are inherently bad things. They are all fantastic. What I am saying is that when we allow any one of these things (or more often, a combination) to eat into our sleep time, it will crush us eventually. You put in a little extra time working, go out for some drinks, then "unwind" by watching TV in bed. Sure, you are going to have only six hours *in bed* (not necessarily asleep), but that's enough, right? No, it's not. Just an hour or two here and there makes a big impact on our health, our cognition, and our waistline.

WHAT CONTROLS SLEEP?

Many ancient religions worshiped the sun as the primary steward of life and wellness. This is not a misplaced sentiment, as the sun controls the biological rhythms of every organism on the planet. Be ye bacteria, plant, fungi, or animal, the sun drives the cellular clocks that determine hunger, reproduction, and aging. Stepping back from the metaphysical considerations of the sun, in practical terms the amount of time in the sun or light (our photo-period), and the intensity of light exposure are the prime determinants of our metabolic processes, especially sleep. Cells in our eyes that are not involved in sight actually register the amount of light, particularly blue light (found in both natural and artificial light), entering the eye and communicates this information to a portion of the hypothalamus. This process sets our wake/sleep patterns, which have profound impacts on our metabolism.

Let me strip this down further. I could make an argument that our "normal" state of consciousness is sleep. A number of metabolic processes cause us to essentially accumulate "sleep pressure" throughout the day, but bright light tends to work against this process, thus keeping us awake. It blunts the production of melatonin, the primary neurotransmitter involved in sleep initiation. If we are getting the right amounts of light at the right times (bright light during the day, little to no light after sundown) we tend to produce a reasonable wake/sleep pattern, and a healthy, insulin-sensitive metabolism. However, our modern lives have compromised our natural rhythms.

Think about how little time we spend outside. We're most often either at home, in the car, or at the office. If we do get outside, it is for brief stints that are not enough to properly regulate our wake/sleep cycles. This means we tend to be sleepy and lethargic all day due in part to the lack of light fighting our normal sleep pressure. Light exposure suppresses melatonin production during the day, which is good. As we will see, this is not what we want at night.

Once the sun does go down we tend to be in environments that have too much light. Ambient lighting, TVs, computers, and smartphones all provide sufficient light to suppress the production of melatonin, which should occur at this time in the evening. Now we feel tired but "wired." We are fidgety, have short attention spans, crave junk food, and decide that a couple of glasses of wine will help us sleep.

You may think sleeping midnight to eight A.M. is as good as ten P.M. to six A.M., but studies show this is not the case. Many things in life only work if the sequencing is correct, and we have deep biological wiring expecting to get light on our person throughout the day, then to go to bed not long after the sun goes down. To the degree we deviate from this plan, we begin stacking the deck against ourselves.

As I said previously, whole libraries of books have been written on these topics, so this is by necessity a cursory exploration. As important as general light exposure is for our health and waistline, we also need sun *on our person*. It's more than just "light in the eyes"—we need sun on us. Part of this story is that sunlight has historically been an important source of vitamin D, which is critical for a dizzying number of metabolic processes, from modulating immune response to suppressing tumor growth. That story is only now gaining some prominence within the medical community. Research also indicates sun exposure may reduce our likelihood of a host of cancers, cardiovascular disease, autoimmunity, and neurodegenerative disease by mechanisms outside of vitamin D.

This may be another point at which you are thinking, *This is madness! If I go out in the sun, I'll get skin cancer!* Well, not really. People who work outside, such as construction workers, tend to have comparatively low rates of skin cancer relative to indoor workers. We have been lathering up with sunscreen to go outside, yet skin cancer rates continue to go up. The problem appears to not be sun exposure, per se, but sunburn. If one ramps up at a safe, moderate pace, one tends to get all the benefits of sun exposure with little of the downsides. What I'm suggesting is go slow, don't burn. We want a therapeutic effect, not to turn you into a leather handbag.

Our ancestors did not have SPF 100 sunblock. They lived with the seasons, mainly outdoors, which meant a lot of sun exposure. Observation of contemporary hunter-gatherers and non-Westernized populations indicates these folks gradually ramp up sun exposure with the changing of the seasons, which allows for incremental adaptations. This appears to foster health versus disease. The bottom line is that we need more, consistent sun exposure during the day to entrain our circadian rhythms. In application, this means getting out in the sun and then covering up before you get much more than a bit of pink to the skin. Folks with darker skin pigmentation can and will burn if not ramped up to sun exposure, so do keep that in mind. You will have a bit more challenging time gauging your maximum dose based on color change so you may need to rely on a clock to gradually ramp up your exposure.

When you hit your sun limit for the day, I prefer hats and clothing over sunblock as the clothing tends to provide complete UV protection, whereas many of the sunblocks may prevent burning but still allow for skin damage. Clearly certain situations will require some creativity in this regard; use your common sense.

HOW TO GET AWESOME SLEEP

Hopefully I've sold you on the idea that sleep is important for a number of reasons, ranging from your health to your waistline. Let's look at how to get the best sleep possible while still living a normal life.

1. Get more daytime sun on your person and in your eyes to establish a normal circadian rhythm. If possible, get outside first thing in the morning, even if only for a few minutes. If you have a chance to go for a walk or eat lunch outside, do it!

2. Our evenings need to be darker, cooler, and not the equivalent of a rock concert if we want to get the best sleep possible. Dim your lights in the evening if possible, and so long as you are not on the dating scene, get yourself a pair of "blue blocker" sunglasses. There is a massive variation

in how much these cost, but price is not always an indicator of efficacy. Grab a $10 pair and put those on in the early evening, just as the sun is setting.

3. Limit evening tech. If you want to watch TV, use your blue blockers. If you *must* use your computer, smartphone, or tablet, wear those blue blockers and also install one of the many light-monitoring programs that remove the blue wavelengths of light from your screen. Most Apple tablets and smartphones now have a setting called Night Shift that allows you to pick when this screen change occurs. For computers you can find programs, such as F.lux, that allow you to set your location and the program automatically changes your screen at sunset. Yes, *Game of Thrones* will look a bit different when programs like this are running, but better sleep will help you avoid the fate of most of the Stark family.

4. Sleep in a cool room. Studies have shown that an optimal sleeping temperature is about 64 to 66°F (about 19°C). Yes, that's a bit on the nippy side, but for good sleep our body temperature must fall a degree or two, and a cool room facilitates this process. Make the room cool, get a blanket, snuggle in, and be amazed at how much better you sleep.

5. Sleep in a dark room. Strive to have your room as dark as a broom closet in the center of the Great Pyramid. You may need to spend some money on blackout curtains, or you can go trailer-park chic and just aluminum foil your windows. Your call. Just make that happen. Ideally, you do not have a clock with a glowing display in your room, but if you must, put it in a drawer or place it across the room and keep a towel handy to cover it. When I say dark, I mean dark. This is a funny topic, as folks will nitpick what exactly this means and wonder if it's really worth it. Do it for a week and let me know how things go.

6. Keep a journal. If you ruminate before bed, keep a journal handy and jot down the things you need to do the following day. At this point, there is

nothing you can do that will help you be more productive than getting a good night's sleep.

7. Get a good mattress. If you have an uncomfortable bed, you are not likely to sleep well. Now, what is comfortable for one person may not be comfortable to another. I've tried several beds and finally settled on a Sleep Number mattress, which allows you to dial in your desired level of firmness. This has been a game changer for me. Interestingly, what is "best" for me changes depending on how much I'm working out and a number of other factors. I will run with my bed nearly as firm as a cement floor for a few weeks, then shift it to the consistency of a marsh-mallow. You can't do that with any other bed that I know of. I have no financial tie to these beds; I just think they kick ass. I actually recommend the lower-cost version of these beds, as it relies on the inflatable bladder to regulate firmness, not foam, which will break down over time.

8. Alternating hot/cold shower. I use this technique at home when I am very busy and my mind is racing. I'll start with a hot temperature that is just at the level of my tolerance. I do hot for 10 seconds, then shift to cool/cold for 20 seconds. I will alternate back and forth five to ten times, finishing on cold. I then hop out of the shower, dry off, and barely make it to my bed before I pass out. This process appears to reset our circadian rhythm to some degree, which helps us to unwind and go to bed. It also facilitates reducing our body temperature, which is a key feature of sleep. If your room is chilly and dark, and if you are a bit cold after your showers, your bed will feel like heaven when you dive into it. Clearly, keep the "cold" portion reasonable. If you dump a bucket of ice water down your back before bed you may not sleep for a week.

9. Make a consistent schedule and stick to it. If you have kids, you know they sleep better when they have a set bedtime routine. Not surprisingly, we do, too. I only half-jokingly say that people need to be "serial

killer" consistent with their bed routine. If you play with this stuff, you will see that the consistency pays off.

10. Stable blood sugar. Good food and good sleep work in a virtuous cycle that helps keep you strong, healthy, and lean. The opposite is also true. I do not recommend eating immediately before bed, as this makes it hard for our body temperature to drop and can make getting into deep, restful sleep more challenging. On the other hand, if our blood sugar drops too low during the night, we can wake up due to the release of cortisol, which is working to bring our blood glucose back up. Some people do better with some good-quality carbs in their dinner, while others (myself included) tend to sleep better with a meal that was mainly protein and fat. Tinker with this and find what works best for you.

This may seem like an overwhelming list of things to do before bed, but it's really not. Once you get your room squared away and into a pattern, this all becomes habit.

Other Sleep Challenges

Most people who follow my basic diet recommendations achieve rapid, easy success in losing fat and getting lean. Almost all the folks who struggle with losing fat have some kind of problem with their sleep. Virtually to a person. Occasionally, this is due to some of the facts I talked about above. Often, however, the problem is a specific profession. Police, military, firefighters, medical personnel, and new parents generally have trouble sleeping due to the demands of their situation. Most people cannot bail on their profession to get better sleep, and parents can't tell a new baby to stop teething so everyone in the house can get some shut-eye. I don't have perfect solutions, as this is legitimately tough. It really boils down to when you can sleep, *sleep*! If your sleep schedule is erratic, if you work nights and sleep days, you *must* prioritize your sleep. All of the sleep hygiene tricks I listed are nonnegotiable. You *must* do them. Sleeping during the day is never going to be as restful and restorative as sleeping at night, but it is better than nothing. The sleep you do get needs to be the best quality possible.

SUPPLEMENTS

Most over-the-counter sleep aids and alcohol do not make you sleep, they make you unconscious. A good alternative is to use 1 to 3mg of sublingual melatonin about 20 minutes before you go to sleep. You will need to play with the dosage, as individual response varies wildly from person to person. Magnesium and vitamin D are critical cofactors in the sleep process, and although a well-constructed diet as detailed in the meal plans in this book should provide adequate magnesium, it would not hurt to take 200 to 400mg of magnesium citrate with your last meal before bed. Most people should supplement with 2,000 to 4,000 IU of vitamin D daily, as even folks who judiciously get out in the sun tend to have suboptimal vitamin D levels.

I do not make many product recommendations, but if you struggle with sleep I highly recommend the Sleep Remedy developed by Dr. Parsley (robbwolf.com/sleepremedy). It contains magnesium, vitamin D, and the cofactors involved with both initiating sleep and maintaining it. This is a solid supplement for anyone, as we all find ourselves either traveling or in a situation in which sleep is less than optimal. If you fall into the shift work category, something like this product is a must-have.

Although this section does contain a lot of information on sleep, we are only scratching the surface of the details. If this is an area that interests you, it is not hard to find incredible amounts of information not just about sleep specifically, but about the effects of inadequate sleep on a host of diseases. Let's shift gears and look at another component of health that has gone awry: stress.

GOT STRESS?

If you asked a large group of people, "Is stress an important factor in health?," most would correctly say yes. That stress is a factor in both health and disease has been understood for more than seventy years, particularly after the work of Hans Selye, who developed the General Adaptation Syndrome (GAS) model of stress. In simple terms, the GAS model suggests that any organism that is subjected to a stress, be that physical, chemical, temperature, or psychological, will go through a predictable process of either adaptation or burnout. If the stress is of sufficient magnitude and duration, we will see first an "alarm" stage followed by adaptation. If the stress is too much, again either in amount or duration, the organism can suffer a host of health problems, not the least of which may be death. It is well understood that all living things need some amount of stress in order to be healthy, but there are clearly thresholds which once passed, can manifest in insulin resistance, suppressed immune function, and increased inflammation.

Because of my Ancestral Health orientation, I long subscribed to the notion that the stress part of our story was another genetic discordance example. Our ancestors likely evolved in an environment in which most stressors were short in duration and relatively infrequent. This idea is likely correct in many regards but it misses the fact that humans are incredibly adaptable. This "caveman" orientation is not particularly helpful given that most of us live in urban centers and face traffic jams, rude drivers, taxes, and the horrors of modern reality TV shows. Most of us neither want nor actually need to move to a small family farm and practice some kind of neurotic "stress control" to be healthy and happy. What we need to do boils down to two simple things:

1. Recognize what really constitutes stress.
2. Reframe our perceptions of everything else that we *think* is stress.

SO, WHAT *IS* STRESS?

In my twenty years of coaching and working with people, I've narrowed down a few areas in which people can, legitimately, beat themselves to a pulp via stress. This typically involves too much exercise, eating too much or the wrong types of foods, inadequate sleep, and work and relationship stress. Additionally, immunogenic foods such as gluten can cause an increase in systemic inflammation that impairs immune function and insulin sensitivity. Most of these stressful issues are a problem of our own making, based on our perceptions. That may come as a bit of a shock, but there is good news: this means we have far more control over what we perceive to be stress than any of us might have thought.

RECOGNIZING AND REFRAMING STRESS

Several years ago, I saw a review of a TED Talk given by psychologist Kelly McGonigal titled *How to Make Stress Your Friend*. My initial response was "bullshit." I was very much in the camp that stress was an insidious disease that could only be remedied by moving to a coconut farm in Central America. Dr. McGonigal actually starts off her talk relating a similar world view.

She had spent years working with her patients to help them "de-stress" using a number of meditation and relaxation techniques. Although somewhat helpful, she wondered if she was really helping people as much as she could. What made Dr. McGonigal question herself was a large study that looked at stress and health outcomes. More than thirty thousand people were asked, "In the past year, have you experienced a significant amount of stress?" These same people were also asked, "Do you believe these stressful events have any impact on your health?" Of the people who responded that they had been both under stress and that they believed stress could negatively impact their health, these folks were 43 percent more likely to die relative to the respondents who experienced significant stress, but who did not feel this should have a negative impact on their health. The latter group appeared to have a "resilient" mind-set, which appears to dramatically alter how they internally perceive and react to stress.

It may seem incredible, but the difference in whether stress impacts us positively or negatively may largely boil down to our perceptions. Andrew Bernstein echoes these concepts in his book *The Myth of Stress*. I actually had the good fortune to talk with Andrew on my podcast, and his work and that of Dr. McGonigal have been nothing short of transformative for me. Let me give you an example.

I'm not generally the most patient driver. I'm a courteous driver, but this has actually been a source of significant self-imposed stress, as I've found people often drive like assholes. Getting cut off in traffic and tailgated has historically made me crazy. As an exercise, I worked to be aware of how I was feeling while driving and, in particular, how I *chose* to react to the drivers around me. If I got cut off, instead of seething internally, I just backed off, gave the person room, and focused on getting from point A to point B with my life and limbs intact. The result? I was not a cranky mess while driving. Yes, clueless drivers are annoying, but I can't control that. I can control how I respond. I've learned to extend this to most areas of my life. Certain things that might have bothered me in the past are really not a big deal now. This may not sound like a very type-A, go-getter way to handle challenges, but a few interesting things have happened:

1. I am a happier person. If I am not pissed off and feeling slighted every time I stand in the long, slow, inefficient line at the airport, I am a much better person to be around. (Okay, the airport line still drives me crazy, but I'm working on it.)
2. As a happier person, when it comes time to get work done, enjoy my family, or just relax and have fun, I am actually in an effective state to do that. Stress does not do our memory or cognition any favors, and it makes us not much fun to be around. If I am not habitually stressed, I get more work done in less time, and that means I have more elective time to enjoy the people and things I love.

I've been pretty consistent in my efforts to reframe what I perceive to be stressful, and the results have not only been impressive but have improved my quality of life. I am more aware of the triggers I perceive to be stressful, and in the moment I ask questions like, "Is this really a problem?; Why do I feel stressed about this?; If I relax, is that going to make this situation easier or harder?" Asking these questions has made a huge difference for me. Andrew Bernstein has a phenomenal online course you can find at http://resilienceacademy.com. This program walks you step by step through how to reframe your situation and create a resilient mind-set. If you need some help getting started and mastering this process, I highly recommend you check out this program.

Given that reframing is key to building a resilient and consequently "low stress" mind-set, there are a few areas that seem to pop up again and again for folks. Let's look at those and consider some strategies for how to better address them.

KEEPING UP WITH THE JONESES

In surveys of stress, people often list "finances" as the consistent number one stress they face. There are a lot of factors here. What we do have control over is how we tackle our personal finances day in and day out. Although you may get cranky at what I'm about to say, I think you'd be hard pressed to shoot holes in the fact that most people suffer financial stress because they live beyond their means. When I was living in Northern California during the first years of the twenty-first century, I saw housing prices go up and up for the better part of a decade. I'm not the sharpest tool in the shed, but my interest in economics coupled with "having a pulse" told me we were in a massive real estate bubble. We were doing pretty well financially, but my wife and I always spent far less than what we made. This was, oddly enough, a bit stressful, as all the folks "in the know" insisted we should be buying real estate, flipping houses, and buying as much car and gear as we possibly could. They thought we were missing out. Then the rapid growth simply slowed down a little. We were still a year or two from the whole system coming unraveled, but the *rate* of growth slowed. A number of our clients were so extended that although we were still technically in a growth phase, they needed the high rate of growth to maintain their standard of living. This put a number of these folks into a legitimate panic as they were too leveraged to survive even a modest downtick in their business.

As the crisis got into full swing, we saw people lose houses, cars, relationships, and their dreams. I'm not laying judgment on this; I'm simply relating what I've observed, and this all dovetails into one of the greatest sources of stress people place upon themselves. These folks never planned for a rainy day, and bought as many houses, cars, boats, and $20,000 wine country weekends as they could. I think it's great if folks work hard, and if they really want X, Y, or Z, by all means, go for it. But what I noticed in talking to folks is this became a game of feeding the ego. If I have more house, then I'll prove to my parents that I amounted to something. If I have the next-level-up car, I can show the people I went to school with that I'm doing all right for myself. When I do consulting, be that for large corporations or police, military, and fire, I talk about all this. It is not popular at first, and I tend to get significant pushback from the hard chargers. My intention is not to tell anyone how to live their lives, but to just ask a simple question: Do you own your shit, or does your shit own you? If you are experiencing financial stress, it may be due to self-talk that has no bearing on reality. Sometimes "proving yourself" is the motivation you need to push through hard times; just don't let that story become a net which drags you into the abyss. Again, you may be wondering what this discussion of personal finances has to do with a health and diet book. All I can say is, if this part of your life is not buttoned up, it will negatively affect every other aspect of your life.

COMMUNITY

It's not news to most people that smoking, excessive alcohol consumption, and carrying too many pounds are not great for one's health. But what if I told you there is one feature of the modern world that increases your risk of going to an early grave as much as obesity, smoking, and excessive drinking? The problem goes by the clinical term "social isolation" but in common parlance this heartbreaking phenomena is simply called "loneliness."

Numerous studies have shown that inadequate social support, simply lacking meaningful relationships with other people, may be as harmful to our health as a pack-a-day smoking habit. How can this be? The mechanisms are complex and not well understood, but our Ancestral Health model may be informative. Humans evolved in tight-knit social groups that entailed an interesting mix of both conflict and love. If you come from a large family, you have seen this up close and personal. Interacting with people appears to stimulate certain centers of the brain in a way that makes us happy and healthy, even if our interactions are not always smooth sailing. A lack of this interaction, including physical touch and even conflict, appears to pose a legitimate stress to our system, a stress that can suppress our immune system and increase our likelihood of developing a number of modern diseases. Our modern world is interesting in that we have nearly limitless options for work, where to live, and how to spend our time, yet these very options tend to take us away from our family and friends, placing us in situations where we do not know most of the people around us. Our social circle constricts to the people we work with, and that may not be a good fit for us.

This is not an easy situation to remedy. Once we have wrapped up our work obligations there is often not much time to attend to our social needs. I honestly struggle with this myself. I do the bulk of my work remotely, so if I do not make a dedicated effort to connect with people I know, I can go weeks or months without spending time with anyone outside my family. The fact I have a "virtual" community is helpful in some ways, but research indicates this may itself be a problem. Online interactions do not provide the same benefits of the real thing. My strategy for dealing with this is I try my best to do activities that take care of multiple needs at once. For example, I do Brazilian jujitsu, which is a fantastic workout, but it also brings me in contact with some wonderful people. I highly recommend you consider something like this, and I'll provide you with some ideas later. Some are pretty active, others less so, but the key point is that you like the activity and enjoy the community: yoga, martial arts, CrossFit, a walking or running group, an art class, a language class, volunteer work, etc. I don't know what the right fit is for you, but I strongly encourage you to find ways to improve your social connectivity. This is an area both my wife and I are working on, but the effort has certainly been worth it.

MOVEMENT

No health or diet book would be complete without at least a cursory treatment of exercise, but I'd argue that most people tackle "exercise" the wrong way. News articles and fitness gurus typically talk about how many calories you burn while exercising, and make the case this will help you to lose weight and feel better. You do burn calories while moving, and you should generally feel better after you exercise, but thinking about exercise as a means of burning calories is focusing on the entirely wrong end of the story. In simple terms, we cannot out-exercise a bad diet. An hour of running can easily be undone with one poorly conceived meal, so please don't fall for the notion that exercise is for burning calories. The reality is, many people around the world live very long lives without "exercising" a day in their lives. They were typically active—they walked, gardened, and danced—but they did not put on a set of gym gloves and lift weights five days per week. I recommend exercise, which I will henceforth call "movement," for the following reasons:

1. We enjoy the activity for the sake of doing it. The activity makes our lives better.
2. We can live our lives more fully due to more strength, flexibility, and endurance.

That's it. You should move because you like it and it makes your life better. Movement can improve how you look, there's no denying that, but if aesthetics are important you need to focus on "forks over barbells." So what type of movement should you do? In short, you need to do what you like to do, as (not surprisingly) that is what you are likely to stick with. Hiking, dancing, gardening, swimming, martial arts, yoga . . . there are a lot of options. If you have never done anything like these activities, check out several of them and decide which one you like the most. Do you like the community? Do you feel safe and welcomed? You should! Shop around and find something that is a good fit for you.

Now, all this said, I will make a soft pitch for doing some specific work a few days per week to help improve your quality of life. This is not a time-consuming process, and you will be shocked at the benefits you gain from just a few minutes a few times per week. You may be backing toward the door saying, "Thanks, but no thanks. I don't like the gym!" Okay, I get it, but let me tell you why this may be important to you. As we age we tend to lose:

1. Muscle mass (and also bone density)
2. Endurance (due to a loss of mitochondrial density)
3. Mobility (the ability to raise our hands over head, to squat, and to get up off the floor, to name but a few movements)

After our mid-thirties, we tend to start losing muscle mass, mitochondrial density, and mobility due to changes in our hormones, and also because we tend to become more sedentary. Muscle mass appears to be one of the best predictors of how long you will live. Now, I'm not suggesting that you become a 300-pound bodybuilder, but if you have any plans of hanging out on this earth for a decent amount of time, you want to maintain your muscle mass to the best of your ability. Mitochondrial density is important, as this allows us to have a flexible, largely fat-fueled metabolism. As we lose mitochondrial density with age, our metabolism shifts more and more toward a carb-centric process. This is not a good thing due to the many factors detailed in earlier chapters. We want metabolic flexibility, and encouraging the growth and health of mitochondria via exercise, and occasional bouts of fasting and/or ketosis, is a fantastic way to facilitate this.

As to mobility, if we become stiff and unable to move properly, we increase our likelihood of injury and wearing out our joints. Keeping our car in proper alignment is important for the mileage we can get from the tires. Keeping our hips, knees, and shoulders in proper alignment is important for the same reason: you do not want that stuff to wear out! Here is a fantastic schedule to shoot for:

1. Most days: Get out and move. As much as you can, doing as many things as you can. You don't need to exhaust yourself. Make it fun and "leave a little in the tank" so you are not so tired and sore that you either do nothing for a week or give up entirely. A good goal to shoot for is 10,000 steps, which is not an insignificant amount given our ability to walk from our house to our car, park a few feet away from our work, and have food delivered to our door, but this is easy to obtain with a little forethought. When I go to get coffee, I park a little ways away from the coffee shop and hoof it to my java fix. A short walk can easily be 1,000 steps each way, and all of a sudden, I have whittled a significant amount off my 10,000/day goal. I use a free steps counter app on my smartphone that just tracks my basic movement. There are also paid apps that link up to you via GPS and give exacting details on your movement. If you want to go full geek on this, that's fine, but if the technology piece is a pain, just get out and move as much as you can.

2. A few days per week, do a full-body resistance training program. This could be weights or just calisthenics using your own body weight. When I am pressed for time, I will hit the gym and do a very quick (5-minute) general warmup, and then start doing a circuit of pressing, pulling, squatting, and lunging. I start off with very light weight, and each pass through the circuit I add a little more. I take as little rest as I can between each movement and after 10 to 15 minutes, I am *done*. My last few sets tend to be fairly heavy, which is what we want to maintain muscle mass. My whole time commitment to this process is about 30 minutes twice a week. That's it. The quick pace allows you to build endurance while also building the muscle mass you need to prevent the ravages of aging. Hate the gym? No problem. Get a few dumbbells and exercise bands and follow one of the thousands of free workouts you can find online. You may not think this little work will really get you any benefits, but all I can say is, try it—you'll like it.

3. Occasionally get a little "froggy" with your movement. If you have mainly been walking, find a hill or steep incline and power up the hill at a good clip. If you have been running, step up the rate on an incline or hill. You only need to push for 10 to 30 seconds, then dial your intensity back to a comfortable level. Once you recover, do it a few more times. Challenge yourself, but there is no need to get it all done in one day. As I said, leave a little in reserve, especially if it's been a while since you've done much in the way of physical activity. Why do this on a hill? The impact we have on our joints is less when we are going up a hill, so if you are carrying extra weight or your movement mechanics are not great, the hill can save you wear and tear. The other reason is that jamming up a hill is *hard*! *Walking* up an incline at a decent pace is as hard as *running* on the flats. What you are effectively doing here is sprint interval training. Research has shown that short intervals can get you

into fantastic cardiovascular shape while also increasing mitochondrial density.

4. A few days each week, do some kind of stretching or yoga. It'd be great if you joined a yoga class (remember the community piece above?), but if you do not have time, resources, or inclination, there are a dizzying number of yoga and stretch routines and videos available online. Some are free, others cost a little, but the quality is remarkably good on many of these programs. I have a stretch routine I follow and tend to do that a few days per week while watching one of my favorite sci-fi shows. This makes my TV-watching a little less lazy, and it makes the stretching a lot less boring, all the while being pretty damn time efficient.

In addition to a few Brazilian jujitsu classes each week, the schedule I have detailed above is pretty much what I have done for the better part of fifteen years. I try to get a lot of low-intensity activity by walking and hiking, but I maintain my strength, muscle mass, and mobility with a few dedicated sessions each week. My time spent in the gym is typically less than an hour each week, yet for a forty-four-year-old guy, I'm in pretty good shape. I will not set any age group records in anything, but I am also able to tackle almost anything I want to do. You do not need pills, potions, or tons of gear to get in really good shape. What you do need to do is find things you like and consistently play at those activities.

Being a bit of an economics geek, I like to think about things from the perspective of return on investment (ROI). I have found incredible ROI in focusing on my sleep, reframing how I view stress, cultivating meaningful relationships, and following an approach to movement as detailed above. I get a lot done, I have the energy to get things done, and I enjoy the whole process immensely. I am not a fan of extremism, and although what I am recommending to you may seem new (and possibly extreme), it's really not. Prioritizing sleep, a resilient mind-set, meaningful relationships, and a fun movement practice will give you far more than it takes. That's a good ROI. That is also setting up both healthy habits and the rewards that will make those habits stick.

CHAPTER 9

Cheating, Morality, and Food

While our hormones, the neuroregulation of appetite, and Optimal Foraging Strategy (OFS) are critical factors in why we gravitate toward certain foods, it is our mental state that ultimately derails efforts the most often. This is the realm of internal dialogue, rationalization, and, unfortunately, self-sabotage. The trap I see people fall into again and again is the notion of "cheating" on their food. Related to this is the notion of having a "relationship" with food. You cannot cheat on your food, and if you are seeking a healthy relationship with food, that very process may be at the root of your problems.

If you struggle in these areas, this short chapter may piss you off so thoroughly that you will take this book and set it on fire. I have had people storm out of consults in tears when I started walking them through a process of self-awareness on these topics. This is not pleasant for either myself or the people I'm working with, but it is critical to get this out in the open if the person seeking help is to succeed. So, although you may have strong emotional response to this material (you may already be mad about that opening paragraph), please keep in mind that I am not laying blame or judgment. I am trying to help you. I have a lot of experience working with people, and I have seen these topics ensnare folks who were otherwise making good progress. If we can get a handle on the psychology of cheating and the misguided notion that we have a relationship with food, we will be liberated from a vicious cycle not dissimilar from escaping a toxic relationship.

CHEATING: SAVE IT FOR YOUR TAXES

So, what exactly does *cheating* mean? The dictionary definition is something like: "to act dishonestly or unfairly in order to gain an *advantage*, especially in a game or examination." (The emphasis is mine.)

File that away for a moment while we go through a hypothetical scenario in which people misapply the term *cheating* to the food they eat. Our hypothetical person (let's call him Sven) has embarked on a program of eating (let's say something like Paleo or low carb), and Sven is motoring along just fine. Then a coworker brings in a plate of incredible treats and somehow these treats make it from plate to mouth. Sven noshes on the treat, gets back to work, and then has a horror-stricken moment in which he says (internally, most likely), "I cheated on my *diet*! I'm such a shit! How could I do this?! Why can't I be stronger, or better . . . I'm doomed to failure. I might as well give up." Sven then stands up, walks to the remaining treats, and eats them all.

Okay, back to the definition of cheating: Did Sven do something underhanded? Did he gain an "unfair advantage"? Was he in any way dishonest? No, no, and no. The terminology does not apply, but the *guilt* of dishonesty hangs over him. This guilt comes from a sense of moral failure. If Sven was only a "better" person, he'd be strong enough to avoid temptation.

Let's take a quick look at the dictionary definition of *morality*: "principles concerning the distinction between right and wrong or good and bad behavior." All societies have complex systems of what is right and wrong, what is moral, and occasionally this extends to certain foods or eating practices. Even hunter-gatherer groups have a list of foods that should or should not be eaten. Looking at the moral considerations of food from a scientific perspective, we do see potential wisdom in some moral guidelines governing food laws. The biblical prohibitions on pork and shellfish might have been a good idea in the past due to the possibility of parasitic infection in the case of pork and death or illness from toxin accumulation in shellfish caused by certain types of microorganisms. People manifest guilt from a number of different perspectives, sometimes secular, sometimes based on religious experience. What I'm trying to get across to you is dead simple:

1. You cannot "cheat" with food.
2. You "eat" food.
3. There are consequences to what we put down our pie hole.
4. That's it.

If you have established a pattern (consciously or unconsciously) of moralizing the food you eat, you are likely going to have a rough time with this change. Based on my experience, you will likely take any minor "transgression" on the plan as yet another sign of weakness or failure and bail on the process entirely. How do I know this? I've seen it thousands, if not tens of thousands, of times in my twenty years of working with people. I'll talk about some strategies for coping with this in a bit, but we need to dig a little deeper into this topic to really put things in the proper context. Hopefully, you now understand that modern hyperpalatable foods are tough to resist. We've talked about Optimum Foraging Strategy, and how we are genetically wired to "eat more, move less." If you really understand and embrace those realities, you are extremely close to liberating yourself from any type of morality or guilt you may feel around food. Perhaps that information, and the realizations that come from processing the implications, are enough for you. If so, fantastic. If not, if you still have this niggling sense that anything less than perfection with your food is failure . . . you have something else going on and it has *nothing* to do with food. Let me share a story to make this point.

Several years ago, I was hired to manage the food and physical training of a *highly* successful businessman. Let's call him Dan. Dan's incredible intellect and near fanatical work ethic have produced products from which all of us have benefited. This guy is literally a world mover, and he has also been seriously overweight most of his life. Dan's weight was reaching a breaking point. After he'd crush a gallon (or two) of ice cream, he would suffer vision loss and a number of other problems. He was likely diabetic but unwilling to go to a doctor lest he be forced to change what he was doing.

We were introduced via mutual acquaintances, and he quizzed me on what my plan would be for him, all the while working his way through two half gallons of ice cream. I think he did this to gauge my reaction and to see if he could get a rise out of me, but I'm pretty Zen about this stuff. I'll do just about anything to help someone who is motivated to do so, but I can also border on callousness if the person is hell-bent on self-destruction. Whatever the case, I impressed Dan enough that he hired me to work with him 24/7 for six months. I'd handle his food and physical training and would do my best to get him to sleep more than four hours per night. The game was on.

I cleaned out the pantry, provided a meal plan for the chefs who prepared the meals for Dan's family, and set up a schedule to meet Dan for physical training. All seemed to be progressing fine, until one evening when I was walking through the house and smelled what could only be . . . doughnuts. I knocked on Dan's office door, and sure enough, he was working his way through a bag of doughnuts. He was evasive about where the food had come from, but with a little digging, I found out that Dan had paid some of his house staff to drive to the doughnut shop and, at a specific time, throw the bag of doughnuts over the security fence ringing his property. On the inside of the fence was another staff person who was waiting to intercept the flying bag of fried dough. Once acquired, they delivered the goods to Dan. Not one to be outdone, I went to Dan's wife and explained the situation and said, "I need a budget for a counterinsurgency campaign." I now had a pool of money to pay the staff to *not* do Dan's bidding with regard to hooking him up with junk food. This worked for a few days, until Dan got wise to our work and simply threatened to fire anyone unwilling to follow through on his requests. I confronted Dan about this, and he just smirked. "It's not my job to make your job easy." He was enjoying this and rather liked the game of spy vs. spy. I was a bit stumped about why this guy was making it so hard for me to help him not eat himself to death. In addition to the tactics I just described, Dan would routinely moralize his food "failures" and turn these minor deviations into an excuse for multiday benders.

I noodled on what the hell was going on and finally had what proved to be an important insight: none of this had to do with food. Food was a symptom, not the problem. I noticed a pattern: Dan was emotionally distant from everyone, including his wife. The only people he really had no barriers against were his kids. In a flash of insight, I knew exactly what was up, and I had a plan for how to address it. The following day, Dan and I were talking, and I told him how incredibly grateful I was for the opportunity to work with him. I was getting paid very well, and this money was helping my wife and I get a number of projects off the ground much faster than we would have been able to otherwise. I was sincere in this feeling, but was also softening him up to get through his nearly impregnable barrier. I then said something like this: "I'll be able to help so many people as a consequence of my work with you, but I have to admit to feeling a sense of failure, as I have not really been able to help you." This caught Dan off guard, and in a very uncharacteristic moment, he was at a loss for words. I then asked him, "Dan, who didn't love you?"

The color drained out of his face and he replied with a barely audible "What?" I repeated the question, and he became really agitated, angry, and flustered. He yelled at me in about six different languages. He was mad. And scared. I asked the question again: "Dan, who didn't love you? This has nothing to do with food. You know it and I know it." He sat back in his chair and I was not sure if he was going to respond, but finally he related the story of his childhood. His parents were hard chargers and did not have the time to raise him. This duty fell on his nanny. He rarely saw either of his parents and was a bright, precocious child who needed love. His nanny knew this on some level, and in addition to her normal caregiving, she prepared elaborate breakfasts of pancakes, crepes, and, not infrequently, ice cream. She would talk and laugh with Dan, they would sing and play games, all the while celebrating with food. For Dan, the association was set: food was love.

I took all this in and then told Dan that was to be my last day working with him. He needed to work with a therapist. He needed to get his whole family involved. Dan was pretty taken aback and brought up the fact that I wouldn't be making the money, which I had just said was so important. Money was a major point of control for Dan, and he defaulted to it immediately. I told him I was not going to take his money and continue to facilitate his situation. Knowing what I knew, I felt that would be amoral. I would be *cheating* him. I would be extracting benefit from his continued suffering.

Dalliances with junk food is not cheating. Gaining financial benefit from another person's suffering is. Do you see the difference? Can you *feel* it?

Dan is doing pretty well now. He has lost a lot of weight, and he is a much more pleasant person to be around. He nearly went through a divorce during this process, but he and his wife managed to motor through things. Dan is *not* perfect. He has better and worse days, but his new normal is a far cry from what it was, both with his eating and his relationships. Speaking of relationships, Dan did not need a "healthy relationship with food." He needed to connect with his friends and family, and he needed to heal from being abandoned as a kid. Focusing on food was a distraction, not a solution.

If you moralize your eating, if you think you still need to find a "healthy relationship with food," I am 99.99 percent sure you are focusing on the wrong things. It's not about the food—it's about something else, and that something else likely boils down to love and connection. This book is damn long and I cover a lot of ground, but I laid all this out with the end goal of actually helping you. *Seven Days to Hollywood Abs* would be an easy book to write and would likely sell like hotcakes, but it's also bullshit. I had to lay out the story about who we are (eat more, move less), how we got here (the changes in our food system and the emergence of the junk food catastrophe), and what our modern world can do to us. I had to talk about sleep, exercise, and community to put all this in perspective. In the opening paragraph of the book, I told you the cards are stacked against us. They are. We have to figure out how to eat, move, and love in a way that is effective in the long term for each of us. None of the changes I am recommending are likely to be easy (initially), but if you can understand that none of this is about morality or failure, that all this is about a mismatch between our genes and our environment, that we have been socially conditioned to loathe ourselves for just being who we are supposed to be . . . we have a chance. People only change when the pain of their current situation is greater than the pain of change. It is my hope that this information, this opportunity for a different perspective, can act as a catalyst. In chemistry a catalyst reduces the energy necessary for a chemical reaction to occur.

In our case, the information and mind-set we can cultivate using this Ancestral Health model can act as a catalyst to help us make the changes we want.

That's a lot of rah-rah, and it's important, but let's look at some practical steps for addressing "cheating" and the supposed morality of eating.

1. I recommend that folks stick to the guidelines of the 30-Day Reset for the full thirty days, evaluate how they look feel and perform, and decide if the process is "worth it." I recommend this because folks get remarkable results and that success is contagious enough to stick with the program long term. I have found more gradual approaches do not produce particularly good results, and given that they also limit the foods people like to eat it bugs them. Poor results plus annoying is not a good recipe for success. Okay, so that's all good advice, but what if you "cheat"? What if you do not navigate the first thirty days flaw-lessly? You have two ways to look at this: it is either a soul-crushing failure and you might as well quit (possibly sell all your worldly pos-sessions and join an obscure religious sect to work off your sins . . .), or you put on your big-kid britches and realize that you are one meal away from being back on track. Those are the options. You can turn this event into a reason to bail on the progress you have made *or* you can look at it for what it is: one "less good" meal out of weeks or months of "very good" meals. Now, if you are having one "good" meal out of weeks or months of pretty poor choices, then you need to ask yourself what you're up to. Is changing what you are doing really important to you? If not, no worries, but let's just be honest and clear and not turn this into a bunch of guilt and drama. If you choose to moralize the event, remember, it's not about the food—it's something else. It's easier to just focus on the next meal than it is to bail on your

progress. It is harder to take the moralized path, so if you do that you have to ask yourself why.

2. People often ask if they will ever be able to eat bread or cookies again, particularly if they have an issue with gluten or a similar food sensitivity. The short answer is, you can have any of that food anytime you want, but there are going to be consequences. I am so reactive to gluten that whatever momentary enjoyment I might have is vastly outweighed by how bad I feel afterward. A piece of bread would make me feel like crap for a week. So although fresh-baked French bread smells pretty damn good, it's just not worth it for me, especially given that there are fantastic gluten-free options these days if I want to kick my heels up. That said, those gluten-free foods are still refined carbs. I save them for occasional use. In the end, eating them doesn't help me work toward my larger goal of seeing my children grow up and hopefully meeting my grandkids.

In marketing there is a saying "facts tell, stories sell." I've tried to give you facts and stories so we can address both the logical and emotional components of your decision-making process. If you give the program and, more specifically, yourself a chance, you might be shocked by what you can achieve. Just remember to take things one day at a time, one meal at a time. You do not need perfection; you need to make a few more good decisions than dodgy ones.

PART 2

Rewire and Reset for Weight Loss and Health

CHAPTER 10

Get Testy! The Plan for Success

L et me float an idea by you: with better information we can make better decisions. To this point, a quote from William Thomson, 1st Barron Kelvin (yes, as in kelvin the measurement), is educational, "If you cannot measure it, you cannot improve it." Lab testing can be incredibly valuable. From your smartphone you can order tests that give you a far deeper insight into your genetics, gut biome, and physiology than doctors were able to order for their patients just a decade ago. We have nearly limitless options to track our health, but we need not and should not take out a second mortgage to finance a ridiculous assortment of testing that does not better inform us about what to do. We need to test what matters—that's it.*

To that end, this chapter looks at the tests and subjective observations that really do affect how we do things day to day that influence our appetite, blood sugar, weight, and health. We will start by establishing where you are

---

* Lab testing is valuable, but it can go to Crazytown pretty quickly. With a little searching on the Internet, one can find health gurus who brag about spending hundreds of thousands of dollars "hacking their biology." These folks are certainly hacking something, but it's generally not health. It's more akin to taking a machete to a cow pie.

currently (health and weight, for example) and then determine goals to help you focus your efforts. We will use a mix of subjective measures like how you feel between meals as well as basic testing like blood pressure and blood glucose levels. This information will help you establish reasonable goals, stay on task, and, perhaps most important, determine which of the options offered in the meal planning section is best for you.

A JOURNEY OF A THOUSAND MILES STARTS WITH A SINGLE HAMSTRING PULL

When I work with people who are looking to make performance, health, or weight-loss changes, I like to ask the following questions:

1. Who are you?
2. What are your goals?

These questions help create a map. Who are you? (Starting point.) What are your goals? (Destination.)

Asking "Who are you?" is not a "What type of tree would you be?" question. It relates to things such as your age and health status. Are you overweight? Do you suffer from diabetes, GI problems, or autoimmunity? Is there a family history of cardiovascular disease, cancer, or neurodegeneration? Do you just feel like death warmed over?

Many of these problems, although seemingly unrelated, have significant overlap. For example, if you are overweight, you are more likely to develop cardiovascular disease, neurodegeneration, or diabetes. Similarly, we have learned that autoimmunity has an element of intestinal permeability, but we also know that intestinal permeability impairs our insulin sensitivity, which increases our likelihood of weight gain, cardiovascular disease, and diabetes! These health challenges are remarkably interwoven, which is why the reductionist approach to medicine has produced lackluster results in dealing with chronic degenerative disease. Fortunately for us, however, our knowledge of the Ancestral Health template, built around sleep, food, movement, and community, addresses all these concerns.

The background work of detailing your subjective situation (how you feel, how resilient you are when going without food for a period of time) coupled with some basic lab work gives us a very accurate picture of your health status, particularly your glycemic tolerance and insulin sensitivity. This information will give us a good starting point from which to gauge the efficacy of the program you are soon to embark upon. I can't emphasize sufficiently how important this is. Although I wish I could make all of this effortless for you, the reality is that for some of you, making the recommended changes will be a struggle, either physically, socially, emotionally, or some combination of the three. But if you track your progress and have a solid starting point, you can look back and say, "Wow . . . that was not easy, but look what I've accomplished." That may make all the difference between you making this change stick and you bailing on the process partway through.

Let's begin by getting familiar with the subjective measures of insulin resistance. The subjective measurements will help you notice how you are feeling with your new program from day to day. The objective measurements such as blood pressure and blood work will provide concrete evidence of how your health is improving.

ARE YOU OVERWEIGHT?

The research on "overweight" is complex. There are some indications that being overweight may improve certain health outcomes, but this is juxtaposed with strong correlations between excess weight, the beginning of insulin resistance, and what is called metabolic syndrome. Although health is clearly important, let's face facts: people are vain. Given this fact, I like to explore this from a different perspective: are you happy with how you look naked? We can cut off a leg and have "substantial, rapid weight loss," but I don't think many people will sign up for the "lose a leg" diet plan. Similarly, folks who begin eating well and exercising may lose significant amounts of fat, but they will also gain muscle and bone mineral mass. The net shift in the scale may not be that impressive, but the person looks fantastic and may need a line of credit to buy new clothes due to dropping pant sizes almost daily. *That* is a good outcome!

Let me share an example of how fixating on weight instead of aesthetics and health can lead us astray. Most visits to the doctor entail a number of measurements, including our height and weight. From this information we can calculate our body mass index (BMI), which looks at how much you weigh relative to your height. BMI can be a helpful number for folks who are significantly overweight, but like most medical measurements, we need to consider it in the proper context. When I was sick due to malabsorption, I weighed 135 pounds, putting me at a BMI of 19.9, smack in the "healthy" range of 18.5 to 24.9. But I was anything but healthy. Currently, I weigh 175 pounds, which puts me at a hefty 25.8, technically "overweight" in the arbitrary BMI range from 25 to 29.9 (obesity is technically 30 to 39.9). I'm forty-four years old, do old-guy Brazilian jujitsu, and motor along pretty well with a decent set of abs. I don't look like Brad Pitt in *Fight Club*, but I just remind my wife that does not matter once the lights are off . . . My point here is this: arbitrary BMI measure puts me in the overweight category when I'm pretty damn healthy and happy. I don't want you to get too wrapped around the axle of your weight, but instead focus on how you look (in the mirror, in photos, etc.) and, most important, how you feel.

If you have a significant amount of weight to lose, we will certainly celebrate your milestones of progress, but I don't want you to be a daily scale watcher. Folks who get in this habit can be psychologically derailed by a few pounds of water retained after one salty meal. Remember: A watched pot never boils; a watched scale never budges. After you take your starting weight, wrap up your scale, put a bow on it, and give it to someone you do not like—let it mess with their minds, not yours. If you have a long way to go, monthly weight checks are plenty. This will keep you focused on your food, movement, and enjoying your life, but will allow you to check in frequently enough to document progress. Let's celebrate inches lost and pants donated, not the daily fluctuations of the scale.

ARE YOU INSULIN RESISTANT, PREDIABETIC, OR DIABETIC?

Although estimates vary, it appears that between 30 and 50 percent of the US population shows signs of insulin resistance and the cryptic indications of metabolic syndrome. Let's first look at some of the subjective signs of insulin resistance to see where you are on the spectrum.

- Do you find that you are extremely thirsty and need to pee "all the time"?
- Does your vision sometimes blur after a carby meal?
- If you cut yourself, is your skin slow to heal?
- Do you generally feel fatigued or "foggy headed"?
- Do you feel hungry less than two hours after having a meal?

I recently performed genetic testing via the online genetics and ancestry lab 23andMe, and was not surprised to find that I am (based on my genetics) "much" more likely than the average person to develop type 2 diabetes and insulin resistance. For years I have noticed that if I do not pay attention to the amount and types of carbs I consume, I suffer fatigue, foggy headedness, and occasionally even blurred vision. I have experimented with keeping carb levels higher than I'm really comfortable with, and interestingly my body composition deteriorates (I gain fat in my abdomen) and my blood work shifts from great to "meh." Many doctors and researchers will dismiss these subjective experiences as anecdotal. Anecdotal they are, but technically, dropping a hammer on your foot and disliking the effects is anecdotal. We don't need a randomized controlled trial to gain insight into every facet of our lives.

If you experience any of the above symptoms, if you get "hangry" (hungry/angry) between meals and/or can only go an hour or two without eating, we have some problems brewing. Let's now shift from the highly subjective to something a bit more concrete: your belly!

TALE OF THE TAPE: WAIST-TO-HIP RATIO

If we consume more calories than we need, we will tend to gain fat. If we are insulin sensitive, this fat will tend to be evenly distributed around the body. If, however, we are insulin resistant (for whatever reason—lack of sleep, stress, inflammation) *and* if those excess calories come in the form of refined carbohydrates, this fat tends to be stored around our internal organs and is called visceral fat.

For reasons that are only now being unraveled, visceral fat appears to be particularly nasty for health and disease potential, releasing a disproportionately large amount of pro-inflammatory signaling molecules, which further impair leptin and insulin sensitivity and appetite regulation. Visceral fat is bad. Given the connection between excessive carbohydrate and visceral fat, your waist-to-hip ratio (WHR) can shed some light on your insulin sensitivity status. As the name implies, the waist-to-hip ratio is a number we obtain by dividing the circumference of your waist (measured at the midpoint between your bottom rib and the top of your hip bone—this is usually about an inch below your belly button) by the circumference of your hip (at the greatest circumference of your behind). In general, the hips are wider than the waist, so we should end up with a number less than one. As an example, a small, reasonably lean female might have a waist measurement of 26 inches and a hip measurement of 37 inches with a W/H (26/37) ratio of 0.70. Let's consider another female who has the same hip measurement of 37 inches but a waist measurement of 28 inches (28/37). This provides a ratio of .75. Now let's check out the WHR chart most medical professionals use to assess cardiovascular disease risk, which is closely tied to insulin sensitivity.

WAIST-TO-HIP RATIO (WHR) NORMS				
Gender	Excellent	Good	Average	At Risk
Males	<0.85	0.85–0.89	0.90–0.95	≥0.95
Females	<0.75	0.75–0.79	0.80–0.86	≥0.86

Studies of pre-Westernized populations have a waist-to-hip ratio in the "excellent" category for most of the individuals studied. Again, this is correlative, but it has also been well documented that as these cultures shift to more modern eating and lifestyle patterns, this profile shifts to match what is the norm for modern populations. It's worth mentioning that the chart above shows the average to be very near what is clinically understood to represent a higher risk of insulin resistance and therefore a host of metabolically driven diseases. "Average" is not a number to emulate.

So grab a measuring tape and let's figure out where you are on this spectrum. If you need a little guidance on taking this measurement, do a search for "waist-to-hip measurement" on YouTube, as there are several videos demonstrating how to do it. Similarly, if the prospect of dividing one number by another number is a bit daunting, search for "waist-to-hip ratio calculator" You will still need to measure your own belly and backside—technology can't do *everything* for us!

HYPERTENSION

Elevated blood pressure (hypertension) is a common early indication of insulin resistance. As insulin levels increase, the hormone aldosterone is also increased. Aldosterone causes us to retain sodium, and the retention of sodium causes us to retain water. Hypertension is nasty in that it accelerates damage to the vascular beds, worsening the atherosclerotic process while also damaging the kidneys and heart directly.

It's pretty easy to get your blood pressure checked, either by buying an electronic device that takes it for you or dropping by one of the many pharmacies that have an automatic device, which will set you back a dollar to use. Here is a chart that shows the general ranges deemed "okay" or "holy cats!" by the medical establishment.

BLOOD PRESSURE CLASSIFICATION SYSTOLIC DIASTOLIC	
Normal	<120 and <80
Pre-hypertension	120–139 or 80–89
Stage 1 Hypertension	140–159 or 90–99
Stage 2 Hypertension	≥160 or ≥100

Your blood pressure reading is composed of two numbers. The larger number (systolic) shows your blood pressure when your heart beats, and your diastolic, the smaller of the two numbers, is the pressure of your arterial system between heartbeats. The graph is largely what you will find in most medical circles. Again, the "normal" numbers have problems, in my opinion. Looking at pre-Westernized populations it is not uncommon to see the norm nearly 20 points less than what is described for both systolic and diastolic blood pressure, often even less than this. There is some literature that suggests a diastolic reading above 75 may be causing low-grade kidney damage. Whatever the case, if your blood pressure is anywhere above the normal range listed here, you want to take that seriously.

Most doctors are stumped as to how to affect BP changes in their clients. Diet and exercise rarely seem to work. As I described above, hypertension causes an up regulation of the hormone aldosterone and the tendency to retain both sodium and water as a consequence. Reducing dietary sodium has a modest influence on this process but this practice seems to work in only a small number of people, and it is not addressing the root cause, which is an abnormally elevated insulin level. A diet with carbs set at a level that works for the individual causes rapid loss of water, which also brings down BP almost immediately. One of the criticisms of low-carb diets goes something like this: "Much of the weight loss is just water weight." Yes, that's true. The formerly insulin-resistant individual just peed out their heart and kidney disease risk, literally down the drain.

If you are at all hypertensive, I do recommend that you perform weekly monitoring. Blood pressure is one of the first things to improve with better diet and lifestyle, so this can provide you with a real sense of accomplishment early in your process. Once you get healthy, I recommend checking your blood pressure at least twice per year to make sure you are not drifting into the danger zone.

THE 'BETUS

The diagnostic criteria for diabetes are surprisingly arbitrary. With malaria you either have it or you don't. Similarly, you are either pregnant or you aren't. These are binary yes/no scenarios. The processes that lead one to diabetes are a long time coming. This is both good and bad. It's good in that if we know what to look for, we can make simple changes to avoid it altogether. However, the often slow progress of diabetes means that most medical professionals are not moved to action until we are quite sick. If you do a yearly physical, you and your doc will likely look at your blood glucose climbing slowly upward and briefly discuss better diet and lifestyle choices before shifting the topic to the new wine bar in town. There is no sense of urgency. Then, one day you get . . . The Diagnosis. It's panic and drama, and all of a sudden you get a bunch of prescriptions to aggressively tackle this problem. But there should be no surprise here. The signs were as clear as a fuse burning toward a stick of dynamite.

Hopefully, we can help you catch all this before a diagnosis of diabetes, but even if you are currently in the thick of dealing with type 2 diabetes, we can still alter its course. What will be critical to your success is a desire to change and serious self-advocacy. I'm honestly a bit frustrated by how ineffective the medical establishment is in dealing with the condition. People on the interwebz and in research circles just muddy the waters arguing over whether too many calories, too many carbs, or too much insulin (or something else) is the cause of diabetes. By this stage of the game (as in being insulin resistant or type 2 diabetic), it does not matter. The most effective way to reverse the condition is to reduce the amount of glucose (carbs) you put in your body to a level that is nontoxic. This may mean a very low-carb diet for some, or simply a qualitative shift in carbs for others. Whatever the ultimate path, at this point the diabetic individual has lost the ability to either produce or respond to insulin in an effective way. Glucose can quickly accumulate to toxic levels, and this can easily spin into a life-threatening situation on an acute level. It most assuredly will affect longevity and quality of life on a longer timescale.

Okay, all that cheery stuff aside, what are the diagnostic criteria* for diabetes?

BLOOD TEST LEVELS FOR DIAGNOSIS OF DIABETES AND PREDIABETES			
	A1C (percent)	Fasting Plasma Glucose (mg/dL)	Oral Glucose Tolerance Test (mg/dL)
Diabetes	6.5 or above	126 or above	200 or above
Prediabetes	5.7 to 6.4	100 to 125	140 to 199
Normal	About 5	99 or below	139 or below

Definitions: mg = milligram, dL = deciliter.
For all three tests, within the prediabetes range, the higher the test result,
the greater the risk of diabetes.

A medical diagnosis of diabetes may be arrived at by using one or several of the following criteria: A1C, fasting glucose, and oral glucose tolerance test. The hemoglobin A1C shows the amount of advanced glycation end products that have accumulated on red blood cells over the past few months. This is likely the most valuable test, as it gives us a sense of blood glucose over time. There are some limitations to the A1C, however. Folks eating a low-carb diet may see relatively high A1C levels, as their blood cells actually live substantially longer than when blood glucose levels are more elevated. Unfortunately, most doctors are not aware of this story, so they may see an elevated A1C in an individual who eats reasonably low carb and

---

* From Standards of medical care in diabetes-2012. *Diabetes Care.* 2012; 35 (Supp 1): S12, table 2.

thus erroneously assume the individual is knocking on the door to diabetes. Fortunately, we do have a slick biomarker, in this case the advanced glycation end-product fructosamine, to validate if the A1C is the real deal or leading us down the wrong interpretive road. If an individual has an A1C on the high side but fructosamine on the low to normal side, we really don't have much to worry about in this specific case. If, however, we see elevated A1C and elevated fructosamine, we have two biomarkers that point toward unhealthy levels of glucose for that individual.

The fasting glucose test indicates one's blood glucose levels after an overnight fast. The medical community puts the cutoff for diabetes at 126mg/dl, while fasting numbers of 99 to 125 are considered prediabetic. In general, I find these numbers to be set far too high. There are caveats, which we will get to in a moment, but these numbers are driven not from the perspective of what is optimum or healthy but what is "normal." That means, normal is the average fasting blood glucose of the folks walking through the door. If everyone going through the system is in fact sick, this may be normal, but not necessarily what we'd like to emulate for better health and a more svelte backside. Don't get me wrong. The fasting glucose test is quite valuable, but stress or infections can skew the number upward, so we need to consider the context of that particular test. Unfortunately, this is also typically the singular test used to make a diagnosis of diabetes or prediabetes. I would be reticent to hang my hat on any one lab value, particularly fasting glucose. If this is elevated, I'd certainly like to see A1C to use as a separate validation.

The oral glucose tolerance test (OGTT) involves an individual consuming 75g of a glucose solution and then checking blood glucose one and two hours post-consumption. This tells us what type of glucose disposal (if any) the individual has. If one has a blood glucose level greater than 199mg/dl at the two-hour mark, you have "the 'betus." If the blood sugar is 140 to 198, you are prediabetic. Again, from a health standpoint, these numbers are likely too high. Studies of pre-Westernized populations show "normal" OGTT results in these populations to be 90 to 110mg/dl! All this considered, I'm not actually a fan of the OGTT for a few reasons and situations. The primary reason is that I do not view the consumption of nearly 100g of sugar as a "healthy" process. The philosophical underpinning of medicine (in theory) is "First, do no harm." If you happen to be insulin resistant, this test will make you feel awful, as it will push blood glucose levels into clearly unhealthy ranges.

Here are what I'd recommend tracking:

1. A1C
2. Fructosamine
3. Fasting glucose levels

As I explained previously, the A1C and fructosamine give us a sense of what glycemic control looks like over the past few weeks and months while also letting us know if elevated A1C is an artifact of actually eating a lower-carb diet. The A.M. fasting glucose number can tell us what our insulin sensitivity/insulin efficacy looks like between meals. Any one of these tests individually can be misleading, but taken as a whole, they can point us in a good direction. Some people who are wound tight ("type A") may have relatively elevated morning glucose levels, but this may not be a big deal if their A1C and fructosamine are telling us the overall blood glucose picture looks favorable.

In addition to the tests listed above, I recommend tracking the following:

1. Total cholesterol, which will include HDL and LDL cholesterol
2. Triglycerides

3. LDL-P, which measures the number of LDL particles that actually carry your LDL cholesterol

Most routine blood work will include total cholesterol as well as HDL/ LDL cholesterol and triglycerides. In the case of triglycerides, we'd like to see those on the "low" side. The generally accepted ranges are:

- Normal: less than 150mg/dl (less than 1.7 mmol/l)
- Borderline high: 150 to 199 mg/dl (1.8 to 2.2 mmol/l)
- High: 200 to 499 mg/dl (2.3 to 5.6 mmol/l)
- Very high: 500 mg/dl or above (5.7 mmol/l or above)

But again, these numbers are an artifact of testing a population that is generally not healthy. Normal is not good enough for our purposes. Triglycerides are an indirect measure of insulin sensitivity and a direct measure of circulating blood fats. I'd like to see triglycerides at least below 100mg/dl and more in the 50 to 75 range. There are genetic variations in this, but if folks get the glycemic load of their diet "right," triglycerides generally plummet.

Cholesterol is a highly contentious topic, and whole books have been written trying to untangle the relationship between cholesterol and cardio-vascular disease. The problem with cholesterol as a predictor of cardiovas-cular disease is that it is at best an imperfect fit. Not everyone with high cholesterol develops cardiovascular disease (specifically, blocked arteries), nor does everyone with low cholesterol levels avoid cardiovascular disease. Science has told us that HDL cholesterol is "good" and LDL cholesterol is "bad." In our work with police and firefighters at the Specialty Health Clinic in Reno, Nevada, we have seen many relatively young people with choles-terol numbers that looked okay but who were ticking time bombs. These folks had what is called discordance. They had low-normal cholesterol levels but quite high lipoproteins, specifically LDL-P. HDL and LDL cholesterol are shuttled around the body inside lipoproteins (HDL-P, LDL-P) and when we look at lipoprotein numbers, we see a much better fit with cardiovascular disease potential. Unfortunately, most doctors, even cardiologists, are unfamiliar with this test. In general, we'd like to see LDL-P below 1,000mmol/l. Folks with numbers in the 1,500 range are considered to be at borderline risk, while those with LDL-P over 2,000 are considered to be at high risk. This is the best of our understanding to date, but I must add a bit to all this. There are *many* factors that can affect LDL-P numbers. Low thyroid, infections (gut permeability), and insulin resistance can all push numbers up. I have seen people change their diet and dramatically reverse insulin resistance and systemic inflammation—these folks felt better than they had in years, and their LDL-P went up! This is a rare situation, but it does happen. Bringing down blood glucose from diabetic or prediabetic levels is clearly good. Reversing insulin resistance and inflammation while also increasing LDL-P levels is a less clear story. My gut sense is that this is still a net win, but we simply do not have the information to make a definitive case. As the takeaway, please understand that basic cholesterol testing is not telling much about cardiovascular disease risk in most cases and it would be smart to ask your doctor to include the test for LDL-P.

Also, keep in mind that the reason we want to know these numbers is so we really know where you are in the insulin resistance/diabetes story. This has huge implications for a remarkable number of health conditions and is often a critical piece in the weight loss story, because when we fix insulin resistance we tend to also repair the neuroregulation of appetite. Additionally, this number will be important to check at the end of the 30-Day Reset so you can correlate your improved blood markers with how much better you are feeling. Thirty days may not seem like long enough to see significant weight loss or improvements in blood work, but you will be amazed by what you can accomplish in this time. This is long enough to see profound improvements (and help to motivate you to stick with the program for a lifetime), while it is short enough that you will be willing to give it a shot.

In talking to folks about goals, the most common areas of interest are weight loss, addressing health concerns, and performance improvement. There can be a lot of specific reasons for these goals: "I want to improve my health so I can keep up with my kids/grandkids," for example. Whatever your goal, I do need to make a point: although the primary motivation for many people is aesthetic (typically weight loss), if we do not address health first, we are less likely to succeed. If you have GI issues or a specific health concern *and* are interested in losing weight, the health issues take the front seat. This is not to say that you will not lose weight in this process—you almost certainly will—but the additional caveats that come with many of the health concerns will be doubly important for you.

ARE WE THERE YET?

All right, friends, neighbors, loved ones! The 30-Day Reset is only *pages* away! Grab a low-carb (preferably caffeinated) beverage and let's get rolling!

CHAPTER 11

Phase One

The 30-Day Reset

Before we launch into Phase One of the 30-Day Reset, I need to give you a virtual high-five and congratulate you for plowing through what is clearly a lot of material. If you've picked up a fraction of what is covered in the book, you now have a remarkably better picture of how food and your environment influence your health and wellness.

As you now know, we have a bit of a challenge as we begin our health and weight loss journey, in that our normal human tendencies (eat more, move less) are quite at odds with our modern world. This is a legitimately complex problem. Therefore, our simple solutions must address this reality and involve eating, sleeping, moving, and loving in a way that works with, instead of against, our genetic wiring.

Easy, right?! It may not seem so at first, but it is. It may be different than what you've done before, and it may require going outside your comfort zone or changing some habits, but trust me, this is doable. The nice thing about this change is that although there may be challenges, there are immediate rewards. You will look, feel, and perform better from the get-go.

Clearly this is a book and not a one-on-one consult, which means I need to strike a balance between offering general information and providing a sufficient framework to help you customize this plan for your individual needs. That said, our approach will likely be fairly familiar for most folks, at least in the beginning. We will focus on nutrient-dense whole foods to rewire your appetite, heal your metabolism, and get you looking and feeling your best.

EATING ON THE 30-DAY RESET

Phase One of the program primarily deals with discovering where you are on the insulin resistance spectrum, which will be important for weight loss as well as a number of other factors. The problems associated with insulin resistance and type 2 diabetes are enormous, but also remarkably easy to fix if we can get folks eating, sleeping, and moving better. As we learned in Part One of the book, our eating is governed by the neuroregulation of appetite. Our brain and our hormones are the real players in determining if we eat to a reasonable satiety level or we take on the job of Professional Eater. Along with the lifestyle considerations of sleep, stress, and exercise, there are three primary dietary components we can control that govern our neuroregulation of appetite:

1. Protein
2. Fiber
3. Appropriate carb content

Protein, particularly protein from lean animal sources, is remarkably satiating. Not to say you should avoid fat from animal products, but things like chicken breast and pork loin are difficult to *overeat*, as they send a very strong "done" signal to the brain.

Fiber is satiating for several reasons beyond simply the "bulk" of the food, but likely relating to the feeding of our gut microbiota and the intrinsic nutrients found in these plant products. Finding the "right" carb intake allows us to dial in our specific carb tolerance and therefore keep our hormonal profile in a state that is favorable for fat loss while repairing our metabolism. There are anthropological examples of pre-Westernized folks who ate both the high and low end of the carbohydrate spectrum. This is interesting and should tell us there may be very different approaches we can take depending on our unique situation. By paying close attention to our subjective measures of satiety, energy, and mental clarity, we can dial in the amount and types of carbs that work best for us.

Appropriate carb content is a bit variable, but I find the 75 to 150g range to be a good place to start for most folks. What does that look like? If we are talking about white rice, it's about three cups, which may sound like a lot, but it's not. Most people can easily down that much rice in a sitting. If we are talking about fruits and vegetables, getting 75 to 150g of carbs requires eating a remarkable amount of food. This is why sticking with Paleo carbs in the beginning of your reset is so important. These foods are nutritious and filling, which makes them hard to overdo.

Given all of the above, for the next thirty days, you will eat three meals per day (crazy, right?) built around the following:

- 4 to 6 ounces of protein at every meal (larger folks may do a bit more; smaller folks will likely stay on the lower side of that general recommendation)
- 75 to 150g of carbohydrates per day, from as wide a variety of fruits, vegetables, and roots as you can manage
- Added fat for flavor. Don't be afraid of fat, but don't drink it through a straw.

If your primary goal is fat loss, or if you are prediabetic, Phase One will help you lose weight quickly and easily. This is due to the fact that this plan is highly satiating and reduces insulin load, yet provides relatively few calories relative to the volume of food consumed. Although the calories in, calories out idea has many flaws, there is a reality that if we reduce caloric intake (assuming our hormonal profile is favorable), we can lose weight, specifically body fat, relatively easily. So, the "fat for flavor" recommendation is to provide variety and nuance to your meals while not overdoing the calorie intake.

Before we get to the meal plans and basic meal construction, we need to cover a few more things to set you up for success.

GETTING STARTED

I've mentioned a few times that facts only motivate a few folks to change. To really see a new behavior stick, we usually need some kind of motivator that touches us at an emotional level. Similarly, a major roadblock to effecting change is the lack of a plan, which leaves us only one option: defaulting to what we know. The old cliché "Failure to plan is planning to fail" may seem trite, but it's true. The following tips and tricks are as important as blood work or a spiritual aha moment.

Clean Out the Pantry

If you don't want to get into street fights, don't go to biker bars. If you don't want to be tempted by junk food, don't have it in the house. Clean out all the bread, cookies, pasta, juice, snacks, ice cream, and your secret stash of treats, whatever those may be. Bag this stuff up and give it to a food bank or homeless shelter. I'm not clear as to the ethics of feeding other folks this stuff, but it seems a waste to throw it away, and we can discuss the moral nuances in the afterlife. I cannot sufficiently emphasize how important it is to *not* have dodgy food options in the house. We are not wired for self-control, so if you want to make things as easy as possible for yourself, don't have trigger foods on hand. Of equal import is what *should* be in your pantry, refrigerator, and freezer. We should have as many spices and spicelike options you can think of. I'll explain why this is important in just a moment when we look at the Food Matrix.

You need to keep lots of varieties of protein in the freezer. In my house we have a medium-size chest freezer so we can buy beef, lamb, fish, and other items in bulk and freeze them for future use. This saves money and allows us to always have good options on hand. The refrigerator should be stocked with perishable items like fruit, veggies, and smart condiments. Again, it's hard to give you specifics here as I do not know what your particular tastes are, but you should shop in bulk and cook in bulk (as is described in the meal plans) so you save money and always have food readily available. Getting caught with no food is an easy way to derail your process, but if you keep your provisions topped off, this will be easy to navigate. If you live in a larger urban area, you can order a lot of groceries to your door with programs like Amazon Fresh. Regardless of where you live (so long as it's in the US) and for nonperishable items, I recommend you check out Thrive Market (thrivemarket.com), as you can order most of what you'd get from a higher-end grocery store but at 30 to 40 percent off retail.

You should always have a mix of nuts such as almonds, cashews, walnuts, and pistachios on hand. Your palate will shape what you stock in this regard. Not everyone likes canned fish, but this is a staple in our house. We always have tuna, salmon, and sardines in the pantry, and I recommend you do the same. Sardines are inexpensive and can be incredibly tasty if you find the right varieties. Look for options packed in water or olive oil instead of soybean oil.

Take this seriously, as your moments of indecision, fatigue, or frustration will make defaulting to old habits easy. What will the kids eat? Same stuff as you. They need the crap formerly living in your pantry even less than you do.

Go Shopping

Take the book with you and reference the shopping list in the appendix or print out the shopping guide at robbwolf.com/shoppinglist. And get shopping. Now that you have no food in the house, you have a choice: either do an extended fast, or provision your digs with chow that is tasty *and* healthy. What to buy? Follow the recipes and foods that fit with the plan, and remember, we do not want to stock the house with items that are going to derail your process. Don't "Euroshop" (buy tiny amounts of food that you run out of in a day), as this will again leave you with inadequate options and increase your likelihood of throwing in the towel before you even get started. Stock up for at least a week—pack the freezer with meat, seafood, and even frozen veggies.

THE FOOD MATRIX

Here is a chart I call the Food Matrix to give you a sense of what most meals will look like. You can download the full Food Matrix chart at robbwolf.com/foodmatrix.

This is by no means meant to be an exhaustive list, but it will give you a pretty good idea of how your meals should go together. Protein, veggies, fats, spices . . . BAM! The recipes in this book largely follow this format. Just as a side note: If you made a meal with one item from each column, you would have 81,000 meal options from this short matrix. Some people complain that changing their eating is boring. I'm not sure how 81,000

PROTEINS (27)	VEGETABLES (24)	FATS (5)	HERBS & SPICES (25)
Chicken breast	Asparagus	Coconut oil	Allspice
Chicken thigh	Avocado	Olive oil	Basil
Flounder	Artichoke hearts	Macadamia oil	Cardamom
Snapper	Brussels sprouts	Avocado oil	Cinnamon
Trout	Beets*	Lard	Celery seed
Halibut	Carrots		Dill
Mackerel	Celery		Fenugreek
Bass	Daikon		Garlic
Salmon steak	Zucchini		Ginger
Salmon fillet	Fennel root		Curry-red
Shrimp	Kale		Curry-green
New York steak	Chard		Curry-yellow
Rib eye steak	Dandelion greens		Oregano
Round steak	Spinach		Cilantro
Ground beef	Acorn squash*		Nutmeg
Beef ribs	Butternut squash*		Rosemary
Rump roast	Yam*		Thyme
Beef stew meat	Sweet potato*		Garam masala
Pork loin	Red pepper		Bay leaf
Pork chop	Yellow pepper		Salt
Pork ribs	Green pepper		Herbes de Provence
Baby back ribs	Red cabbage		Chili powder
Bacon	Green cabbage		Paprika
Pork roast	Napa cabbage		Cumin
Lamb chops			Black pepper
Lamb rack			
Venison steaks			

*Dense carbohydrate—eat in moderation until leanness goals are reached.

meal options are boring. It may not be ice cream and pizza, but it's not boredom. Let's build a few sample meals so you can get a sense of how easy this is and how much variety is waiting for you.

For our first example meal, we'll simply take the first item from each of the columns: chicken breast + asparagus + coconut oil + allspice

Here's how you put it together:

Heat some coconut oil in a skillet, add the chicken breast (cut into cubes or chunks), then add the asparagus and allspice and cook until the chicken is cooked through, about 5 minutes.

From start to finish this is perhaps a 10-minute process at most. If you cook a double portion (which I highly recommend) and pack some for later, you will save yourself the time of preparing another meal. Want a totally different meal experience? All you need to do is tweak the seasoning from allspice to the next item down the list, basil. Or ginger, or garlic, etc. The Food Matrix is helpful both in getting you going and also in helping you over the long term. The most spartan of kitchens likely has a couple hundred food combinations when we look at the cooking process through the lens of the Food Matrix.

The real magic, though, is not in the proteins or the veggies; it comes with things like herbs and spices. I use some fairly off-the-beaten-path items like ancho chiles, green and red curry paste (available at your local Asian grocery or in the Asian food section of most supermarkets), and fish sauce. All this is in addition to the old standbys: salt, pepper, garlic, ginger, mustard, etc. I also lean heavily on things like salsa and taco sauces, as they impart amazing flavor and pack a powerful antioxidant punch. Let me give you an example of how having these items on hand can enhance a meal: Scrambled eggs and cantaloupe is not a bad breakfast by any means, but what if you add a zingy salsa to the eggs and sprinkle some herbes de Provence (savory, marjoram, rosemary, thyme, and oregano) on the cantaloupe? There is no comparing the two meals, and with just a little twist you have completely changed your taste experience, transforming a somewhat ho-hum meal into "hell yeah!"

I released the Food Matrix idea many years ago, and it has helped a lot of people navigate their eating from the kitchen to the restaurant, as the basic format is how we construct most of our meals. Once you "get" that we always have a protein, lots of veggies, and some good fat, the rest is easy. Although there is an outstanding assortment of recipes and meal plans in this book, I have both an option and a suggestion for you. It would be a fantastic idea for you to spend several weeks, if not the entire 30-Day Reset period, building your own meals using the Food Matrix. My reason for suggesting this is twofold: it will get you in the kitchen (not a bad skill to have) and you will understand on a deeper level how easy it is to make (or order) simple, tasty meals. Let's build this up from scratch and see how it works.

PROTEIN	VEGGIE	FAT	SPICE
Egg	Carrot	Olive oil	Salt
Italian sausage	Broccoli	Butter	Pepper
Chicken breast	Spinach	Bacon fat	Garlic powder
Steak	Asparagus	Coconut oil	Basil
Ground beef	Cauliflower	Red palm oil	Chili powder

I have listed five different proteins, veggies, fats, and spices, which give us 625 *different* meals. This is a remarkable amount of variety, and I think you have to admit that a kitchen/pantry with only those ingredients would look pretty skinny.

To put this into play, let's build a few more meals, starting with breakfast. As you will learn in the meal plans, it's wise to lose the arbitrary idea that there are certain foods that "must" be eaten for any given meal. People usually get excited about breakfast because it often looks like dessert wrapped in the guise of healthy eating. Breakfast cereal, croissants, and the like are certainly tasty, but when consumed regularly are doing nothing good for you. All that said, I get that people are creatures of habit and we need to take all this in baby steps. With that in mind we will focus on egg and sausage options for breakfast. Looking at our chart, let's go straight across the top:

egg + carrot + olive oil + salt

Let's get started: Shred a carrot or two on the large holes of a box grater (might as well get a pre-breakfast workout, right?). Heat a generous amount of olive oil (say 1 to 2 tablespoons) in a skillet. Add the grated carrots and cook, covered, for about 5 minutes.

In a bowl, whisk together a few eggs and add them to the skillet. You could mix all this as it cooks and end up with a scramble *or* you can cook it covered and end up with an open-face omelet (or frittata). As to the salt, you can add it at the end or at any point in the cooking process.

Simply doing a scramble versus an omelet or frittata changes the whole meal . . . the experience is entirely different. Now let me add another simple tweak: Instead of scrambling the eggs, just crack them on top of the carrots and cook, covered, until the eggs are over-medium or over-hard, you call it. We now have three simple meals that are remarkably different, and we have not even changed a single ingredient, just how we handle them. Not a fan of eggs? No problem—use Italian sausage and add it at the same point you would the eggs.

I'll digress a moment and shine a spotlight on how easy this process is. This is also how you can order meals when you are eating out. Not sure what is compliant on a given menu? Ask to have some veggies cooked in a pan with eggs on top, either scrambled together or cooked over-medium. Or ask for sausage instead of eggs. Or bacon. Or chicken. Or steak. Have some fruit on the side with a cup of coffee. Or two. That's it. People will occasionally complain this way of eating is "boring." It's not boring. I find that folks who complain of boredom are really just cookie addicts, or pining for bread and cereal. I get it, but let's be honest and call all this what it is. Boredom is defined as "the state of being weary and restless due to lack of interest." If meals like this do not appeal to you, it's because we need to do some basic rewiring of your palate. People do not get "bored" with cocaine; they do, however, need more and more of it to reach the same psychological highs they have achieved in the past. Same deal with refined carbs. We will talk later about how and when you can kick your heels up and have some items that do not follow this basic template, but you need to understand not every one of your meals is going to be like a Julia Child cover band. *Not* if you want to get a handle on your health and waistline. You can and will rewire your palate to appreciate simple meals like this—heck, I dare say you'll even come to love them!

What about lunch and dinner? Follow the same process. If you need hard guidelines to follow, make sure you have all the ingredients listed in the chart above (five each proteins, veggies, fats, and spices) available at all times. Use only those ingredients for a few weeks to a month, then start adding other items, particularly spices (or jump into the meal plans on page 178), preparing them in the same basic way. If you find the options from the chart not to your liking, make sure you have at least five items you *do* like from the protein, veggie, fat, and spice categories. The Food Matrix has many more ingredients than I have listed here, so please do use that as a starting point. Something to consider: I'm keeping all this perhaps overly simplistic. You can clearly go wild and use both salt *and* pepper in a meal! Or pepper *and* basil, or broccoli *and* asparagus. I'm not saying that every meal you ever eat must follow this exact format, but I am making the point that there is a staggering amount of variety awaiting you even if you just stick to a stripped-down meal prep strategy like this one. I can think of a number of ways to make this process more complex and cumbersome. I *cannot* think of any way to make it easier and more effective. The Food Matrix is interesting in that it is both training wheels and "teaching a person how to fish instead of giving them a fish." If cooking is a challenge, I'd stick to this degree of simplicity for several weeks to a month. Like I said, you could easily run your entire 30-Day Reset using the Food Matrix alone. However, if you're handy in the kitchen and not intimidated by slightly more complex meals, the meal plans that follow are a great place to start.

MEAL PLANS

A quick note on meal plan structure: Most people will follow the basic Phase One meal plans as outlined here. This approach is incredibly powerful for losing weight, reversing insulin resistance, and getting healthy. If you have an autoimmune disease or suffer from chronic inflammation or serious GI problems, you might consider jumping into the Autoimmune Paleo (AIP) plan, which I've also included here. It is a bit more restrictive than the basic plan, but is also exactly what some folks need to address more complex issues. Alternatively, you could follow the basic plan, then reassess, and if the results are not optimum, step up to the AIP protocol. People have followed both paths and had good success. Two additional meal plans can be found in the Ketosis chapter. This includes the Transitional Ketosis plan, which allows for a modest amount of low-glycemic load carbs to be consumed alongside generous helpings of MCT oil, which helps folks achieve a therapeutic level of ketosis. There is also the nutritional ketosis plan that can be used for serious health concerns including certain types of cancer, neurodegenerative disease, or weight loss that has not responded to the Phase One approach, due largely to an inability to fully resolve issues related to the neuroregulation of appetite. If you have eaten a Standard American Diet for years, you may find jumping straight into ketosis to be as pleasant as rolling naked on broken bottles. It *might* be a good idea to follow the basic Paleo approach for 2 to 4 weeks, then use the transitional ketosis and nutritional ketosis plans as appropriate. Since relatively few people will need those tools, I have put all that material in a later chapter and explain the pluses and minuses of the various options in much greater detail.

There are *lots* of folks out there begging for meal plans. Having things explicitly spelled out—"eat this today, eat that tomorrow"—can be helpful to get some people going, but it is also a very rigid process. For each person that approach helps, however, there are ten people asking what they can substitute for the recommended meal. I'm going to provide you with some loosely based concepts and some killer recipes to help you with what to put in your pie hole. To that end, I've taken a middle-of-the-road approach here and instead of telling you that *you must eat salmon for dinner on Monday*! I'm giving you a template to help you plan your week, subject to change based on your life and your schedule. There are some nifty websites and apps out there that can help you stay sane with your shopping lists and favorite recipes. I particularly like the free app called Wunderlist. You can share your lists with significant others and make coordinating your shopping a breeze. People who have food to come home to—either something already made or something they can easily put together—will see the most success and will be a little more apt to avoid dodgy food choices.

A few things to keep in mind:

1. If you don't like a recipe, don't make it. Don't try to force yourself to eat salmon if you know you don't like it. Along that same vein, if you have a thousand appropriate recipes pinned on Pinterest, use those! What I've provided here is a loose template to help those who need some hand-holding along the way.

2. A word on breakfasts: At our house, we don't pigeonhole certain foods into only being for certain meals. That might mean Thai coconut soup for breakfast or scrambled eggs for dinner. If you simply must have eggs and "breakfasty" foods for breakfast each day, then go for it. But a leftover burger with some slaw for breakfast is pretty darn tasty and satisfying. Think outside the *huevos*.

3. Sit down at some point during your week (many people do this on Saturdays or Sundays) and plan your meals for the week. Once you

have a plan, do your shopping so you aren't running to the store eighty-seven times during the week or, worse, resorting to SAD foods.

4. "The best is the enemy of the good." I think Voltaire said that. If you're struggling with finding time to cook, get a rotisserie chicken. If your budget constrains your grocery shopping, do the best you can. It's great to have pie-in-the-sky aspirations, but not if it means completely derailing you. Do what you can, where you are, with what you've got.

5. Portion sizes. Here's where things can get a bit dodgy. If you're John Welbourn (a 300-pound NFL lineman), you should be eating a heck of a lot more at a meal than one of the Olsen twins. For all intents and purposes, and for your sanity and mine, too, let's figure on an average of 4 to 6 ounces of protein per meal (about the size of your palm). It's super easy to increase your portion sizes at a meal: just eat more. However, when it comes to planning, if you and someone else in the house are eating like Mr. Welbourn, you're likely going to need to double or triple recipes as needed. These weekly plans assume two grown people in the house. Got kiddos running around? Maybe double some of the recipes.

Regarding the recipes, all the nutritional estimates are just that—estimates—based on the website Calorie Count. Recipes were not sent to an independent lab for analysis. This info serves as a rough guideline for you to estimate your macros if you are following things that closely and whether you need to dial up or dial down certain things in your meals. In my opinion, it's super easy to up your calorie/fat intake by adding some avocado or an extra dollop of coconut oil, butter, or ghee. If a particular recipe has you not quite hitting your macros, adjust as you need. Carb counts reflect net carbs (total carbs minus dietary fiber). A benefit of eating this way is that it's generally difficult to overdo either calories or carbs. Dense carb sources like bread and rice are pretty easy to overdo, whereas Paleo carb sources (as we use in this plan) are naturally satiating.

NOTES ON INGREDIENTS: GRASS-FED SOURCES, PASTURED, ORGANIC?

Ideally I'd like to see everyone eating grass-fed meat, organic produce, and sustainably caught fish. If you have the bandwidth to take that extra step, great. If not, don't let this be a deal breaker for you. Conventional meat and produce are still better for you than soda, bagels, and sugar.

Okay, now on to the weekly templates. Let's operate with the understanding that there are twenty-one meals in a given week (breakfast, lunch, and dinner). Now, I'd say that the average person probably eats about five or more of those meals away from home (see pages 192–193 for some dining-out options). These plans figure on sixteen to eighteen meals consumed at home each week. If you eat fewer meals at home, then now you have more leftovers to tide you over in your next week, or you can freeze some portions for emergency use—think homemade Lean Cuisine.

These plans help guide you for two weeks, and we just repeat this template to round out the thirty days. I've included handy shopping lists for each week in the Appendix, so be sure to copy those when you're planning for the week. If you're the kind of person who can eat the same thing every single day, then do what works for you. On average, you have five different "main courses" each week and some sides to tinker with. That means if you cook up two or three of the meals over the weekend, you're only back in the kitchen two other times the whole week (not counting reheating leftovers). If you watch one hour of television every day, maybe swap that out for some cooking time, or better yet, cook while you watch TV!

PHASE ONE—WEEK 1

Here you go. Your first week at eating in Phase One. If you're coming from a typical standard American diet, you may need to up your carbs more than what's listed here to keep you from feeling wonky. Add a baked sweet potato, some roasted winter squash, or a banana or other fruit to help you make this transition. Please keep in mind that the recipes listed here are *suggestions*. You can use this same basic format and pick other recipes. I'm trying to strike a balance between giving you enough structure to succeed and not overwhelming you with rigid details. All that said, these recipes were developed by Julie and Charles Mayfield, authors of the bestselling *Paleo Comfort Foods* and other cookbooks. They are fantastic, and I think you will love them.

On the Menu

- Chicken Tikka Masala (page 259) served with Cauliflower Rice (page 254)—yields 6 servings
- Flank Steak (page 271) served with Twice-Baked Sweet Potatoes (page 318) (or plain baked sweet potatoes), Roasted Broccoli and Cauliflower (page 294)—yields 8 servings
- Cioppino (page 263)—yields 8 servings
- Sausage and Egg "Sandwiches" (page 299)—yields 4 servings
- Rotisserie-Like Chicken (page 295) with Asian Slaw (page 243)—yields 4 servings
- Scrambled eggs with veggies, if you just can't stomach "non-breakfast foods" in the morning.
- Staples: Chicken Stock (page 258), made with the chicken carcass from the rotisserie chicken

Plan of Attack

It's up to you how you want to attack this week. Could be that you do most of your planning and shopping on Saturday, then Sunday you choose to make:

- Rotisserie chicken (slow cooker) with Asian slaw
- Flank steak with sides (grill and oven)
- Cioppino (stovetop)

While you're prepping veggies and items for what you'll be cooking that day, might as well chop up what you'll need for the Chicken Tikka Masala. Then, later in the week on a night you know you have more time, cook up the Tikka Masala, and cook the Sausage and Egg "Sandwiches" on a morning that works for you. After the rotisserie chicken is cooked, remove the meat from the chicken carcass, place it in a container, and refrigerate it, then use the carcass to make the chicken stock overnight. In one day, you have cooked enough food to get you and one other grown person through ten meals this week, and you're on your way to making stock. Feel like you're going to need to eat more this week? Increase how much you make of the recipes.

PHASE ONE—WEEK 2

On the Menu
- Chicken Alfredo (page 255)—yields 8 servings
- Guac-Stuffed Burgers (page 279) with Mashed Cauliflower (page 284) and Bacon-Wrapped Asparagus (page 245)—yields 8 servings
- Thai Coconut Soup (page 317)—yields 8 servings
- Tomato Meat Sauce (page 337) served with zucchini noodles—yields 8 servings
- Satay Skillet (page 297)—yields 8 servings

Plan of Attack

On Sunday, brown the ground beef for the tomato meat sauce and make the sauce, put the Thai coconut soup in the slow cooker, and make the guacamole and the guac-stuffed burgers, mashed cauliflower, and asparagus. Later in the week, make the chicken alfredo one night and the satay skillet another. You've just been cooking in the kitchen three times in one week, but you've created enough food for about twenty meals for you and someone else. And again, if you won't eat a burger for breakfast, fry or scramble up some eggs and bacon, maybe with a nice sweet potato hash.

AUTOIMMUNE PLAN—WEEK 1

Now's the time to eliminate nightshades, eggs, and a whole host of things that could be causing an inflammatory response in folks with autoimmune disease or serious GI problems. While that task might seem daunting, these recipes will show you that despite those omissions there is still a lot of flavor in the world.

On the Menu

- Weeknight Chicken Breasts or Thighs (page 320) with Mashed Cauliflower (page 284) and Sautéed Greens (page 301)—yields 8 servings; you can use some of the cooked chicken to make a salad with the Caesar-Like Dressing (page 328)
- Shepherd's Pie (page 306)—yields 8 servings
- Kitchen Sink Sauté (page 281)—yields 8 servings
- Fish Packets with Lime-Coconut Sauce (page 269)—yields 4 servings
- Greek Kabobs with Tzatziki Sauce (page 276) with Mashed Cauliflower (page 284)—yields 8 servings

Plan of Attack

Fire up the grill and cook up those chicken breasts and kabobs, along with the fish packets and mashed cauliflower. Brown the ground beef you'll use later for the kitchen sink sauté. Later in the week, use some of the chicken along with the Caesar-like dressing to make a basic Caesar salad (just get some romaine leaves and toss everything together). Make the shepherd's pie and kitchen sink sauté on days that fit your schedule.

AUTOIMMUNE PLAN—WEEK 2

On the Menu

- Beef Tacos using AIP seasoning (page 249) with Guacamole (page 334)—yields 6 servings
- Chicken Soup (page 256)—yields 8 servings
- Pork Chops with Peach Chutney and Roasted Okra (page 288)—yields 6 servings
- Shrimp Stir-Fry (page 309)—yields 4 servings
- Prime Rib (page 292) with Sautéed Mushrooms (page 302) and Roasted Broccoli and Cauliflower (page 294)—yields 8 servings or more

Plan of Attack

Prime rib screams "Sunday night" to me. While that's cooking, brown the ground beef to use later in the week for some tacos, and get that chicken soup cooking (slow cookers are always great if you don't want to use the stove). Go ahead and prep the vegetables that you'll need for the stir-fry and pork chops—this will make cooking those on a given weeknight super fast.

HOW MUCH SHOULD I EAT?

In my early years of coaching folks, I had a client who took my recommendation to eat "Paleo foods to satiety, regardless of amount" to a remarkable

Keeping Track

You may find it odd that a biochemist (that would be me!) is not generally a fan of weighing and measuring food. I mean, that's what chemists do—weigh and measure stuff, right? From a psychological perspective I've found the process of weighing and measuring food to be, well ... a bit neurotic. I've relied on general guidelines with most of the folks I work with and we have achieved incredible results ranging from profound fat loss to elite-level athletic performance. I really like this "seat-o'-the-pants" approach, but there are compelling reasons to get both specific and quantifiable about not just our food but many areas of our lives.

If we want to effect change, sometimes we need to be a bit meticulous and set up our process such that we know what our inputs and outputs are. Without an understanding of inputs and outputs—that is to say, what we are doing and what type of results we produce—our results are at best a guess. If things are going well, no problem. But if we are getting subpar results, not having a plan means we can't know how to fix things. One of my mentors, Coach Greg Glassman (the founder of CrossFit), drove this point home in an interesting way. At nearly every Cross-Fit seminar, someone would ask Coach Glassman, "How do I get more pull-ups?" To which Greg would reply, "How many do you have currently?" Without fail, the person would say something like, "Well, it's between eight and ten pull-ups." Greg would reply, "The reason you are not making progress on your pull-ups is because you do not care about them. If you really cared you would know exactly how many you can do. You would tell me you can get eight solid pull-ups, with the attempt on the ninth being able to get your eyebrows over the bar."

When we care about something that we want to improve or change in a significant way, we need to track what we do. Otherwise, success is at best random, and even if things are going in a favorable way, we don't know why.

extreme. The guy started with us at more than 400 pounds, and although he was making some progress on the program, it was not at the pace I'd expected. When I looked at his food log, I noticed that he had a mid-afternoon snack of "nuts." I asked him how many nuts he was eating and he said, "Oh, you know, one of those Costco containers of cashews . . ." Yeah, that tub of nuts contained almost 3,500 calories! The same number of calories many hard-training athletes consume in a given day. This was on top of his breakfast, lunch, and dinner. I acknowledged that I'd perhaps provided too much latitude on this plan and instructed him to weigh out a few ounces of nuts and stick with that. Almost immediately he began losing weight at a good clip, and we got him back to his athletic high school weight of 220 pounds. In general, folks can eat to satiety with these types of foods, but clearly, a heroic effort to consume massive amounts of food may derail weight loss efforts.

HOW ABOUT SNACKS?

For each meal, you'll follow the guidelines I mentioned earlier, but when it comes to snacks you'll want to literally check your gut. Ideally, you should be able to go multiple hours between meals—this is a sign of a healthy metabolism and indicates that we got the amounts of protein, carbs, and fats "right." We should not need food the way someone with emphysema needs an oxygen tank. So, if you *really* need a snack, by all means go for it, but first ask yourself the following: Why do you need the snack? Is this just fidgety eating due to boredom, or are you really hungry? If you are truly hungry, what type of hunger are we talking? Are you hungry but functional (good cognition, clear headed), or are you *hangry* (nervous, shaky, foggy headed, ready to kill someone and eat them).

Hangry means we might not have our air/fuel mixture quite right yet. So before you reach for the snack, consider this:

1. Did you eat enough in total at your last meal? If you are a bit hungry but functional, you likely got the carb amount right but did not eat enough.
2. Did you eat too many carbs? If you are hangry, this is most likely the problem.

Although insulin is far from the sole controller of appetite, it plays a big part, particularly if an individual is insulin resistant. I don't want to belabor the hunger point too much, but I have some perspective on this that I think is helpful, even though it may seem a bit counterintuitive. On one hand, folks need to learn to be comfortable with a little hunger. It won't kill us and if we can get a handle on that process we become more resilient and life is just easier. Our genetics and metabolism are designed to withstand frequent, small bouts of fasting ranging from a few hours to several days. This is not a comfortable situation, but it should not be crippling. Under these conditions our bodies should easily transition into and out of ketosis, which, as you learned in the previous chapter, offers such amazing benefits when food or carbohydrate are scarce.

If we are insulin resistant, however, we do not seamlessly transition into ketosis, and the blood sugar crashes we experience are of a magnitude and type that are almost druglike. They are superphysiologic. Our brains do not like blood sugar swings, and the low blood sugar one experiences while insulin resistant produces a profound drive to "fix" the problem. This is "hanger." I experienced this process for the better part of twenty years and, to be blunt, it sucked. I was planning my next meal before my current meal was eaten, because I was so anxious about what would happen if I found myself going more than a few hours without eating. I now have fantastic resilience in this regard, and if I get really busy, I may not get in breakfast and only do late lunch at two P.M. and then a dinner at five or six. I don't do this every day, as it is a bit stressful, but when I need to do that or if I'm traveling and my food options are terrible, going without a meal for many hours is no big deal. I get hungry, but this is not the panicky, dysfunctional state you find when you're hangry. So, if you are hangry between meals, dial down your carbs and dial up your fats, or possibly even do a system reset using a period of ketosis.

ROBB, ABOUT THOSE SNACKS!

So you understand that we should generally not *need* snacks, but what if the spirit grabs you and you just want a little something around midday? Jerky (make sure it's gluten-free—watch out for varieties that contain soy sauce!), nuts, and fruit are fantastic options. It's hard to overdo jerky due to jaw fatigue, but as we learned on page 183, folks can easily overdo nuts, so weigh out 1 to 2 ounces and call it done. With fruit, use your good judgment. I'm hard pressed to eat two apples, but I can sit down and eat just about a whole watermelon. That does become somewhat self-limiting, as afterward I'll use every square of toilet paper in the house, but for weight loss, eating huge amounts of fruit is not going to help your cause. Dried fruit of all kinds needs to be treated like nuts: weigh out an ounce or two and call it good. As I said, I can barely eat two apples, but I could easily eat ten apples' worth of dried apple chips. In a perhaps surprising suggestion, given my caveman predilections, I think dark chocolate is a great occasional option. Here is the caveat: That dark chocolate needs to be dark—at least 80 percent cacao—and you should limit it to a few squares per day. Yes, you can have some dark chocolate daily, as long as it is not a gateway drug to bagels and ice cream every day.

BEVERAGES, BOOZE, AND BEYOND

So, what should you drink to support your new way of life? In general, we are talking about unsweetened beverages like coffee, tea, and this amazing stuff called water. How much of that should you drink? With water, my wacky suggestion is to drink when you're thirsty, and stop when you're not. The health industry is fraught with quasi-mystical information surrounding water. Our thirst is generally a good indication of when we need to drink—let's rely on that. With regard to caffeinated beverages such as coffee and tea, the scientific literature is pretty clear that these beverages offer a host of health benefits, likely due to their antioxidant content. The only real caveats I have here are to try to develop a taste for these beverages without sweetening them (I'll tackle sweetened beverages in a moment), and be mindful that caffeine can and does negatively affect sleep in some folks. Recent genetic research indicates some people clear caffeine from their system almost as fast as they can drink it. Other people may take thirty-six hours to fully remove the caffeine from one cup of coffee. You likely intuitively know where you are in this story but just be mindful that too much of a good thing is still too much.

How badly a given person freaks out about the recommendation to ditch sweetened beverages gives me immediate insight into how much of a battle this change will be overall. Sweetened beverages seem to be on par with cocaine and heroin with how "frisky" folks are in their consumption. You now know how powerfully processed foods can hijack our neuroregulation of appetite, and drinking calories is a fantastic way to catch an Uber to downtown Chubbyville. Consider this: What is a common practice among bodybuilders, strength athletes, and folks who want to be *big*? Shakes. Liquid calories. Using liquid calories, these folks can consume far more than if they stuck with chewable food. If you want to be *big*, take in lots of calories in liquid form. Otherwise, stick to water, plain tea, and black coffee.

ARTIFICIAL SWEETENERS AND SUGAR

Sigh . . . I've had the sugar-and-artificial-sweetener conversation many, many times. I've mellowed a bit in my old age, but part of that is just getting tired of arguing with folks. In my experience, sweetened beverages, be they artificial, natural, or supernatural, are "gateway drugs." They contribute to poor compliance. So my recommendation is to avoid these items until you are at a point where you are happy with how you look, feel, and perform. Even then you need to moderate your intake lest you spin out and make other poor food and lifestyle choices. You likely know if sweetened beverages are a trigger item for you, so use your best judgment.

ROBB, WHAT ABOUT BOOZE?!

Alcohol is not particularly healthy, but let's face it: it's a lot of fun. The big problems I see with booze (aside from liver failure) are calories and sleep disturbance. Stick with hard alcohol with a bit of lemon or lime juice, floated in some soda water. My NorCal Margarita (2 shots of tequila, juice of 1 lime, soda water) has become pretty popular in the past five years; if you have not tried it, give it a shot. Beer is problematic due to the calories it contains and its gluten content. This makes me incredibly sad, as I truly love beer, but if you are gluten-reactive, I suggest steering clear. Dry wines are not a bad option, and I love the folks at Dry Farm Wines (robbwolf.com/dryfarmwines).

As we learned in chapter six, alcohol is not a sleep aid. It makes you unconscious, but it does not promote restful sleep. The best I can offer in this regard is to consume your booze as far away from your sleep as possible. Some see this as a recommendation to have booze with breakfast. I can't really get behind that, but it's a better idea for your health than a nightcap right before bed.

ASSESSING PROGRESS

How do you know if this nutty (and meaty) schtick is working? In addition to the objective and subjective measures we discussed in the previous chapter, I'd like you to do the following:

1. Take before pictures and update those every two weeks. Take these in the same clothes (or none—just keep those off the Internet!) in the same light and in the same relative positions. If you need to do a selfie to pull this off, I won't begrudge you that. Take a picture showing your front, side, and southbound profile. The transformations folks have achieved on this program are nothing short of amazing. If you spend a little time documenting this process, it'll be a hell of a motivator when you face your moments of doubt.

2. Pick a performance goal. I'll talk about the specifics of movement and exercise later, but I want you to think about a goal that is easy to measure and that you actually find more fun than threading barbed wire through your nose. I *hate* running, unless you are talking about doing sprints. I'm kinda fast twitch, so a goal for me might be to see how many 100-meter repeats I can do in 10 to 15 minutes. Your goal could be as simple as doing a short walk to your mailbox. Time that walk as you begin the program and just try to consistently improve on that time. Never been able to do a push-up or pull-up? Those are all worthy goals. When that goal gets too easy, pick a new goal. I'm okay with you picking more than one goal; just don't overwhelm yourself when you're getting started. What we are trying to do is give your brain that little cocainelike hit of dopamine we get from achieving a goal. I'm writing this book with a program called Scrivener, and I can set a little box in the corner with a daily word count goal. At the beginning of the day, the box is an angry

red. As I make progress, it shifts to orange, then yellow, and I get to wrap up my day with a dopamine-gasm of a little green box telling me I've met my goal. It may sound lame, but it works! Similarly, if you see consistent improvements in your performance goal, it'll help keep you in the fight.

WHAT IF MY RESULTS ARE NOT UP TO PAR?

After about thirty days, you should see some significant changes in your health and physical appearance. A small percentage of people will not get the "brochure experience." This means they are not losing fat or experiencing improved sleep, energy levels, and performance. Perhaps blood work is not improving. This is where we will need to do a little investigation to figure out where the problems may lie. Here are a few common problems I see again and again:

Are you *really* following the plan?

I'll ask folks this question and usually get an emphatic yes, but upon further digging I find that maybe one meal per day was from the plan, while the birthday cake at lunch and "special treat" from a family member have popped up consistently.

If you are in debt and want to get out of debt, you have only two options: make more money or spend less. Often a combination is smart, as it pushes things from both ends. Similarly, if you want to look and feel better while losing weight, you will need to alter your eating, especially in the beginning. When you get to a healthy place with your metabolism, eating, and lifestyle habits, you will have a little latitude in what you can get away with, but in the beginning we need to gain momentum, and eating food not on the plan will simply not facilitate that goal. I wish I could sugarcoat this, but I'd be lying to you, and hey, no one needs more sugar!

How much sleep are you getting?

I've thought about writing a book called *Sleep Your Way Skinny*, as this can be the most important part of the whole story. If you are not getting into bed reasonably early, waking up without an alarm (ideally), and getting at least eight hours of *sleep* (not just time in bed), weight loss is going to be hard, if not impossible. Be honest with yourself. Have you prioritized sleep? If not, this is a good place to look.

Are you actually insulin sensitive?

There is interesting literature that suggests that folks who are insulin resistant do better on lower-carb diets. Folks who are insulin sensitive (but still overweight) likely do better on lower-fat diets. This program is designed with the *assumption* that you are insulin resistant, as a remarkable swath of the population is insulin resistant, either from poor diet, sedentariness, gut issues, poor sleep, or an unholy combination of these. If you are insulin sensitive (which can be determined by your fasting insulin levels, A1C, and a generally favorable waist-to-hip ratio), you will need to tweak the dietary plans toward more whole, unprocessed carbs and add less fat to your meals.

What If You Need More Help?

The vast majority of people following the plans detailed in this book will see dramatic improvements in their blood work, energy, and waistline. But some may have specific issues that go beyond the ability of any book to address. If you find that you are not making the progress you want, or if you have lab values that are confusing or just not moving in a favorable direction, it's time to get additional help. Go to robbwolf.com/healthresources for a list of practitioners and further testing options.

GET A BUDDY, AND OTHER STRATEGIES FOR SUCCESS

Misery loves company! Seriously, though, accountability is important, and if you can find a friend or coworker to do this with you, that will keep both of you on track. If you falter, this is your person to lean on for support. Join a CrossFit gym, martial arts class, yoga studio, or walking group and bamboozle someone into doing this program with you. If you can rope a spouse or significant other into doing the program, that's great, but I find this to be a tough sell at times. Marriage and relationship counseling are unfortunately outside the scope of this book, but I'll just throw this out there: If this person who theoretically loves you is a pain in the ass about helping you live a better life, is this person friend or foe? Really. Think about it.

KNOW YOURSELF

Most dietitians tell us to simply "eat in moderation." Although it's unclear what exactly that means, it *is* clear that this advice fails more often than it succeeds. Bestselling author Gretchen Rubin provides some insight on this topic in her book *Better Than Before*, as she details that people tend to fall into one of two camps: abstainers and moderators. Abstainers need to steer clear of a certain food or behavior, like playing video games, or they tend to slide into unhealthy patterns. Moderators, by contrast, can take or leave a food or activity. This is a great book, and I can't recommend it enough. Gretchen also has a fantastic website to support the book, which can help you figure out if you are an abstainer or moderator by taking a simple quiz.

Gretchen makes the point that the population is about 50/50 with regard to the moderator/abstainer categories, but interestingly, about 90 percent of registered dietitians are moderators. In an act of incredible confirmation bias: these well-meaning RDs make a recommendation (eat in moderation) that is set up to fail at least 50 percent of the time. When considering food, particularly hyperpalatable food, this story likely changes even more in that ice cream, pastries, and other hyperpalatable foods bypass our neurological "off switch" while we are consuming the food, and we tend to fixate on those foods if they are at all available. Adding another wrinkle to this: I have noticed that folks can be either a moderator or an abstainer depending on the food at hand. My wife will eat any and all chocolate in the house in quick order. I'll have a piece every couple of weeks. By contrast, a bag of potato chips will meet a quick end at my hands (or teeth), whereas Nicki barely touches them. The point here is that the general recommendation of "clean out your pantry" is a good one, but it's particularly important to keep trigger foods out of the house. We can moralize, hand-wring, and argue about this topic until the chocolate-covered cows come home. Or we can understand how we are wired to eat and make plans that set us up for success.

EATING OUT

Eating out with friends and family is a nice time to kick your heels up, but it's easy for this to turn into a "hookers and cocaine" binge versus just having something a bit different than your usual fare. That said, here are some guidelines I'd like you to follow:

1. Stick with the program for at least thirty days. You can do anything for a month—hang in there, get amazing results, then make an informed decision about how tightly you want to run things in the future. You can easily build a meal compliant with the 30-Day Reset at just about any restaurant.

2. I generally recommend that you stay gluten-free both at home and when eating out. Every day there are more and more research articles indicating that this is a smart move for many people. Is it *really* a terrible prospect to have a chocolate torte or ice cream instead of a pastry? This is all I'm suggesting. Once you get through your thirty days, you can kick your heels up occasionally. But more often than not, go for gluten-free options.

3. If you eat out for most of your meals due to travel or not knowing how to boil water, clearly we need to modify this recommendation. If the former, let's limit your heel-kick-upping to once per week. If you don't know how to cook, the Food Matrix (pages 168–169) is an amazing resource for how to navigate that forgotten room of the house called "The Kitchen." I think a lack of cooking knowledge, as well as the lack of desire to prioritize cooking at home, is a huge problem, as it tends to leave us earlobe deep in easily accessible, low-quality food. As much as I might finger wag about needing to fix that, I am aware of the social trend toward preparing and eating less food at home. I have spent upward of thirty weeks per year on the road, for years at a time, and all this really boils down to is making better choices. Even when my options are not great, I can make better choices. You can, too.

WORK AND SCHOOL

Work and school can be places of rough peer pressure coupled with far too many bad options. The work environment really goes beyond peer pressure to outright sabotage on a scale that would make a CIA spook jealous. If you let folks know you are eating better, the person who would barely talk to you now hand-delivers cupcakes to your desk. How thoughtful! I don't know how to say this tactfully, so I'll say it bluntly: people are (occasionally) jerks when someone is trying to make a change, whether that change is climbing out of debt or getting healthy. Many people are helpful and supportive, but for some, the notion that one of their coworkers is trying to improve themselves is somehow interpreted as a judgment against the folks who are not participating. That is someone else's problem—do not let them make it your problem. The best advice I can offer here is the same advice that will save you most of the time: plan ahead. Have your meals prepped and know who is going to try to undermine your efforts. The buddy system is also a good way to get some folks on your team, as is just letting people know that you are trying to make a change and you'd appreciate help, not subterfuge to derail your process.

EMBRACE THE BROWN BAG

Have nuts, jerky, and apples handy (I like apples because they are reasonably tough relative to other fruit). At the clinic, I have a couple of bags of jerky and nuts in a drawer in my office. I keep a couple of apples on the desktop so I do not forget them and find a pile of mold a few months down the road. In general, I try to bring fresh meals, but if I get busy, I know I have these foods as a fallback. I highly recommend you do the same. Additionally, figure out the restaurants you like that either deliver or are easy to get to. Have menus for those places handy, and have their numbers on speed dial! Some restaurants have apps where you can order and choose pickup or delivery in seconds. Just make those meals based around our basic Paleo template (veggies, protein, healthy fat), and you are set. Any perceived challenge to getting yourself fed increases your likelihood of making suboptimal decisions. You need to do a little preparation to make sure when those inevitable surprises pop up, you are ready to deal with them.

MEALS DELIVERED

As much as I'd like to see folks cooking more of their meals, the trends are not painting that as a likely outcome. People are eating out and ordering in more than ever in history. Fortunately, there are phenomenal programs that now offer amazing meals delivered either fresh or frozen and at a price point that is not much different than what you would spend to cook at home. I do not recommend that you rely on these services exclusively, but rather use them to help fill the gaps in your planning or to reduce stress on particularly busy days. If you keep a few frozen meals handy at home and work (if possible), you will always have an easy fallback if you get too busy to prep a meal. If you know that, say, Tuesday and Thursday evenings are particularly challenging due to family obligations, have meals delivered for those days and get signed up on an auto-ship program so at the beginning of every week you have your "big day" meals ready to go. If you are hankering for a fantastic meal-delivery option, check out the Good Kitchen: robbwolf.com/mealsdelivered.

Shortcuts?

Feeling overwhelmed by all this? I recommend that folks jump into this process with both feet, as the results are honestly amazing. People lose weight, reverse inflammation, and generally feel fantastic. But I'll be the first to admit that this whole process can be a lot to tackle. If you are feeling overwhelmed, here is a "program minimum" that will provide huge benefits while making change as easy as possible.

Sleep: Follow every recommendation from the sleep and stress chapter to the letter. If folks did just this, they would be amazed by how much better they look and feel.

Food: Remove all liquid calories from your diet. Ditch the sugary coffee drinks, juices, and smoothies. Get a palm-size piece of protein at every meal and as many veggies as you can handle, and avoid white carbs. Potatoes, rice, and bread are the big no-no's.

Move: I don't care what you do, just get out and move as much as you can, as often as you can. Get sun on your skin.

If you follow these simple guidelines, you *will* make progress. Your palate will change and you will feel better. Perhaps this will be all you need to feel more confident about starting the 30-Day Reset.

After completing Phase One's 30-Day Reset, you will be ready to implement Phase Two of the program: the 7-Day Carb Test plan detailed in the next chapter. For folks following the basic Paleo plan, this is your likely next step so you can see what type of latitude you have with carbs that generally do not fit under the Paleo umbrella. If you still do not have great blood glucose control or lab numbers, you might consider sticking with the basic plan until those numbers look great.

CHAPTER 12

Phase Two

The 7-Day Carb Test Plan

The general guideline of "eat whole, unprocessed foods" will always be valuable. However, as we learned earlier, there are massive differences in how different people respond to various amounts and types of carbohydrates and food in general. Do you respond well to rice? Bananas? Beans? Without testing these foods, we must rely on subjective measures such as how we feel between meals to get a sense of how various foods affect us. In order to truly create a personal nutrition blueprint (and shun one-size-fits-all diets), we need to take our eating to the next step. This will allow us to potentially find much more latitude in what we can eat and still stay slim and healthy. In Phase Two, we will learn how to dial in to our optimum carb intake. We can accomplish this via the 7-Day Carb Test. Before we get to the details of that process, I want to hit a bit of an exculpatory clause (i.e., cover my ass).

When folks read this book, there will be those who say I'm an idiot for recommending low-carb diets at all. They will cling tenaciously to the calories in, calories out model and largely dismiss the influence of hormones and the neuroregulation of appetite in the process of health and weight gain. There will also be folks who say I'm a dullard for *not* recommending a low-carb diet to *everyone*. They will say the whole story here relates to insulin control *only*, and calories are inconsequential. Now, let me ask you something: How can I be an idiot about both of these polar-opposite situations? I'm going to make a possibly self-serving statement: both of these camps—the low-carb jihadis and the calories in, calories out canards—have opted for a one-size-fits-all approach in lieu of the messy process of individual truth. Despite the fact that we have more information at our disposal than ever in history, everything from the political process to environmental issues and what is the "optimum" way to eat has been reduced to two warring ideologies with little room for nuance and individual needs. Here is my incredibly controversial proposition: people are different and they may need to use different approaches to reach certain goals.

Pretty crazy, right? People are different, and nothing works for everyone. I know parts of this book read like a legal disclaimer, but when folks embark on a process of change, they are frequently assailed by friends, family, and Internet keyboard warriors who have strongly held opinions based on a pretty flimsy understanding of this material. My goal is to provide a path that allows you to find what works for you. There *is* a process that will work for you. Despite the fact that the process *does* work for you, there will be people who can make compelling cases for why it's the wrong move. All I can offer is to let the results drive the process and bugger the naysayers.

STEP ONE: BUY, STEAL, OR OTHERWISE OBTAIN

1. Blood glucose monitor. This is what we will use to test our blood glucose response to meals. There are a remarkable number of options ranging from as little as $10 to as much as $200. Traditionally, blood glucose

monitors involve using a lancet (a small needle) to extract a small drop of blood from your finger. This is not as bad as it sounds, but I get that this is a daunting prospect for some folks. As I am writing this book, a number of wearable blood glucose options are emerging—literally each week it's a different story as to the latest and best option. In Europe, there is a version that is worn like a temporary tattoo and communicates with one's smartphone. Instead of putting info here that will be out of date well before the book is even published, I'll direct you to robbwolf.com/monitors to stay up to date on the best options. If you are not needle-phobic I recommend something like the Accu-Chek models, which can test for both blood glucose and blood ketones. If you need a little help getting going with your glucometer, just search the Internet for "using glucometer." There are a number of short videos, usually produced by the glucometer manufacturers, on how to use your device.

2. Basic meal tracker. We need to track what we eat, when we eat it, and what our blood glucose response is. You could go old-school on this and just use pen and paper, but there are fantastic free apps for this process as well. Check out the app store for the best-rated food tracker for your mobile phone. I'm assuming that if you are taking this more detailed, tech-intensive path, you have a smartphone that will accomplish what we want to do here! If not, there are online trackers you can use to input your info from a desktop computer.

You will need to record the amount of a particular food you eat (50g of rice, for example). Remember, we are only concerned with the effective carbohydrates—the total carbohydrates minus the fiber—and on page 202 you will find a list of foods and the amount necessary to reach 50g of carbs.

STEP TWO: TEST YOUR CARBS

The path to personalized nutrition is simple: you will test a specific amount of carbohydrate every morning at breakfast for seven days. This means you *just* test that food—you don't have coffee with a bunch of creamer, or some kind of pre-breakfast snack. If you want to have plain coffee, tea, or even water before or with your test meal, that's fine, so long as you do the same thing with each meal you test. Don't do coffee one day and water another day. Based on how you respond to each of these foods, you will know if they are a good or bad option for you, in regard to both the amount and the type. You will:

1. Start by eating a food with 50g of effective carbohydrate. This is the *whole* meal. We do not eat other foods at this time, as we just want to track the effects of this singular food.

2. Track your blood glucose response two hours after your meal (just your carbohydrates test food) using your blood glucose monitor. This literally means eat your test food (meal), set a timer for two hours, then take a blood sugar test as per the instructions associated with your glucometer. Ideally, your blood glucose will be between 90 and 115mg/dl at that point. If it is higher than this range, I'd like you to retest that food on a different day at breakfast again, eating 25g of effective carbohydrate (just cut that original 50g portion in half). Retest your blood glucose response two hours after this meal. If it is still above 115mg/dl, then this particular food is likely not a good fit for you.

Let me give you a personal example and share how this information has changed my eating. I tested my response to both white rice and lentils. I cooked a small pot of rice one evening, let it cool, and then stored the rice in the refrigerator overnight. When I got up the following morning, I weighed out my prescribed amount of rice (a food scale actually works better than measuring cups, as it tends to be more accurate). I ate the rice, set a timer for two hours, and then checked my blood glucose. The result was a whopping 155mg/dl. This is effectively diabetic blood sugar levels. I had blurry vision and felt like crap the rest of the day. I waited a few days to recheck the white rice with 25g of effective carbs, and the result was 118. Better, but still higher than what I'd really like to see. For the lentils, I used a canned variety, and due to the fiber and protein content of the lentils it actually required almost two cans of lentils to reach the 50g amount. At two hours, my blood glucose was 94mg/dl!

I now include lentils and other beans pretty frequently in my meals, as I both feel good with these (the subjective measure) and my blood glucose is fantastic. I rarely eat rice, as I honestly prefer other carb options, and I don't care to flirt with diabetic blood glucose levels. If I do a very hard work-out I occasionally have a small helping of rice as part of my post-workout meal.

Given that you may be retesting a few (or several) foods, this may in fact be longer than a seven-day test, but within that time span you should have a better idea of the carbs that work for you. This process will let you know precisely how you respond to various foods and will allow you to find a per-meal carb load that works for you. In addition to the blood glucose response, I want you to be aware of subjective responses that may be a sign of intolerance or sensitivity (which could include skin issues or joint pain) to certain foods, such as clouded mental clarity, low energy, or "hanger" after a meal.

This means you might have a decent glycemic response to a food like corn, but because of an allergy or sensitivity, you may not want to eat it very often due to the immunogenic properties of the food. As you look through the list of recommended foods below, you might notice that I do not include any gluten-containing foods. I consistently see folks do better by avoiding gluten, and I highly recommend you tinker with that, again for at least thirty days, and then, if you want to, reintroduce and check your response. Gluten avoidance seems to be an incredible return on investment for many people, but I'll leave it up to your personal experience to decide what the truth is for you. But for crying out loud, give it a solid thirty days! People constantly whine and complain about gluten avoidance. I know those foods are tasty, handy, and likely part of your routine. If I could find a scientific way to get folks to eat bread, bagels, and crackers and not suffer serious problems, I would sell so many books, *Wired to Eat* would be better known than Harry Potter. I would not recommend avoiding gluten if there was not a compelling reason to do so.

Here are several common carbohydrate sources with the quantities needed to provide you with 50g of effective carbohydrate.

FOOD	VOLUME MEASURE	WEIGHT (G)	WEIGHT OZ.
GRAINS AND PSEUDOGRAINS			
white rice (cooked)	1.14 cups	180	6.35
brown rice (cooked)	1.03 cups	210	7.4
oats (cooked)	2.1 cups	485	17.1
Cream of Rice	1.8 cups	440	15.5
polenta	1.4 cups	360	12.7
corn tortillas	5.5 tortillas (small)	130	4.6
grits (cooked)	1.4 cups	360	12.7
buckwheat (cooked)	1.75 cups	290	10.2
quinoa (cooked)	1.47 cups	275	9.7
amaranth (cooked)	1.25 cups	310	10.9
gluten free bread	3.5 pieces	120	4.2

FOOD	VOLUME MEASURE	WEIGHT (G)	WEIGHT OZ.
LEGUMES			
lentils (cooked)	2.18 cups	430	15.17
black beans (cooked)	1.95 cups	335	11.82
pinto beans (cooked)	1.73 cups	295	10.4
chickpeas/garbanzo beans (cooked)	1.55 cups	255	9
lima beans (cooked)	1.55 cups	290	10.2

FOOD	VOLUME MEASURE	WEIGHT (G)	WEIGHT OZ.
VEGETABLES			
white potato (baked)	2 cups or 1.6 potatoes	250	8.82
sweet potato (baked)	1.45 cups, or 2.5 medium	290	10.2
parsnips (cooked/boiled)	2.4 cups sliced	370	13.1
cassava/yucca	0.7 cups	140	4.9
taro (cooked)	1.3 cups	170	6
yam (cooked)	1.6 cups (cubes)	220	7.8
butternut squash (cooked)	3.4 cups (cubes)	690	24.3
carrots (raw)	5.8 cups chopped	740	26.1
lotus root	3.25 cups	390	13.8
onion (sweet, raw)	2.3 onions	755	26.6
beets (cooked)	3.7 cups (slices)	630	22.2

FOOD	VOLUME MEASURE	WEIGHT (G)	WEIGHT OZ.
FRUITS			
mango	2.3 cups pieces	375	13.2
bananas	1.1 cup (mashed)	250	8.8
grapes	2 cups	300	10.6
grape juice	1.4 cups	350	12.3
watermelon	4.6 cups (diced)	700	24.7
oranges	2.9 cups (sections) or 3.5	485	17.1
orange juice	2 cups	490	17.3

continued...

FOOD	VOLUME MEASURE	WEIGHT (G)	WEIGHT OZ.
apples	3.9 cups (sliced) or 2 medium	425	15
applesauce	2 cups	492	17.35
blueberries	2.85 cups	420	14.8
cherries	4.6 cups with pits (3 cups)	475	16.8
cantaloupe	4.4 cups diced	690	24.3
honeydew melon	3.55 cups diced	605	21.3
pineapple	2.6 cups (chunks)	420	14.8
peaches	4.1 cups	625	22
papaya	3.8 cups (1-inch pieces)	550	19.4
plantains	1.15 cups (slices)	175	6.2

National Nutrient Database for Standard Reference
Release 28 slightly revised May, 2016 Software v.2.6.1
The National Agricultural Library

Can you use other carb sources? Yes, but you will need to figure out how much of that food you need to eat to get 50g of effective carbohydrate. I've done the work for you on a number of carb sources, but if you have some specific favorites, you can certainly run with that.

SO, ROBB, REMIND ME WHY I SHOULD DO THIS?

Some of us won the "genetic lottery" by having super-healthy parents who imparted to us a low likelihood of problems such as diabetes, cardiovascular disease, or neurodegeneration. Some of us were additionally lucky in that we had all the early life experiences that seem to set us up for success. Then we have people like me, who appear to come from the "shallow end of the gene pool." The good news is that even though I do not have optimal genes or a perfect early life story, it may no longer matter. Using our knowledge of

Can I Do This at a Time Other Than Breakfast?

You may want to do your testing at a meal other than breakfast, but this is begging for problems. We tend to have fairly fixed schedules in the morning and do roughly the same things. By contrast, our exercise, stress, and meals vary quite a lot throughout the rest of the day relative to the time between waking and eating breakfast. If you do run the test at a non-breakfast time, just shift your test carb to the appropriate time. The main point is that we want the same time of day, the same spacing between meals. For consistency, I recommend that you eat a consistent meal before your test meal. For example, if you use lunch as your test meal, eat the same breakfast and try to keep all your other variables the same, such as amount and timing of exercise, coffee intake, etc. I strongly encourage you to stick to the breakfast option for testing, but I know this question will come up. The results will almost certainly be subpar relative to a breakfast test, but if you follow these steps, it should help reduce the variables that can give us confusing readings.

Personalized Nutrition, I can monitor my carb intake such that my metabolism functions as well or better than the most genetically talented person. How is this possible? By finding the foods I do best with and largely sticking with those options, I will maintain an optimum blood glucose level while ensuring my gut biome remains healthy and strong.

The information we gain about problematic food is also valuable beyond simple avoidance. Let's say you don't do well with bananas, but you really like those golden fruits. You could keep bananas mainly as a post-exercise carb source, as we tend to require less insulin to regulate blood sugar after vigorous activity.

It's perhaps worth mentioning that the information surrounding Personalized Nutrition is quite new and we are just learning about this story. It's probable that once you have improved your gut health by sticking mainly with more favorable foods for three to six months, you may be able to better tolerate problematic foods. A bit later I make the case for retesting certain foods every three to six months as a type of mini reset. This may be a good idea for several reasons, not the least of which is reassessing your overall tolerance to both favorable and previously unfavorable foods.

At no point in history have we had this type of information literally at our fingertips.

WHERE DO WE GO NOW?

You now understand how you are wired to eat, and we have used the 30-Day Reset (which includes modifying your lifestyle factors such as sleep, stress, movement, and community) to fix your neuroregulation of appetite. You should be feeling great and losing weight, as we have stacked the deck in your favor, perhaps for the first time in your life. From here we have used the 7-Day Carb Test to go from the general to the specific and find out precisely which carb sources you do best with and which you should avoid.

In general, you should stick with the guidelines of the 30-Day Reset. This is more or less the template we will follow from here on out. What I'd like you to do is to start adding variety in your carb sources based on those you do well with. For most people, under most circumstances, 50g of effective carbs is a pretty safe upper limit. You can certainly play with that, but unless you are training at a very high level, you really do not need more.

A lot of questions come up about how one maintains success over a lifetime. In the next chapter, I'll give you some concrete rules to follow as well as some general guidelines. Again, one size does not fit all, either in food or in approaches to change.

CHAPTER 13

Phase Three

Riding into the Sunset

If we look at the statistics around weight loss and dietary change, we see that people are fairly good at the initial steps. They stick with things for a few weeks or months, but then they slide back into old habits. I think you likely understand now that it's not just sliding into old habits—folks are assailed by the lure of hyperpalatable foods at every turn, and our social interactions are largely built around food and drink. It should be no wonder that maintenance is tough. This understanding is helpful, but it also sells us short. If you have stuck to the program through Phases One and Two, you did most of the hard work. Long-term maintenance boils down to the following: doing more things "right" relative to "wrong." Are you sleeping enough? Getting outside and playing? Making generally good food choices? When things go sideways, it's usually not just one thing—it's everything. We start staying up late, skipping our morning walk, and somehow or another, we start buying and keeping dodgy food in the house, which—surprise, surprise—we eat too much of. There are lots of ways to try to keep things on track, and developing healthy daily habits is likely the best option. But what if those daily habits slide to such a degree they become counterproductive to our goals? Something I have found helpful for many folks is the seasonal reset. At the beginning of summer, fall, winter, and spring, people reevaluate their progress and goals and make an honest assessment of how they are doing. This is only helpful if we are honest about this process and hold ourselves accountable. Although much of the focus of this book is related to health and weight loss, let me share an example of what I've been struggling with and how assessment and accountability have helped me.

I had a pretty severe back injury about fifteen years ago, which can still get cranky at times. So long as I stay active and hit some specific stretches, my back is great. *But.* If I get busy and push my mobility work off to another day, every once in a while I end up with a really "spicy" lower back that will lay me up for a week. I can make all kinds of justifications about being busy with work, the kids, and what have you, but the reality is, my *goal* is to be as healthy as possible and as active as possible with my family, particularly with my two young girls. If I let my mobility suffer such that my back goes out, I have effectively shot myself in the foot (or back) and set myself both off course and backward relative to my goals. What I did recently was set a goal for getting a solid backbend (again) and maintaining that indefinitely. A well-done backbend requires that my hips, shoulders, and back are all strong, but also mobile. I set reminders in my smartphone to keep me on task, and I even enlisted my wife and a few friends to do this with me so we can keep one another accountable. The results have been fantastic. I'm close to having a really good backbend, and more important, my back feels great.

If you have lost a lot of weight, improved your health, or hit a certain pant size, that is clearly fantastic. But what should you do if you start sliding out? You need to honestly assess what you are doing that is derailing your success. Getting inadequate or poor sleep, skipping exercise, and making dodgy food choices are the main causes of folks backsliding. You may find it helpful to do another 30-Day Reset and also to run another 7-Day Carb Test to get you back into your good habits and the routine that worked in the first place.

I do want to address folks who have a significant amount of weight to lose and/or some health issues to resolve, but this same information applies even if you are at your goal and just looking for how to make all this work over the long haul. If you are in one of these camps, stick to the basic Paleo template (modified with the carbs you do well with from the 7-Day Carb Test) and get as much variety as you can within those bounds. It can take a little time, but you can and will make incredible progress by sticking to this plan. Even though that's my recommendation, I know folks will want to know how or if they can fit in a bit more "latitude." Latitude usually boils down to the following question: "How often can I have 'bad carbs'?" I'll give you an arbitrarily concrete answer to that, but I'll also give you a real-world answer that I think is much more valuable. First, the real-world answer: It depends. What is your situation? Your goals? Do you still have a significant amount of weight to lose? Do you tend to spin out if you eat trigger foods? Do you have big goals for your health and wellness? Let me use myself as an example again. I am pretty healthy at this point, as I've been tinkering with my eating and lifestyle for a long time, but I also have genetic predilections toward things like type 2 diabetes. I did wound care for one of my parents due to this disease and I *refuse* to subject my kids to that process. I have two amazing daughters, and I want to be a part of their lives for as long as possible—and I'd really like to live to play with my grandkids. Given all this, I do not get all "hookers and cocaine" with my food very often. Maybe once per month I'll have some gluten-free pizza or ice cream. Here is an important point: I just let these diversions from my normal eating happen. I do *not* plan these things out days or weeks in advance like a heroin addict getting ready to tie off for a hit. All that anticipatory stuff, the planning and scheming for the off-the-rails meal, plays into the neural wiring tied to addiction. Talk to a drug addict and they will tell you the anticipation and planning are often far better than the act/drug itself. There is a lot to learn from that with regard to building up to some kind of epic meal. Some people can make this type of behavior work (with food or drugs). Most cannot. So, I caution against doing this. What I'd like you to do is get to a place where you can be out at dinner, a family function, or a cocktail party, and when pie, ice cream, or similar items are available, you can eat them and enjoy them and it does not matter one damn bit with regard to your health, psyche, or waistline. If the bulk of your meals are on point, your sleep is good, and you are active, these occasional dalliances will not matter. Based on my blood work and how I look, feel, and perform, this approach is working very well for me, and the effort is absolutely worth the relative sacrifice. I've been sick before, and I really prefer health. All that said, I have greatly increased the variety of carbs I take in by mapping my blood glucose response, and either eating the types of carbs I do well with, or generally keeping the serving size small (recall my lentils versus rice example). I recommend you do the same.

Some folks will read the above and still pester me about how often and how many "bad carbs" they can have. My response to the people in this camp is this: you can have two meals per week to do with pretty much what you want. In theory we should be eating roughly twenty-one meals per week, so two meals make up 10 percent (well, technically 9.52 percent, but who's counting, right?) of that, which means you are sticking to the plan about 90 percent of the time. As always, here are my caveats to this:

- I generally recommend that you stick to gluten-free options. If you are convinced gluten is not a problem for you, then by all means, include it, but as I've said many times in this book, I'm shocked by how many people do better without gluten.
- Know yourself. If this off-the-rails eating takes on the appearance of a college drinking binge in Tijuana, this is likely not a good option. You need to decide if the cost-benefit ratio is worth it to you.

- If you turn these events into the equivalent of the Kitchen Sink Challenge I described early in the book, consuming 8 pounds of ice cream in a sitting, we have a problem. I am *not* advocating that. Eat a portion that you'd be comfortable being filmed eating and having the footage placed on YouTube.

If you are following the basic guidelines of the plan, you should be getting a decent amount of protein each day, good fats, and a carb level that is not problematic for you. In general, we are likely talking 100 to 150g of carbs a day from Paleo sources like fruit, yams and sweet potatoes, squash, and a mix of other carbs that work well for you, as you discovered via the 7-Day Carb Test. There are some special circumstances where you may need more (hard-training athletes) or fewer (folks who, for whatever reason, are carb intolerant). But most people will find a pretty good sweet spot here that gives them latitude while also maintaining health and weight. This type of eating leverages the neuroregulation of appetite in a way that works for us instead of against us.

Let's look at a practical example of how all this seemingly disparate information might come together in real life.

Amelia's Story

Amelia is a thirty-two-year-old professional who hails from a family of incredible culinary depth: her mom is Italian; her father is from Mexico City. Amelia was rail thin in her youth and most of college, but in her early twenties she started gaining weight. A lot of it. She also developed some odd skin conditions including eczema and vitiligo (loss of pigmentation to the skin). She crushed her graduate program, finishing top of her class, all while working part time to put herself through school. Although she had always been active, playing volleyball in high school and college, her activity and time outdoors became less and less frequent as she worked her way through academia, eventually entering the pressure cooker of "real life." Amelia worked long hours and was, not surprisingly, under a lot of stress. Her one consolation, the one thing she felt she had control over and that gave her consistent satisfaction, was eating, particularly eating those comfort foods from her mixed-culture childhood. This story progressed until Amelia was 100 pounds heavier than she had been in high school. She now found sleeping difficult and woke up exhausted, regardless of how long she spent in bed. Amelia knew she had some serious problems brewing and finally went to her doctor to get some help. Her doctor was not one of the run-of-the-mill MDs who spends five minutes with each patient; she had a background in Functional Medicine and was a fan of the Paleo diet and thus did extensive intakes to understand the full picture of each of her patients. She ran blood work on Amelia, and the results indicated that Amelia was knocking on the door of type 2 diabetes and sporting shockingly high inflammation levels. Amelia and her doctor talked about where her health status was and what her goals were. She was in a serious relationship, planning on getting married and starting a family soon. She knew that with her weight and already being close to diabetes, pregnancy was likely to pose some problems both for herself and the baby. Her doctor recommended Amelia follow some strict sleep-hygiene practices and embark on a Paleo diet for thirty days, then return for a follow-up. Amelia focused first on setting up her kitchen for success. In this case, that meant clearing out all the refined carbs, cakes, cookies, ice cream, and other pseudo-foods. She then went shopping, and instead of sticking to a super-rigid program, she pulled recipes that were both Paleo and had elements of her childhood comfort foods. She made a huge pot of marinara sauce on Sunday and instead of putting this on pasta, she cooked several spaghetti squash and ladled the marinara over the squash "noodles," freezing these in containers so she could easily reheat them for dinner. One thing Amelia was particularly good at was honestly assessing what she could accomplish in a day or week. Prepping dinner for the week was doable; breakfast and lunch was going to require some outside help. After looking online, Amelia found a meal delivery service that had Mexican-themed dishes that fit Paleo parameters. She placed an order, and on Monday morning, Amelia showed up at work and sure enough, there was a package of meals waiting for her. She put two meals in the refrigerator and three in the freezer, and caught the attention of several of her coworkers in the whole process. The response from her coworkers was mixed. A few people were pretty interested, while others seemed borderline hostile to the whole idea, making thinly veiled quips about "another fad diet." Instead of questioning herself, she roped several of her coworkers into joining her for at least thirty days. These folks all signed up for the meal-delivery service, and they got together on subsequent Sundays to cook food together, and actually swapped meals so they were not eating the exact same dinner every evening. Breakfast was the one meal Amelia insisted on eating fresh each day, as she took this time to have a coffee, eat her meal, and generally get ready for her day. The total prep time for her breakfast was less than ten minutes.

Amelia and her coworkers stuck to this first thirty days and not only enjoyed the experience but also became quite a bit closer as a consequence of cooking and sharing meals as well as taking daily walks at lunchtime and during breaks. Amelia noticed her clothes were fitting much more loosely and that her skin was looking better than it had in years. Her eczema was completely gone, and she was certain that her vitiligo was much improved. At her thirty-day follow-up visit, Amelia told her doctor her energy was great and asked if it was possible her skin conditions could have improved with her dietary changes. Her doctor affirmed that skin issues often resolved when eating this way and that the vitiligo was an autoimmune condition, which seemed to respond particularly well to the anti-inflammatory nature of this way of eating. Amelia was down 25 pounds and her blood sugars (including A1C) were much improved. Her doctor said that if she wanted to tinker with testing certain carbs to see how she responded to them, that would be an appropriate next step. Her doctor did advise that since her vitiligo was improved, it would be wise to stick with gluten-free options. Amelia thought about what to test that was not in her basic Paleo plan and settled on the following: rice, corn (in the form of tortillas and polenta), and beans, both whole and refried. These were the foods she grew up with and were likely to be a challenge when she went home to visit family. The results of her carb testing revealed that Amelia did pretty well with whole beans, corn tortillas, and polenta, but refried beans and rice pushed her blood glucose quite high. If she was going to eat those items, she needed to keep the portions pretty small. Incorporating these "safe" carb sources from these old childhood staples really increased the variety and freedom of her meals. She continued to drop weight, as evidenced by her need to continue buying smaller clothes (she had been counseled against being a daily scale watcher). The holidays were fast approaching, and Amelia was looking forward to visiting her parents for Thanksgiving. When she arrived, everyone commented on how great she looked, how much weight she had lost. She explained that she had been eating "a bit differently" but did not try to make too much of it. When dinner was served, she spied one of her favorite spreads: pasta with marinara sauce and warm toasted French bread. She asked her mom if she perhaps had some polenta cooked, and her mother's face fell. "What's wrong with what I cooked? You love my pasta!" Amelia covered the awkward moment gracefully by saying of course she loved the pasta, but no one made polenta as good as her mom. An hour or so after the meal, Amelia noticed serious discomfort in her stomach. She had often felt this feeling in the past after a meal, but had never thought much of it, as it had been happening for as long as she could remember. She really noticed it this time, as she had not had this problem for the past few months of her new way of eating. She went to bed early and tried to find a comfortable position that made her stomach feel better, but she did not sleep well that night. The next morning, her mom had espresso and biscotti laid out for breakfast, and Amelia was a bit chagrined about what to do. Again, not wanting to create drama, she went ahead and had the biscotti, and again, had pretty bad stomach problems as a consequence. She motored through the rest of her visit.

When she got back to her apartment after her holiday weekend, she felt bloated and her eczema was back with a vengeance. Amelia often talked to her parents via video chat, and later in the week she had a heart-to-heart with them about her health and what she'd like to do during her next visit. Her dad was pretty responsive to the talk but her mom was clearly hurt and took all this information personally. In a future call, Amelia spoke with her mother further and made it clear that this was just the situation she was in—there was no guilt or blame, just something that needed to be worked through. Her Christmas visit was a dramatically different affair, as she had options that worked for her, which meant the rest of the family actually had more options, too.

After a year and a half, Amelia had lost more than 90 pounds, and her eczema and vitiligo were all but gone. She convinced her coworkers to join a cardio kickboxing gym. She got married and is trying to get pregnant. She stays strictly gluten-free but has learned that an occasional gluten-free pizza for dinner, or a breakfast of espresso and gluten-free biscotti is no big deal in the generally healthy lifestyle she has created.

Full Disclosure: Amelia is not one single person, but an amalgam of three people. I've taken elements of their stories and wed them together in this example so you can get a sense of how folks navigate a large number of contingencies, from dealing with autoimmunity to the complexities of work and family interactions. This is as "real world" as it gets. What you should take from this is that success is not about perfection or making things so difficult that you and everyone around you is miserable due to your changes. This is about flexibility, accountability, and honestly assessing what battles are worth fighting, and which are worth some negotiation and modification.

If you are a "read between the lines" kind of person, you likely get the implications of this story with regard to living the rest of your life. We use the 30-Day Reset to get our proverbial ship pointed in the right direction. We then use the 7-Day Carb Test to understand what carbs we do best with and to help us create a truly personalized nutrition plan that will lead to success in the long term. Phase Two of the plan helps us get as much variety as possible into our diets while staying within a framework that ensures our success. From there, it's about exploring and being flexible. Every meal does not need to be perfect, but we cannot fool ourselves that we are "eating well" when most of our meals leave us feeling terrible. We need to really get to know ourselves, particularly from Gretchen Rubin's perspective of abstainers versus moderators. Some people can have some ice cream or nachos and it is no big deal. For other folks, these are trigger foods that lead to weeks or months of poor eating. Additionally, we need to navigate the many social situations where eating well is challenging. Each situation is different, so it seems silly to offer a concrete solution. You need to figure out what your "no go" scenarios are (if any) and fit that into the larger context of your life.

I've racked my brain for some kind of pep talk that will keep you motivated over the long haul, but I come back to the same things. You need a strong "why." You need a reason to make these changes and just keep doing them, even when your motivation is in the toilet. That may sound daunting, but it's not. We are talking about one meal at a time, one day at a time. Instead of fixating on your whole life, just focus on getting the next meal right. You do not need a motivational speech to take your next breath, because it's automatic. If you make this new way of eating and living automatic, it will be as effortless as taking your next breath.

CHAPTER 14

Hammers, Drills, and Ketosis

The Best Tool Your Doctor May Never Use

My dad was a contractor who specialized in electrical installation. He was remarkably good at this and loved figuring out tough problems. He roped me into helping with several jobs, and I found the process of pulling wire, checking voltage, and all that goes into that type of work pretty interesting, albeit a bit scary. I was convinced I'd get my fingers singed sooner or later!

My dad took this work very seriously, and when we started on a job like a remodel, I could almost set my watch by my dad digging into the guts of a building and then bellowing, "What kind of idiot wired this place?!" Being the low man on the totem pole, I had no idea what my dad was talking about. After one of these outbursts, I asked my dad something to the effect of, "How can all this same stuff be done that poorly?" To me, these buildings with wires, electrical boxes, and circuits had all the same stuff my dad was installing or fiddling with. Ah, the ignorance of youth! My dad explained to me that it was not a situation of not using the right wire or circuit, but *how* these tools were used. Often, the previous electrician had laid out shortcuts and bypassed safety issues that my dad could just not abide. He and his coworkers would discuss the relative merits of one process versus another, but there was not a massive amount of dissent in the ranks. No one was suggesting that electrical wire should be made from wood, nor did anyone suggest that one should use a saw when a screwdriver was clearly the tool for the current task.

This experience may seem rather mundane, but it really had an impact on me. I understood there should be general principles that govern a given process, with nuances emerging when we started talking about cost/benefit ratios and details. Although my background is in biochemistry, I started off pursuing an engineering degree. Between that, my natural curiosity, and those early lessons from my dad, I've tended to arrive at solutions by combining the best theory I have at my disposal with a wacky thing called "outcomes." Did the process work? Was it cost effective in terms of application and adherence? In other words, could folks follow the program or would they prefer to run away screaming?

You may be wondering, *What does all this have to do with health and nutrition?* Glad you asked. In this chapter, we will explore one of the most contested topics in medicine: the use of ketosis as a therapeutic agent. Ketosis is a tool, like a hammer or drill, which means it should be used at the right time, for the right job. It should be used with respect, because if inappropriately used, it has as much potential to harm as to help. Perhaps most important, however, ketosis is a tool that should not be maligned or set on a shelf due to the ignorance of the greater medical establishment.

Ketosis and fasting may prove to be some of the most powerful tools in our collective medical kits, yet most doctors are not only unaware of the therapeutic potential of these processes, they wrongly view them as uniformly dangerous. Are scissors dangerous? Yes, that's why we don't run with them! Used properly, they are an indispensable tool, just like ketosis. Depending on your specific health situation, this may be the most important chapter in the book. If you have a serious health concern such as neurodegenerative disease, you will be armed with a tool that may save your life.

Due to the relative challenge of eating a ketogenic diet, I've saved this information for folks who either have particular health issues that may not fully respond to the basic plans covered previously, or for people who may be looking for an edge with regard to cognition, weight loss, and antiaging strategies. I am a bit unique in that I am confident ketosis and fasting are powerful tools when used properly, but I also recognize that they are not panaceas appropriate for all people at all times. Let's dig into what ketosis is (and is not) and critically evaluate if this is a tool you need in your personal tool box.

KETOSIS: WHAT IS IT?

Under "normal" physiological conditions, we tend to fuel a significant portion of our metabolism, particularly the energy needs of our brains, from carbohydrates. I put "normal" in quotation marks because the frame of reference for studying our metabolism is our modern, consistently overfed world. This overfed state is not in fact normal, healthy, or optimal, as the genetics governing our metabolism were forged in an environment in which access to food was inconsistent and the activity level to procure this food was reasonably high. Our distant ancestors embarked on an experiment of sorts in which they traded large guts like those seen in chimps and gorillas for smaller guts and larger brains (the Expensive Tissue Hypothesis). These larger brains were indeed energy hungry, and as Richard Wrangham posited in his work *Catching Fire*, we likely employed the cooking of both animal foods and dense carbohydrate sources such as tubers to fuel our hungry brains.

It has only been for the past few hundred years that our food supplies have truly been stable. For the foraging societies that preceded us, a certain amount of food scarcity was literally "baked in the cake." Not every day was a success with regard to hunting or gathering. Because our brains are so large and metabolically active (only about 2 percent of our weight yet nearly 20 percent of our energy usage), food scarcity could pose a serious problem for our cognitive abilities, arguably the greatest asset humans have relative to other animals. If the brain can *only* run on glucose (as most health care providers claim), we must have a consistent supply of dietary glucose or we will "bonk" (experience serious cognitive problems due to low blood sugar) and cannibalize the proteins in our body to produce glucose for the brain, a process called gluconeogenesis. Fortunately for us, biology figured out an elegant solution to the problem of inconsistent food sources and a large, hungry brain in the form of ketosis.

If you recall from the digestion chapter, when we are either fasting or eating at a significant caloric deficit, our body tends to mobilize our stored body fat for energy. If carbohydrates and proteins are sufficiently limited, fat enters our mitochondria (specifically in the liver) in large amounts. Without sufficient glucose (or protein) to catalyze the metabolism of fats, we shift to a different process, ketosis, which solves several problems simultaneously. Ketosis takes the high-energy fat molecules stored in our bodies and converts them to a form that can fuel the heart, muscles, organs, and, perhaps most important, the brain. This provides an almost limitless supply of brain-friendly fuel in the form of ketones, while decreasing the need for our metabolism to use our muscles and internal organs to produce glucose.

Ketone bodies (beta-hydroxybutyrate and acetoacetate) are water soluble, which is why they are so effective at fueling the brain: they easily pass the blood-brain barrier. Entering ketosis under starvation conditions dramatically slows the loss of muscle and organ mass as the bulk of our energy requirements are met by converting our abundant fat stores into easily metabolized ketones. Additionally, we do not see cognitive impairment as the brain easily shifts to ketone use and this protects the brain from the ups and downs associated with a carb/glucose dependent metabolism. Many people (but not all!) experimenting with ketosis notice that cognition is "fantastic" (I'm one of those people). Check out the following graph of the blood glucose and ketone levels in an obese individual who was tracked over a 382-day water-only fast.

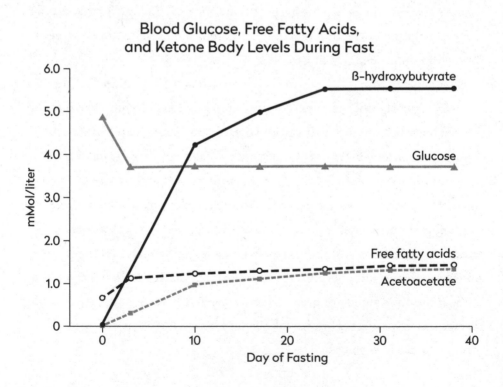

Blood Glucose, Free Fatty Acids, and Ketone Body Levels During Fast

Here is what we see:

1. In the first few days, blood glucose levels fall and then maintain a solid baseline.
2. Concurrently, free fatty acids and ketones increase.

The patient reported feeling "great" during this fast, and yes, that is 382 days, over a year, of medically supervised fasting. The patient was not hungry, as blood glucose levels were consistent, and for many people, ketones themselves appear to blunt hunger in a profound way. If we think about this, it's really smart engineering. If we have to go for extended periods without food, we need to feed the brain, but we do not want to lose an enormous amount of protein from our muscles and organs to keep blood glucose levels consistent. Ketones provide an alternate fuel for the brain and body while making small amounts of glucose from the glycerol backbone of triglycerides (fats). Ketosis also offers an amazing benefit in that it encourages our bodies to evaluate if the cells and proteins in our cells are healthy. Ketosis causes a low-grade stress (hormesis), which causes damaged or sick cells to die via a process called apoptosis. The constituents of these cells get recycled instead of becoming diseased. This helps us in two ways: it provides raw materials to help us during scarcity, and it eliminates damaged cells that have a high likelihood of becoming cancerous or diseased. Much of what we perceive to be aging appears to be an accumulation of damaged cells and cellular components. Intermittent ketosis, either by fasting or nutritional ketosis (a high-fat, low-carb, moderate-protein diet) appears to be an effective strategy to address this problem and may offer profound antiaging benefits.

Another common feature of aging is a loss of mitochondria, which can negatively impact our metabolism and may be a common problem in diseases ranging from cancer to autoimmunity to neurodegenerative disease.

I don't want to get too far into the weeds on this, but one of the benefits of ketosis is that it dramatically increases the mitochondrial density of our muscles and organs. More mitochondria means more energy.

A key failing of the calories in, calories out model of weight loss and health is that it reduces the complexity of human metabolism to something that looks like a furnace or candle. "Stuff burns" is not remotely an accurate description of what happens in our bodies. A better way to look at this process is one of a complex information processing system in which all the inputs and outputs modify our genetic expression via the proteins our genes code, our hormonal status, and even the gut biome, which itself feeds back on the system, providing its own influence. It is likely our genetics are wired for periods of both feast and famine. Our modern world has shifted that story to continual feast, which is a problem from a basic calorie perspective, but calories are just the start. This chronically overfed state sends mixed or unhealthful signals to our genetics and metabolism. Our highly tuned physiology literally does not know what to do with this information.

This is an important point to keep in mind: a healthy metabolism should be able to shift seamlessly between fat and glucose as a primary fuel source. For most people, embarking on a period of fasting or a ketogenic diet can be pretty rough in the beginning. This is not the way it should be. If we are insulin sensitive and generally healthy, we should be able to weather these transitions with just a bit of discomfort, which in our ancestral environment was the driver to seek out food during times of scarcity. Our modern world of easily accessible, hyperpalatable foods has hijacked this process and keeps us perpetually on one side of this dynamic process, leaving us inflamed and insulin resistant. We are awash in energy that causes signaling cascades that actually degrade our health, from the cellular level on up. To be healthy, it appears we need this reset (periods of scarcity) to occur, at least occasionally.

Although the ketogenic state brought about by fasting is not identical to that of nutritional ketosis, they are remarkably similar. But both of these healthy, normal metabolic states are completely different than the rightfully feared condition of ketoacidosis. Ketoacidosis is dangerous—life threatening, in fact—but it is not the same as ketosis brought about by fasting nor nutritional ketosis. Check this out:

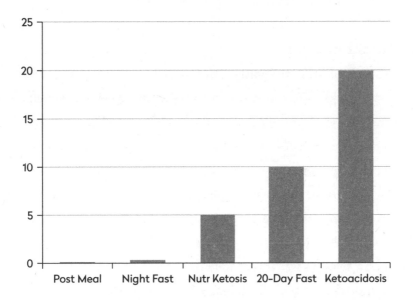

While eating normal mixed meals, we tend to see virtually no ketone production. After an overnight fast, we see a small amount. Under the state of nutritional ketosis, we tend to see a range of 1 to 3, while an extended fast can produce ketone levels as high as 7 to 10. Ketoacidosis, by contrast, produces levels that are much higher than either fasting or nutritional ketosis. The medical community recognizes that blood glucose has healthy and unhealthy ranges, yet there is not the same awareness around ketone levels. Ketoacidosis is most common in poorly controlled diabetes cases, in which insulin usages does not match carbohydrate intake. This can dangerously shift the blood pH, leading to coma and possibly death. So I do not want to make light of the concerns medical professionals have on this topic, but it's also time for them to not just "get through" their biochemistry, but to actually remember it. It is as unreasonable to equate ketoacidosis with fasting and nutritional ketosis as it is to somehow link normal blood glucose levels (in an insulin sensitive individual) with diabetes. Ketoacidosis is too many ketones; diabetes is too much blood glucose.

Nutritional Ketosis

There is some indication that fasting may have been used as early as 500 BCE to treat epilepsy. One must wonder at how early people connected the dots on this process, but it likely looked something like this: An individual who suffered from epileptic seizure improved during times of food scarcity. Food scarcity stops, and seizures come back. Another round of scarcity (fasting), and seizures reduce in frequency or severity or perhaps resolve entirely. Not a randomized controlled trial (RCT), but not everything in life needs an RCT to become valuable information. The knowledge of the effects of fasting and seizures was fortunately not lost to time, and has made its way down through the ages. In the early 1900s, physicians and researchers used a ketogenic diet for childhood epileptic seizures, and the results were (and are) remarkable. The diet did not work all the time, but in an age before antiepileptic drugs, the ketogenic diet worked quite well. This was an important step, as children are one group for whom fasting (nutritional scarcity) is not a good option. With the advent of modern pharmacology, several antiepileptic drugs were developed, but they came with their own set of side effects and were again, not universally effective. A few universities, like Stanford, maintained a ketogenic diet program for years. With the advent of the Internet, people were able to research a wide variety of topics and parents looking for help with their children's epilepsy often found the early work on this topic.

Although still a fringe research area, information about the ketogenic diet has exploded in recent years due to academic interest, but I must make the point: this interest was inspired by grassroots activism on the Internet. When researchers really began looking at the mechanisms of the ketogenic diet, they found that this way of eating:

1. Dramatically reduced insulin levels
2. Reduced and normalized blood glucose levels
3. Provided an alternate fuel for the brain (ketone bodies)
4. Stabilized electrical activity in the brain
5. Reduced inflammation

By understanding these mechanisms, researchers also began looking at a number of other conditions that might benefit from the ketogenic diet, including cancer, neurodegenerative diseases such as Parkinson's and Alzheimer's, and diabetes.

CANCER

In the 1920s, Otto Warburg observed that certain types of cancers shifted to a metabolism built exclusively from glucose fermentation. This is in stark contrast to most normal cells, which use the mitochondria to metabolize protein, carbs, and fat in a process called cellular respiration. It was theorized that mitochondrial dysfunction was the root of most cancers. This theory held sway until the characterization of the DNA double helix in the 1950s. At this time the metabolic theory of cancer fell out of vogue and we have spent the past seventy years looking at and treating cancer from a genetic rather than metabolic perspective. Although outside the scope of this book, it is worth mentioning that given the enormous effort to treat cancer as a genetic disease, we have relatively little to show for the process. This may seem an outlandish claim, but unfortunately, it's not. With few exceptions cancer rates have remained stubbornly consistent over the past hundred years. If you are particularly interested in the history of cancer and the ketogenic diet, I recommend you read *Tripping Over the Truth* by Travis Christofferson.

NEURODEGENERATION

It's tough to imagine a disease more feared than cancer, but neurodegenerative diseases such as Parkinson's, Alzheimer's, and dementia could be contenders. For decades these conditions have been regarded as completely separate disease entities. However, recent research has suggested that inflammation, overfeeding, elevated blood glucose, and gut dysbiosis may be common triggers that then manifest as different diseases based upon individual genetics. Accordingly, ketosis and fasting may be helpful for the following reasons:

1. Ketones offer an alternate energy source for the brain, thus preventing cell death that may occur with these diseases.
2. The state of ketosis may encourage damaged mitochondria to repair themselves, halting the disease process.
3. Cells that are too far gone may undergo apoptosis, thereby reducing inflammation caused by senescent (damaged) cells.

There have been a few small studies in which individuals suffering from neurodegenerative disease were fed a low-glycemic-load diet supplemented with medium-chain triglycerides (MCTs). MCTs are interesting in that we tend to metabolize them preferentially and the result is an appreciable increase in blood ketone levels. This protocol has proven beneficial for certain neurodegenerative diseases, and research in this area is really ramping up. Additional tools that may prove helpful include ketone salts and esters. These substances can produce ketone levels that are quite high and simply need to be mixed with water to be consumed. While these are by no means cure-alls, they are nonetheless exciting opportunities for those suffering from these diseases.

Five years from now, we will know much more about ketosis, fasting, and the potential use of exogenous ketones. Currently we have far more questions than answers. Until we have more data on this topic, I think the following is a scientifically sound way to use what we know about MCT oil and other exogenous ketone sources to help us with nutritional ketosis or even fasting:

1. Shift to a low-glycemic-load diet and supplement with 1 to 2 table-spoons of MCT oil two or three times per day. (Coconut oil is a good source of MCTs, although there are purified MCT sources, which work far better so long as they are tolerated. *Go slow* with these, as your system could have an adverse reaction that will have you headed toward the bathroom.) Follow this protocol for two to three weeks. As an aside, this is effectively the Transitional Ketosis approach for which meal plans are provided a bit later.

2. After that period, shift to a ketogenic diet (carbs typically 30 to 50g per day, not counting fiber) with moderate to low protein (between 75 and 100g per day). If the MCTs are working, then you may continue them.

3. After at least a month of consistent ketosis one could move toward one- or two-day fasts a few times per month. If you choose this path, I recommend you follow the work of Dr. Jason Fung (intensivedietary-management.com) and pick up a copy of his book *The Complete Guide to Fasting*.

This is a largely theoretical template, but there are anecdotal reports of folks using this protocol with good success. This process might be beneficial because the initial stage (transitional ketosis) helps to normalize insulin levels while providing an "easy" source of ketones in the form of MCT oil. This should make the transition to ketosis and possibly fasting much easier. If you have been eating poorly and are insulin resistant, slamming your body straight into ketosis or fasting might be beneficial from a metabolic perspective, but it can be hell. Clearly you should talk to your health care provider about this process if you are considering it, but I will reiterate that most health care providers may not know the difference between ketosis and ketoacidosis and may be unfamiliar with any of the research on this topic; therefore, they may not be in a good position to help you. If your primary care provider is not up to speed on this material, you will need to keep looking and interviewing until you find the right person.

DIABETES

For the type 2 diabetic, I am honestly stumped why a ketogenic (or low-carb) diet plus some amount of fasting is not standard of care. People continue to argue about the cause of diabetes, but this is a moot point once you are sufficiently down the path of diabetes. You have the problem—let's fix it in the most efficient way possible.

The diagnosis of type 2 diabetes is predicated on excessively elevated blood glucose levels (A1C and/or fasting glucose). This means your body does not handle carbs well. The obvious solution would seem to be "reduce carbs to a nonpathogenic level." This suggestion is approached as if the recommendation were cannibalism, not carb control. Nothing drops blood glucose levels better than a ketogenic diet and/or fasting. In the case of the ketogenic diet, you take in very few carbs. In the case of fasting, you take in nothing! In both cases, we dramatically reduce systemic inflammation and insulin levels. Dr. Jason Fung has written another outstanding book on this subject called *The Obesity Code*. He uses a therapeutic fasting routine with his patients and has remarkable success. This process clearly needs to be medically supervised, especially if you are on a number of medications, but again, it'd be helpful if your health care provider is reasonably well versed on this subject. You may be wondering why I recommended following the 30-Day Reset and 7-Day Carb Test plan for most folks, including type 2 diabetics, when ketosis and fasting are so incredibly powerful for this condition. There are a few reasons:

- A Paleo-type diet has been clinically shown to reverse type 2 diabetes and insulin resistance. Ketosis *might* effect this change faster, but we do not really know that for sure.
- Ketosis can be pretty extreme for some people. Heck, just not eating junk food during the 30-Day Reset is a big ask for many people! The basic Paleo template is generally more doable for folks, at least in the beginning.
- Medical professionals lose their minds when their patients say they are following a ketogenic diet. These same people often freak out over the idea of a Paleo diet (if it's called that) but are okay with what it actually is: whole unprocessed food, decent amounts of protein, and prodigious amounts of fruits and vegetables. As I've said, this position is largely due to ignorance of the facts about these dietary approaches, but that does not help the patient much if they are essentially stuck with a doctor who does not know about any of this. Given all that, a basic Paleo approach is generally easier, again, at least as a starting point.

TYPE 1 DIABETES

Perhaps even more controversial is the idea of using a ketogenic (or low-carb) diet for the type 1 diabetic. If you recall, type 1 diabetes is an autoimmune disease that damages the beta cells of the pancreas, thereby halting the production of insulin. This can be a life-threatening disease if not properly managed, but the standard of care has essentially been "eat what you want, control blood sugar with insulin." If you follow that advice with a functional pancreas, you have a good chance of ending up obese and/or diabetic. In the case of the type 1 diabetic, this is even more of a problem, as no matter how well we try to manage blood glucose levels, be that via an insulin pump or frequent blood glucose checks, we never do as good of a job as our pancreas does. There are quite a number of anecdotal reports claiming a ketogenic diet dramatically improves type 1 diabetes management. If you look to the literature, you do not find much. A few case reports that imply the protocol may have merit, and quite a number of review papers warning against the potential problems (again theoretical, as these authors have no more evidence to suggest this is a bad idea than I have to suggest it may be a good one). My goal here is to provide some context and information if you or someone you know suffers from type 1 diabetes. I don't think anyone should be satisfied with the current treatment options for this disease, but it's remarkable how much pushback occurs in even trying to have a discussion on the topic. If you are a type 1 diabetic, I highly recommend you check out the website optimisingnutrition.com, created by Marty Kendall. Marty is an engineer by training but his wife is a type 1 diabetic. He was pretty dissatisfied with the standard of care in treating her condition, so he went in and looked at the problem as apparently only engineers can. Unencumbered by classic medical training, Marty correctly reasoned that if controlling blood glucose is a serious problem for the type 1 diabetic, why not rely on an alternate fuel, namely ketones, thus reducing the complexity of the problem. If you or someone you know are type 1, I strongly recommend considering a path of management that might deviate a bit from the standard of care.

WEIGHT LOSS

Low-carb and ketogenic diets have a long history of success. In the early 1900s, William Banting wrote one of the first booklets on using a low-carb diet for fat loss titled *Letter on Corpulence*. For more than fifty years, it was common practice for physicians to recommend that their overweight patients limit starchy and sugary foods, and there was not much in the way of controversy on this topic. As I described in the early chapters of the book, that story changed rather dramatically in the 1950s, and we are only now circling back to a point where low-carb and ketogenic diets are being adopted by the medical mainstream.

The basic Paleo diet approach (with the inclusion of favorable carbs as discovered via the 7-Day Carb Test) works remarkably well for most people for both health concerns and significant weight loss. As with everything, however, there is no one-size-fits-all approach. For some people, a ketogenic diet is the "only" method that seems to work for them over the long haul. Our best understanding of this situation suggests some people may have suffered significant damage to the regions of the brain that govern appetite. This change in neural activity means that even the highly satiating foods normally consumed in the basic plan are not up to the task of triggering the "off" switch in the brains of certain people. Ketosis may facilitate some measure of rewiring that produces an acceptable degree of appetite control. We do not yet understand the precise mechanisms, but we do understand that for some people for whom other methods fail, the ketogenic diet may be the best (or only) solution.

SHOULD YOU DO SOME FORM OF KETOGENIC DIET OR FASTING?

I have split fasting and ketosis out of the main sections of the book because I approach them as distinct tools. This implies that these tools have both specific applications and concerns. The 30-Day Reset and 7-Day Carb Test will fix *most* of what ails us, but not everything. If you are suffering from a neurodegenerative disease, suspect you may be at risk for certain types of cancer, or have not responded as favorably as you'd like to weight-loss efforts, it may be time to give these tools a shot. I love eating this way, as I have incredible energy in general, and although I do find it hard to fuel my Brazilian jujitsu while in ketosis, my cognition is fantastic and I am literally *never* hungry. But I suspect ketosis is just something that fits my physiology and psychology. This will not be the case for everyone. I've said this before but it is worth repeating: most folks should start with the 30-Day Reset and 7-Day Carb Test Plan. The possible exceptions are folks with serious health concerns (neurodegeneration being perhaps top of the list) that may benefit immediately from a ketogenic approach. If you head down the ketogenic and/or fasting route, here is the suggested process to follow:

- 2 to 4 weeks of the Transitional Ketosis program
- At least 30 days of the nutritional ketosis program
- Ease into fasting by using what's called time-restricted feeding (TRF). This is a fancy term for "have dinner early, eat breakfast late." In practical application, this could mean having dinner around five P.M. (or whenever you can fit it in, but earlier is better), then having breakfast around nine A.M. the next day. That will be a 16-hour fast. Do this a few times per week and see how you feel; pay attention to how you sleep as well as your energy levels. If you are doing okay, then all you do is slowly

increase that time period. If you are doing the TRF twice per week, I'd say just try to add an hour each week. Recently I have tried an early eating version of TRF. I have breakfast first thing in the morning and I make it BIG. I have a large lunch around two or three P.M. and then little if any dinner at five or six P.M. I honestly prefer this method to skipping breakfast. Drink plenty of water, but I'd be careful with how much caffeine you consume at this time, as fasting is pretty stimulating all by itself. I have seen people seriously overcaffeinate, as your tolerance will be less than when you are eating regular meals. At some point you will push this out such that you are essentially doing a dinner-to-dinner fast a few times per week (or month). For most people this is as far as I'd push this process. If you want to go longer durations, you need to find a health care provider well versed in this material to help monitor your progress.

If you decide to embark on any form of the ketogenic diet, be that transitional or the nutritional ketosis approach, here are the meal plans to help get you started.

WEEK 1 KETO TRANSITION

On the Menu
- Creamy Chicken and Vegetables (page 266)—yields 6 servings
- Grilled Strip Steaks (page 278) with Fried Brussels Sprouts (page 272)—yields 8 servings
- Pork with Cauliflower Medley (page 291)—yields 4 servings
- Seafood Chowder (page 304)—yields 8 servings
- Rotisserie-Like Chicken (page 295) with Sautéed Greens (page 301) and Sautéed Mushrooms (page 302)—yields 4 servings

What Are Possible Downsides of Ketosis?

There are a host of other conditions that may benefit from a low-carb diet, ranging from traumatic brain injury to reproductive difficulties. I don't have the space to look at each of these topics, but you can do some great investigative work by searching for a specific condition and "low-carb diets." All this said, there are some folks for whom low-carb or ketosis are not a good fit:

1. Some people see dramatically elevated cholesterol levels and, perhaps more important, LDL-particle (LDL-P) count. This is a concerning development and my friends in the lipidology world do not look at this favorably. Unfortunately, we have few if any studies looking at the specific situation of an individual eating low carb *and* seeing elevated LDL-P. This is a confusing situation as every other biomarker we'd like to consider for heart disease, systemic inflammation, insulin levels, and A1C all improve on a low-carb diet. So, is this a net win or a net loss? We just don't know. For the folks who respond this way to a ketogenic diet, simply upping the carbs to 100 to 150g/day brings LDL-P levels down dramatically. There is clearly a deeper story here that no one has the answer to, but if your blood work shifts toward higher LDL-P while in ketosis yet normalizes on 100 to 150g of carbs per day, I think it's safe to say the latter path is better for you.

2. Athletes. Some ultra-endurance athletes have reported better performance using a ketogenic diet. This makes sense as these folks are generally running on fat due to the relatively low intensity of their training, but I have seen significant problems in folks trying to eat low carb and participate in more intense activities such as CrossFit, mixed martial arts, soccer, and other activities with significant amounts of sprinting and intensity. This is again a hotly contested area, as the pro-keto folks will swear that this way of eating can work for anyone. I cofounded the first and fourth CrossFit affiliate gyms in the world and have worked directly with thousands of people in both that sport and others, and what I have consistently found is that higher-intensity activities do not lend themselves to keto fueling. Folks may do better on generally lower carb levels (I certainly do), but there is an inflection point at which I do not see benefits. There are a number of research projects under way looking at this topic, so we'll

have some hard data in the years to come, but for now I cannot recommend a ketogenic diet for folks who perform large amounts of high-intensity work. Now, all that said, the folks at Ketogains.com and strength coach Craig Preisendorf of superhero-maker.com *have* had success with folks doing a ketogenic diet and high-intensity activity. So there may still be ways to make this work, but as with all things, individual situations and needs will dictate what tool we use.

3. Gut flora. Ketogenic diets are, by their very nature, carbohydrate restrictive. This means we will almost certainly reduce the amount of fermentable carbohydrate the gut bacteria receive to live on. This can be a good thing if one suffers from small intestinal bacterial overgrowth (SIBO). In fact, folks diagnosed with SIBO are generally recommended to eat a low-carb diet to starve back the pathogenic gut bacteria, then they slowly introduce probiotics and quality carbs to feed the beneficial bacteria. At very low carbohydrate levels, the gut bacteria may actually feed on the mucus layer in the gut (which contains significant amounts of carbohydrate), but this is moving us in a bad direction with regard to gut health. The mucus layer acts as a semipermeable "condom" that keeps the intestinal contents out of direct contact with the gut while allowing nutrients to move from the gut into the circulation. If the mucus layer is compromised, bacteria and intestinal contents (poo) have direct contact with the gut lining, and this may be a highly inflammatory process. All this said, it *might* be possible to provide the gut with adequate amounts of fermentable carbohydrates by eating prodigious amounts of vegetables, including onions, leeks, and garlic, all of which provide unique, low-glycemic-load carbs that can also feed the gut.

Ketosis is a powerful therapeutic tool, but like all tools, it needs to be used for the right job. I don't know if it's the best option for you, but it is certainly something to keep in mind.

Plan of Attack

Choose the seasoning you'd like for the rotisserie chicken and get that going in the slow cooker. While that cooks, slice, dice, and chop all the vegetables you'll need for other recipes. Since frying is not often for the faint of heart, perhaps cook (and eat) some of the fried Brussels sprouts and the steak on the same cook-up day. Soups and chowders usually taste better the next day anyway, so why not make the seafood chowder at the same time? And before you head to the grocery store, check out the shopping list for Week 1 in the Appendix.

WEEK 2 KETO TRANSITION

On the Menu

- Asian Short Ribs (page 244) with Mashed Cauliflower (page 284)—yields 6 servings
- Lemon Herb Salmon (page 283) with Cabbage and Onion Noodles (page 252)—yields 6 servings
- Savory Crispy Baked Chicken (page 303) with Asian Slaw (page 243)—yields 6 servings
- Spaghetti Squash Pesto Casserole (page 313)—yields 6 servings
- Shrimp with Coconut-Lime Cauliflower Rice (page 310)—yields 6 servings

Plan of Attack

Short ribs love long cooking times, so get those cooking on your cook-up day. After smelling them in your oven for a few hours, no doubt you'll want to eat some of them the same day. Get the chicken brining for the savory baked chicken, and chop/prep all the vegetables for other dishes. The spaghetti squash casserole is perfect for lunches, so we suggest cooking that up on your big cooking day. Then you've got super-quick and easy lemon dill salmon and shrimp and coconut rice to look forward to later in the week, along with the savory baked chicken.

WEEK 1 NUTRITIONAL KETOSIS

On the Menu
- Breakfast Muffins (page 251)—yields 4 servings
- Crispy-Skin Salmon with Asian-Style Vegetables (page 267)—yields 6 servings
- Ginger Garlic Green Onion–Crusted Fish with Cream Sauce (page 274) with chopped cucumber pieces tossed in rice vinegar—yields 4 servings
- Slow-Cooker Pork Butt (page 311) with Roasted Bok Choy (page 293)—yields 8 servings
- Ultimate Superfood Burgers (page 319) with Roasted Broccoli and Cauliflower (page 294)—yields 8 servings

Plan of Attack
Get that slow cooker out again and cook the pork butt. Consider tackling the breakfast muffins and ultimate burgers and all their accompaniments on your cooking day, too, along with slicing, dicing, and chopping the needed ingredients for recipes later in the week. And before you head to the grocery store, check out the shopping list for Week 2 in the Appendix.

WEEK 2 NUTRITIONAL KETOSIS

On the Menu
- Lamb Chops (page 282) with mixed greens tossed with Creamy Dill Dressing (page 332)—yields 6 servings

- Pork Tenderloin and Roasted Asparagus and Hollandaise (page 290)—yields 8 servings
- Oven-Roasted Brisket (page 286) with Squash Ribbon Salad (page 315)—yields 8 servings
- Whole Roast Chicken and Vegetables (page 322)—yields 6 servings
- Garlic-Cilantro Shrimp (page 273) with Mashed Cauliflower (page 284)—yields 4 servings
- Beef Stir-Fry (page 248) with Cauliflower Rice (page 254)—yields 4 servings

Plan of Attack

This may look like a lot of recipes, but if you started with the 30-Day Reset, you're likely a pro at cauliflower rice and mashed cauliflower, so cross those off the list right away. The garlic cilantro shrimp, pork with asparagus and hollandaise, and beef stir-fry are really quick cooks, so you can save those for later in the week if you'd like (and just get all the chopping and prepping done on your cooking day). The brisket is another low-and-slow one, so get that going on your cooking day. The whole roast chicken and vegetables also require the oven, so you may wish to wait on those. The beauty of that dish is that it's very little preparation time (though it will appear as if you slaved over things for hours). It is a perfect Sunday meal. And before you head to the grocery store, check out the shopping list for Week 2 in the Appendix.

CHAPTER 15

Recipes for Weight Loss and Beyond

RECIPES

Asian Slaw

Asian Short Ribs

Bacon-Wrapped Asparagus

Baked Halibut

Beef Kabobs

Beef Stir-Fry

Beef Tacos

Breakfast Muffins

Cabbage and Onion Noodles

Sweet Cabbage and Onion Noodles

Cauliflower Rice

Chicken Alfredo

Chicken Soup

Chicken Stir-Fry

Chicken Stock

Chicken Tikka Masala

Chicken Tortilla-Less Soup

Cioppino

Coconut Cream Drops

Creamy Chicken and Vegetables

Crispy-Skin Salmon with Asian-Style Vegetables

Fish Packets with Lime-Coconut Sauce

Flank Steak

Fried Brussels Sprouts

Garlic-Cilantro Shrimp

Ginger Garlic Green Onion–Crusted Fish with Cream Sauce

Greek Kabobs with Tzatziki Sauce

Grilled Strip Steaks

Guac-Stuffed Burgers (or Balls)

Kitchen Sink Sauté

Lamb Chops

Lemon Herb Salmon

Mashed Cauliflower

Meatza

Oven-Roasted Brisket

Pork Chips

Pork Chops with Peach Chutney and Roasted Okra

Pork Tenderloin and Roasted Asparagus with Hollandaise

Pork Cutlets or Chops with Cauliflower Medley

Prime Rib

Roasted Bok Choy

Roasted Broccoli and Cauliflower

Rotisserie-Like Chicken

Satay Skillet

Sausage and Egg "Sandwiches"

Sautéed Greens

Sautéed Mushrooms

Savory Crispy Baked Chicken

Seafood Chowder

Seafood Stew

Shepherd's Pie

Shrimp Kabobs

Shrimp Stir-Fry

Shrimp with Coconut-Lime Cauliflower Rice

Slow-Cooker Pork Butt

Slow-Cooker Pot Roast

Spaghetti Squash Pesto Casserole

Spare Ribs

Squash Ribbon Salad

Stuffed Mushrooms

Thai Coconut Soup

Twice-Baked Sweet Potatoes

Ultimate Superfood Burgers

Weeknight Chicken Breasts or Thighs

Whole Roast Chicken and Vegetables

DRESSINGS, SAUCES, AND MORE

5-Minute Hollandaise Sauce

Asian Dressing

Asian Marinade

Caesar-Like Dressing

Chimichurri

Cilantro-Lime Marinade

Compound Butter

Creamy Dill Dressing

Fauxmato Sauce

Guacamole

Pesto Sauce

Tangy Avocado Sauce

Tomato Meat Sauce

Asian Slaw

Serves 4 to 6 · AIP WITH MODIFICATIONS

To make this dish a meal, top with some grilled chicken (page 320), steak (page 278), or other protein of your choosing. If you can tolerate bell peppers, add some as desired.

. . . .

1   small head cabbage (napa, green, or red, or a combination), shredded or thinly sliced

3   carrots, shredded

3   green onions, sliced on an angle

2   cups snow peas, sliced on an angle

¾   cup Asian Dressing (page 326)

½   cup slivered almonds (omit if AIP)

Combine all the ingredients in a large bowl and toss to coat well.

PER SERVING (6 SERVINGS)

Cal: 241
Pro: 5g
Carb: 12g
Fat: 18g

Asian Short Ribs

Serves 4 to 6 · AIP WITH MODIFICATIONS

Short ribs are typically super fatty, and a lot of that fat cooks off into the sauce. As the sauce cools, skim the fat off, if desired. Umeboshi paste is a tart, sour paste made from pickled, unripe green ume plums. You can find it at many health food stores and Asian markets, as well as from Thrive Market and on Amazon. If you do not have umeboshi on hand, use a few tablespoons more rice vinegar or plum (ume) vinegar. Serve these with mashed cauliflower.

. . . .

1 tablespoon coconut oil

4 to 5 pounds short ribs

¼ cup coconut aminos

2 cups beef stock

2 tablespoons umeboshi paste

1 tablespoon rice vinegar

1 tablespoon minced fresh ginger

1 orange, quartered

3 garlic cloves, mashed

1 lemongrass stalk, tough outer layer removed, inner core smashed

1 cinnamon stick

¼ teaspoon whole cloves (omit if AIP)

½ cup thinly sliced green onions

1. Preheat the oven to 325°F.

2. In a large Dutch oven, heat the oil over medium-high heat. Working in batches if needed, add the ribs and brown on all sides. Arrange all the ribs in the pot meat-side down.

3. In a medium bowl, whisk together the coconut aminos, stock, umeboshi paste, vinegar, and ginger; pour this over the ribs.

4. Add the orange, garlic, lemongrass, cinnamon stick, and cloves to the pot and bring the mixture to a boil. Cover the pot and place in oven for 4 to 6 hours, or until the ribs are fork-tender.

5. Use tongs to transfer the ribs from the pot to a serving platter and top with the green onions.

PER SERVING (4 OUNCES COOKED MEAT, NOT INCLUDING RIB BONES)

Cal: 569
Pro: 21g
Carb: 6g
Fat: 51g

Bacon-Wrapped Asparagus

Serves 4 to 6 · AIP WITH MODIFICATIONS

. . . .

12 bacon slices (AIP–
friendly for AIP)

5 garlic cloves, minced

1 pound asparagus,
tough ends trimmed

1 tablespoon balsamic
vinegar

PER SERVING (4 SERVINGS)

Cal: 164
Pro: 12g
Carb: 4g
Fat: 11g

1. Preheat the oven to 400°F. Line a baking sheet with aluminum foil or parchment paper.

2. Place the bacon slices on a flat surface and sprinkle with the garlic.

3. Wrap 3 or so asparagus stalks (fewer if they're particularly thick) with one piece of the bacon (garlic-side in), working in a corkscrew fashion.

4. Place the asparagus bundles on the prepared baking sheet and back for 15 to 20 minutes, or until the bacon is cooked through.

5. Drizzle with the vinegar before serving.

Baked Halibut

Serves 4 · AIP WITH MODIFICATIONS

4 (6-ounce) halibut
fillets

2 tablespoons olive oil

Salt and black
pepper

4 tablespoons
Compound Butter
(page 331)

PER SERVING

Cal: 382
Pro: 46g
Carb: 0g
Fat: 23g

1. Preheat the oven to 400°F. Line a baking sheet with parchment paper.

2. Place the fillets skin-side down on the prepared baking sheet. Drizzle them with the olive oil and sprinkle with salt and pepper.

3. Bake for 10 minutes, or until the fish flakes easily with a fork.

4. Serve immediately, with a tablespoon of compound butter on each fillet.

Note: Omit black pepper and compound butter if AIP.

Beef Kabobs

Serves 6 to 8 · AIP

. . . .

¾ cup olive oil

2 tablespoons minced garlic

1 tablespoon minced fresh rosemary

1 tablespoon minced fresh parsley

2 teaspoons dried thyme

1 teaspoon dried oregano

2 tablespoons red wine vinegar

2 pounds boneless sirloin steak, cut into 1-inch cubes

12 to 15 button mushrooms

3 yellow squash, cut into ½-inch discs

1 teaspoon sea salt

> PER SERVING (8 SERVINGS)
>
> Cal: 397
> Pro: 36g
> Carb: 3g
> Fat: 26g

1. In a bowl, whisk together ¼ cup of the olive oil, the garlic, rosemary, parsley, thyme, oregano, and vinegar to make a marinade.

2. Place the beef in a large zip-top bag or dish and pour the marinade over. Marinate in the refrigerator for at least 30 minutes or overnight.

3. Soak 8 to 12 bamboo skewers in water for at least 30 minutes to prevent burning. Heat a grill to medium-high and rub the grates with oil.

4. Remove the beef from marinade. Thread the beef, mushrooms, and squash on the skewers, alternating between the three and leaving some space between each.

5. Brush the vegetables with the remaining olive oil, sprinkle the kabobs with the salt, and grill for 8 to 10 minutes, turning every few minutes, until the beef is cooked through and the vegetables are tender.

Beef Stir-Fry

Serves 4 · AIP

. . . .

1   pound beef sirloin
    or top round steak,
    sliced into thin strips

½   teaspoon sea salt

1   tablespoon
    arrowroot powder

3   tablespoons coconut
    oil or ghee

1   cup carrots, thinly
    sliced on an angle

2   cups mushrooms,
    sliced

2   bunches baby
    bok choy, coarsely
    chopped

2   garlic cloves, minced

1   teaspoon grated
    fresh ginger

¼   cup coconut aminos

¼   cup beef stock

4   green onions, sliced

1. In a medium bowl, combine the beef with the salt and arrowroot powder. Set aside.

2. In a large skillet, heat 1 tablespoon of the coconut oil over medium-high heat. Add the carrots and mushrooms and cook for 2 to 3 minutes.

3. Add the bok choy, garlic, and ginger, stir, and cook for another minute or two.

4. Transfer the vegetables to a large bowl or plate and add the remaining 2 tablespoons coconut oil to the pan. Add the beef and cook for 3 to 4 minutes. Stir in the coconut aminos, stock, and cooked vegetables. Cook until the liquid thickens.

5. Remove from the heat, stir in the green onions, and serve.

PER SERVING

Cal: 354
Pro: 40g
Carb: 7g
Fat: 18g

Beef Tacos

Serves 8 · AIP USING AIP TACO SEASONING (PAGE 250)

On your prep day, cook at least 2 pounds of ground beef to have on hand for the week. Then, take the cooked beef (or really any cooked ground meat of your choosing—lamb, pork, chicken, etc.) and use it for this dish to make your life easier. Now you'll have dinner on the table in no time flat.

. . . .

2 pounds grass-fed ground beef

2 to 3 tablespoons taco seasoning, store-bought or homemade (page 250)

1 tablespoon coconut oil or olive oil

1 medium onion, finely chopped

Salt

OPTIONAL GARNISHES

Napa cabbage leaves, romaine lettuce leaves, or Siete foods tortillas (almond flour or coconut and cassava flour—the latter being AIP-friendly)

Shredded lettuce

Diced tomatoes

Guacamole (page 334)

Salsa

1. Heat a large skillet over medium-high heat, and add the ground beef. Brown the beef, using a spoon to break apart the meat, and add the taco seasoning, stirring well. Remove the beef to a bowl.

2. In the same skillet, heat the coconut oil over medium heat. Add the onion and cook for 5 to 7 minutes, or until the onion is softened and translucent.

3. Add the meat and ¼ cup water to the skillet. Stir and simmer until heated through.

4. Taste and season with salt.

PER SERVING, WITHOUT OPTIONAL GARNISHES

Cal: 261
Pro: 21g
Carb: 1g
Fat: 18.8g

basic taco seasoning

Makes about 5 tablespoons

. . . .

2 tablespoons chili powder

2 teaspoons ground cumin

1 teaspoon garlic powder

½ teaspoon onion powder

½ teaspoon ground oregano

1 teaspoon paprika

2 teaspoons sea salt

2 teaspoons black pepper

Combine all the ingredients in a small bowl. Store in an airtight container if not using immediately.

AIP taco seasoning

Makes about 5 tablespoons · AIP

. . . .

2 teaspoons ground turmeric

1 tablespoon garlic powder

1 tablespoon onion powder

1½ teaspoons dried oregano

1 teaspoon dried thyme

1½ teaspoons dried parsley

1½ teaspoons dried cilantro (*not* coriander seeds)

2 teaspoons sea salt

Combine all the ingredients in a small bowl. Store in an airtight container if not using immediately.

Breakfast Muffins

Serves 4 to 6 · AIP WITH MODIFICATIONS

. . . .

1 tablespoon coconut oil or ghee, plus more for greasing

½ cup minced onions

½ cup diced mushrooms

1 garlic clove, minced

1 pound ground pork

2 teaspoons garlic powder

1 teaspoon celery salt (omit if AIP)

1 teaspoon dried rosemary

½ teaspoon dried basil

½ teaspoon salt (do not use if using the celery salt)

6 large eggs, whisked (see Note)

1. Preheat the oven to 350°F. Grease the wells of a 12-cup muffin tin with coconut oil.

2. In a large skillet, heat the coconut oil over medium heat. Add the onions, mushrooms, and garlic. Cook for 5 to 7 minutes, or until onions are softened and translucent.

3. Add the ground pork, sprinkle with the garlic powder, celery salt (if using), rosemary, basil, and salt (if using), and cook until the pork is cooked through, about 7 minutes.

4. Evenly distribute the pork mixture among eight of the prepared muffin cups.

5. Divide the egg over the pork in each muffin cup and bake for 20 minutes, or until the eggs are set.

Note: If you're following AIP, replace the eggs with 2 cups roasted squash and serve as hash instead of muffins.

PER SERVING (6 SERVINGS)

Cal: 209
Pro: 27g
Carb: 2g
Fat: 10g

Cabbage and Onion Noodles

Serves 6 to 8 · AIP

Serve as a stand-alone vegetable or a bedding for protein.

. . . .

2 tablespoons coconut oil or ghee

1 sweet yellow onion, thinly sliced

1 small head green or red cabbage, cored and shredded (4 to 5 cups)

Salt

1. In a large saucepan, heat the coconut oil over medium heat. Add the onion and cabbage and cook until softened.

2. Season with salt.

PER SERVING (6 SERVINGS)

Cal: 76
Pro: 2g
Carb: 5g
Fat: 5g

Sweet Cabbage and Onion Noodles

Serves 6 to 8 · AIP

- 2 tablespoons coconut oil or ghee
- 1 sweet yellow onion, thinly sliced
- 1 small head green or red cabbage, cored and shredded
- 1 Granny Smith apple, peeled, cored, and thinly sliced
- 2 teaspoons ground cinnamon

  Zest of 1 orange (optional)
- 1 tablespoon red wine vinegar

  Salt

1. In a large saucepan, heat the coconut oil over medium heat. Add the onion and cabbage and cook until softened.

2. Stir in the apple, cinnamon, and orange zest (if using) and cook for 2 to 4 minutes more, until the apples are softened.

3. Stir in the vinegar and season with salt.

PER SERVING (6 SERVINGS)

Cal: 86
Pro: 2g
Carb: 7g
Fat: 5g

Cauliflower Rice

Makes 6 to 8 cups · AIP

A staple in Paleo and low-carb circles, "riced" cauliflower is a great substitute for times when you want something to help sop up sauces or juices or when you'd like to add a little texture to soups and stews.

. . . .

1 head cauliflower, core and green leaves removed, coarsely chopped

PER SERVING (6 SERVINGS)

Cal: 24
Pro: 2g
Carb: 3g
Fat: .1g

To rice with a food processor:

- Using the chopping blade of the processor: Put one-third to half the cauliflower florets in the work bowl and pulse until the desired consistency is achieved. Do not overprocess into mush. Transfer to a large bowl, then repeat with the remaining cauliflower.

- Using the shredding blade: Put some of the florets in the feed tube of the processor and pulse. Repeat until all the cauliflower is used. If your head of cauliflower is particularly large, you may need to remove some of the riced cauliflower from the work bowl before finishing the entire head.

To rice with a box grater:

- Keep the pieces of cauliflower large, and simply shred on the small or medium holes of the grater (whichever your preference). Be forewarned that this technique usually results in bits of cauliflower going all over the kitchen.

Chicken Alfredo

Serves 6 to 8 · AIP

- 2 cups cauliflower florets
- 2 tablespoons olive oil
- 2 tablespoons coconut oil or butter
- 1 sweet onion, chopped
- 2 garlic cloves, minced
- 1 teaspoon sea salt
- 1 cup chicken stock
- ½ cup coconut milk
- Juice of 1 lime
- ½ teaspoon capers
- 12 ounces button mushrooms, sliced
- 2 pounds cooked chicken, cut into ½-inch cubes
- 4 to 6 medium zucchini, julienned or spiralized
- ¼ cup coarsely chopped fresh parsley

1. Preheat the oven to 400°F.

2. Toss the cauliflower with the olive oil and spread it over a baking sheet. Roast for 10 minutes, stirring once.

3. Meanwhile, in a large skillet, heat 1 tablespoon of the coconut oil over medium-high heat. Add the onion and cook until translucent. Stir in the garlic and cook for 1 minute more.

4. Transfer the onions and garlic to a blender and add the roasted cauliflower, salt, stock, coconut milk, lime juice, and capers. Blend until thoroughly combined and set aside.

5. Return the skillet to the stove and heat the remaining 1 tablespoon coconut oil over medium heat. Add the mushrooms and cook for 3 to 5 minutes, or until softened. Stir in the chicken to heat through.

6. Serve the chicken and mushrooms over a bed of raw zucchini and top with the sauce. Garnish with the parsley.

PER SERVING (6 SERVINGS)

Cal: 293
Pro: 35g
Carb: 4g
Fat: 14g

Chicken Soup

Serves 6 to 8 · AIP

Mix in some kale or spinach if you'd like to add more green veggies to your life. You can also add some cauliflower rice (page 254) to make this more of a chicken and rice soup.

. . . .

¼ cup bacon fat, coconut oil, or other fat

1 large onion, sliced

4 garlic cloves, minced

1 large parsnip, peeled and coarsely chopped

2 carrots, chopped

4 celery stalks, chopped

1 cup fresh parsley, chopped

1 tablespoon dried chives

1 bay leaf

4 cups chicken stock

2 pounds cooked chicken, shredded, or 2 pounds raw chicken breasts or thighs, cut into bite-size pieces

Sea salt

1. In a large Dutch oven or soup pot, melt the bacon fat over medium heat. Add the onion and cook for 5 to 7 minutes, or until translucent and softened.

2. Add garlic and parsnip and cook, stirring frequently, for 1 to 2 minutes more.

3. Add the carrots, celery, parsley, chives, bay leaf, stock, and chicken and bring to a boil. Reduce the heat to low and simmer, covered, for up to 1 hour.

4. Taste and season with salt.

PER SERVING (8 SERVINGS)

Cal: 282
Pro: 34g
Carb: 6g
Fat: 12g

Chicken Stir-Fry

Serves 6 to 8 · AIP WITH MODIFICATIONS

Serve over cauliflower rice (page 254).

. . . .

2   tablespoons coconut oil, avocado oil, or ghee

2   pounds boneless chicken breasts or thighs, cut into strips

1   yellow onion, chopped

1   bunch asparagus, trimmed and cut into 1-inch pieces

1   red bell pepper, seeded and chopped (omit if AIP)

1   garlic clove, minced

1   teaspoon minced fresh ginger

1   jicama, peeled and julienned

1   tablespoon orange zest

    Juice of 1 orange

2   tablespoons coconut aminos

1. In a large skillet or wok, heat the coconut oil over medium-high heat until shimmering. Add the chicken and cook, stirring frequently, for 5 to 7 minutes.

2. Add the onion and cook, stirring, until translucent and softened. Add the asparagus, bell pepper, garlic, ginger, jicama, orange zest, orange juice, and coconut aminos and cook until the liquid has reduced by half.

PER SERVING (8 SERVINGS)
Cal: 293
Pro: 35g
Carb: 5g
Fat: 12g

Chicken Stock

Makes 3 quarts

. . . .

3 pounds chicken bones, necks, feet, wings, carcass

1 fennel bulb, coarsely chopped

4 celery stalks, chopped

3 carrots, chopped

3 quarts distilled water

2 bay leaves

½ cup loosely packed fresh parsley, chopped

4 or 5 sprigs fresh thyme

1. Place all the ingredients in a slow cooker and cook on High for 6 to 8 hours; the longer you cook, the more intense the flavor will be.

2. Strain the stock through a sieve and discard the solids. Store in jars in the refrigerator for up to 4 days, or freeze for later use.

PER SERVING (1 CUP)

Cal: 86
Pro: 6g
Carb: 8g
Fat: 3g

Chicken Tikka Masala

Serves 4 to 6

Try this dish over cauliflower rice (page 254).

. . . .

1½ pounds boneless skinless chicken thighs or breasts, cut into bite-size pieces

¾ cup unsweetened coconut yogurt (or Greek yogurt if you tolerate dairy, or coconut cream if you can't find either)

1 tablespoon plus 2 teaspoons garam masala

2 teaspoons ground turmeric

2 tablespoons ghee, coconut oil, or olive oil

1 onion, minced

1 tablespoon tomato paste

1 teaspoon ground ginger, or 1 tablespoon grated fresh ginger

3 garlic cloves, minced

1. In a bowl, combine the chicken, yogurt, 2 teaspoons of the garam masala, and 1 teaspoon of the turmeric and marinate in the refrigerator for at least 30 minutes.

2. In a large deep-sided skillet or Dutch oven, heat the ghee over medium heat. Add the onion and cook, stirring, for 5 to 7 minutes, or until the onion is translucent and softened.

3. Stir in the tomato paste, the remaining 1 tablespoon garam masala, remaining 1 teaspoon turmeric, the ginger, and the garlic. Cook for 3 to 4 minutes, until fragrant.

4. Add the okra and cook for a few minutes more, until slightly softened.

5. Add the chicken along with the marinade (you will be cooking this), stir to combine well, and cook for 5 minutes to brown the chicken.

6. Using your hands, squeeze the tomato pieces as you add them to the pan, releasing some of the juices. Stir in the red pepper flakes (if using), coconut milk, and salt.

(continued)

1 pound okra, thinly sliced on an angle

3 tomatoes, coarsely chopped

¼ teaspoon red pepper flakes (optional)

1 cup coconut milk or heavy cream

½ teaspoon salt

¼ cup fresh cilantro, minced

PER SERVING (6 SERVINGS)

Cal: 457
Pro: 40g
Carb: 11.2g
Fat: 27g

7. Bring the mixture to a simmer and cook for 8 to 10 minutes, or until the chicken is cooked through. Taste and adjust the seasoning as needed.

8. Serve garnished with the cilantro.

Chicken Tortilla-Less Soup

Serves 6 to 8

. . . .

2 tablespoons coconut oil or olive oil

2 pounds chicken breasts or thighs

2 quarts chicken stock

1 (28-ounce) can fire-roasted tomatoes (you can also fire-roast your own, or use canned tomatoes)

1 large onion, diced

6 garlic cloves, minced

2 jalapeños, seeded and diced

2 poblano peppers, seeded and diced

1 teaspoon garlic powder

1 teaspoon ground cumin

½ teaspoon cayenne pepper

1 teaspoon chili powder

1 cup fresh cilantro, chopped, plus more for garnish

Juice of 2 limes

Sliced avocado

1. In a large Dutch oven or soup pot, heat 1 tablespoon of the coconut oil over medium-high heat. Add the chicken and brown for 3 to 5 minutes on each side. Add the chicken stock and tomatoes and bring to a boil. Reduce the heat to maintain a simmer and cook for 20 to 30 minutes, or until the chicken is cooked through.

2. Using a slotted spoon, transfer the chicken pieces to a cutting board and use two forks to shred the chicken.

3. While the chicken is cooking, in a large skillet, heat the remaining 1 tablespoon coconut oil over medium-high heat. Add the onion and sauté for 4 to 6 minutes, until translucent.

4. Add the minced garlic, jalapeños, poblanos, garlic powder, cumin, cayenne, and chili powder and sauté for 1 to 2 minutes, until fragrant. Transfer the mixture to the soup pot and stir to combine.

5. If desired, to thicken the soup, use a slotted spoon to transfer some of the tomatoes, onions, and peppers to a blender or food processor and puree. Pour back into the broth mixture.

(continued)

6. Add the chicken, cilantro, and lime juice to the pot. Taste and adjust the seasoning as needed.

7. When ready to serve, divide cilantro and avocado evenly among the bowls for garnish.

Note: Instead of the individual spices, you can substitute 1 tablespoon of your favorite taco or fajita seasoning. See page 250 for suggestions.

Cioppino

Serves 6 to 8 · AIP WITH MODIFICATIONS

. . . .

2 tablespoons olive oil
or coconut oil

1 fennel bulb, chopped

1 onion, chopped

1 teaspoon kosher salt

½ teaspoon dried
oregano

½ teaspoon dried basil

3 or 4 garlic cloves,
chopped

2 bay leaves

2 cups diced tomatoes
(see Note)

1 (8-ounce) bottle
clam juice

1 cup dry white wine
(optional)

6 cups fish stock or
chicken stock

1 pound clams or
mussels, scrubbed

½ pound baby scallops

½ pound shrimp,
peeled

½ pound halibut, cut
into 1-inch pieces

¼ cup fresh flat-leaf
parsley, chopped

1. In a large pot, heat the olive oil over medium-high heat. Add the fennel, onion, and salt and cook for 5 to 7 minutes, or until the onion is translucent.

2. Add the oregano, basil, garlic, bay leaves, tomatoes, clam juice, wine (if using), and stock. Bring to a simmer, reduce the heat to low, and cover. Simmer for 20 to 25 minutes.

3. Add the clams, scallops, shrimp, and halibut, cover, and cook, stirring occasionally, for 5 minutes more. Discard any unopened clams.

4. Serve in large bowls garnished with the parsley.

Note: Substitute 2 cups Fauxmato Sauce (page 333) for the diced tomatoes if following AIP.

> **PER SERVING (6 SERVINGS)**
>
> Cal: 243
> Pro: 30g
> Carb: 12g
> Fat: 6g

Coconut Cream Drops

Makes about 8 tablespoon-size drops per variation

Because sometimes you want a sweetish little treat. If you prefer, you can use melted butter instead of coconut oil for any variation.

. . . .

CITRUS DROPS

AIP

2 tablespoons coconut oil

6 tablespoons coconut butter

1 teaspoon orange, lemon, or lime zest

1 tablespoon fresh orange, lemon, or lime juice (use whatever citrus you zested)

¼ teaspoon vanilla extract

PER SERVING (8 SERVINGS)
Cal: 117
Pro: 8g
Carb: 2g
Fat: 11g

CHOCOLATE MINT DROPS

2 tablespoons coconut oil

6 tablespoons coconut butter

2 ounces dark chocolate chips (at least 60% cacao), melted

1½ teaspoons unsweetened cocoa powder

½ teaspoon peppermint or spearmint extract

PER SERVING (8 SERVINGS)
Cal: 150
Pro: 1.6g
Carb: 3.3g
Fat: 14.2g

CHOCOLATE BACON DROPS

2 tablespoons coconut oil

6 tablespoons coconut butter

1 bacon slice, cooked and chopped into small bits

2 ounces dark chocolate chips (at least 60% cacao), melted

PER SERVING (8 SERVINGS)
Cal: 163
Pro: 2.4g
Carb: 3.3g
Fat: 15.1g

1. For each variation, put the coconut oil and butter in a microwave-safe bowl and microwave for about 30 seconds, stirring to combine as they melt.

2. Mix in the remaining ingredients, then evenly distribute the mixture among some small candy molds or mini-muffin cups. Set aside to harden before serving.

Creamy Chicken and Vegetables

Serves 4 to 6 · AIP

. . . .

2 tablespoons olive oil, coconut oil, or other cooking fat

½ onion, diced

2 cups mushrooms, sliced

2 garlic cloves, minced

1½ pounds chicken (breast or thighs)

1 pound zucchini or yellow squash, cut into half-moons about ¼ inch thick

1 cup coconut milk

½ cup chicken stock

2 cups fresh spinach

¼ cup loosely packed fresh basil leaves, chopped

1. In a large skillet or frying pan, heat the olive oil over medium-high heat. Add the onion and sauté for 5 minutes, or until softened and slightly browned.

2. Add the mushrooms, garlic, and chicken and cook, stirring, for about 5 minutes more, until the mushrooms are slightly softened and the chicken is browned on the exterior.

3. Stir in the zucchini, coconut milk, stock, spinach, and basil, cover, and simmer for 10 minutes, or until the chicken is cooked through.

PER SERVING (6 SERVINGS)

Cal: 421
Pro: 37g
Carb: 6g
Fat: 28g

Crispy-Skin Salmon with Asian-Style Vegetables

Serves 4 to 6 · AIP WITH MODIFICATIONS

- 3 tablespoons coconut aminos
- 1 teaspoon sesame oil (omit if AIP)
- 2 tablespoons rice vinegar
- 2 teaspoons fish sauce
- 1 (1-inch) piece fresh ginger, peeled and minced
- 2 garlic cloves, minced
- 1½ pounds skin-on wild-caught salmon fillets (4 to 6 fillets), at room temperature
- Salt and black pepper (omit pepper if AIP)
- 2 tablespoons coconut oil or olive oil
- 3½ ounces fresh shiitake mushrooms, stems removed, sliced
- 4 cups baby bok choy, chopped
- 1 tablespoon arrowroot starch

1. Combine the coconut aminos, sesame oil, vinegar, and fish sauce in a small bowl. Add about 2 teaspoons each of the ginger and garlic and set aside.

2. Place the salmon pieces on a paper towel–lined plate and pat dry on all sides. Liberally season each side with salt and pepper.

3. In a large stainless steel skillet, heat 1 tablespoon of the coconut oil over high heat until almost smoking. Add the salmon pieces, skin-side down, and swirl the pan for 20 to 30 seconds. Press down on each piece of fish to ensure the entire skin is in contact with the skillet (salmon skin will shrink up some upon being in contact with the heat). Cook, undisturbed, for 6 to 8 minutes, or until salmon easily releases from the pan. Flip and cook for a minute or two more on the other side. Transfer to a plate, skin-side up.

(continued)

4. While the salmon is cooking, in another large skillet or wok, heat the remaining 1 tablespoon coconut oil over medium-high heat. Add the remaining garlic and ginger, the mushrooms, and the bok choy. Stir and cook for 3 to 5 minutes, or until the mushrooms are softened.

5. Pour in the coconut amino mixture and stir to combine. Cook for about 2 minutes more.

6. In a small bowl, stir together the arrowroot and 3 tablespoons water to make a slurry. Add the slurry to the skillet, stir, and cook for about 2 minutes, or until the mixture has a silky texture.

7. Serve the salmon fillets over the mushroom–bok choy mixture.

Fish Packets with Lime-Coconut Sauce

Serves 4 · AIP

Top each serving of fish with a pat or two of butter or a dollop of ghee if more fat is needed.

. . . .

¾ cup coconut milk

Zest of 2 limes

1 tablespoon fresh lime juice

2 tablespoons olive oil

2 small shallots, minced

1½ pounds zucchini and/or yellow squash, sliced into rounds

2 garlic cloves, minced

4 (6-ounce) pieces cod or any other mild white-fleshed fish

2 tablespoons chopped fresh basil

Salt and black pepper

1. Heat a grill to medium-high (about 400°F) or preheat the oven to 400°F.

2. In a small bowl, combine the coconut milk, lime zest, and lime juice and set aside.

3. Tear off four 12-inch pieces of aluminum foil. Fold each piece of foil in half and crease down the middle. Open the foil like a book and fold up some of the edges around one of the halves to help hold in the fluids. Drizzle that half with some of the olive oil. Repeat with the other pieces.

4. Evenly distribute the shallots and zucchini among the foil packets and sprinkle each packet with some of the garlic.

5. Place the cod on top of the vegetables and pour one-quarter of the coconut milk mixture over each packet. Divide the basil among the packets and liberally season with salt and pepper.

(continued)

PER SERVING

Cal: 407
Pro: 42g
Carb: 6g
Fat: 23g

6. Fold over the opposite side of the foil, then roll up the edges tightly to seal the packets. Flip over each packet (so the fish is covered with the veggies) and place on a baking sheet.

7. Grill or bake for 5 to 7 minutes, then flip over the packets and cook for 7 minutes more, or until the fish is cooked through and flakes easily (thicker pieces of fish may take longer).

8. Carefully open the packets (or cut a slit right through the middle). Use caution, as a lot of steam will emerge.

Flank Steak

Serves 6 to 8 · AIP

. . . .

2   garlic cloves, smashed

1   tablespoon fresh parsley, roughly chopped

1   tablespoon fresh oregano, roughly chopped

1   tablespoon fresh rosemary, roughly chopped

½   cup olive oil, plus more for the grill grates

¼   cup apple cider vinegar

2   pounds flank steak

PER SERVING (8 SERVINGS)

Cal: 334
Pro: 32g
Carb: 1g
Fat: 22g*

---

1. Put the garlic, parsley, oregano, rosemary, olive oil, and vinegar in a food processor and pulse to combine. Set aside about half the marinade.

2. Put the steak in a large zip-top bag or container and cover with the remaining marinade. Seal the bag or cover the container, and allow the steak to marinate in the refrigerator for 4 to 6 hours or overnight.

3. When ready to cook, let the meat come to room temperature. Heat a grill to medium-high and oil the grill grates.

4. Remove the steak from the bag and discard the bag and marinade.

5. Grill the steak for 4 to 6 minutes per side, depending on your desired doneness.

6. Brush the reserved marinade over the steak and transfer to a cutting board. Let the meat rest for 5 to 10 minutes.

7. Thinly slice the steak across the grain and serve.

The fat amount actually consumed will be far less than this, as half the marinade will be discarded.

Fried Brussels Sprouts

Serves 6 to 8 · AIP

. . . .

1 cup duck fat or coconut oil

2 pounds Brussels sprouts, trimmed, halved lengthwise, and patted dry

3 garlic cloves, thinly sliced

2 tablespoons balsamic vinegar

Sea salt

PER SERVING (8 SERVINGS)

Cal: 110g
Pro: 4g
Carb: 6g
Fat: 7g*

1. In a Dutch oven, melt the duck fat and heat until it registers about 400°F on a deep-fry thermometer.

2. Working in batches, carefully add the Brussels sprouts to the hot duck fat and cook until browned and crisp on the outside. Use a slotted spoon or spider to transfer the sprouts to a large bowl.

3. Repeat to cook the remaining sprouts, adding the garlic to the duck fat with the final batch of sprouts.

4. Pour the vinegar over the sprouts, season with salt, and stir. Serve warm.

Fat is assuming ¼ cup of the oil is retained and consumed (about 1½ teaspoons per serving).

Garlic-Cilantro Shrimp

Serves 4 to 6 · AIP

Adding a few tablespoons of butter and heavy cream or coconut milk makes this a creamy dish, and increases the fat quite a bit.

· ·

2 tablespoons coconut oil or ghee

3 tablespoons minced garlic

1½ pounds shrimp, peeled (tails left on) and deveined

½ teaspoon sea salt

¼ teaspoon ground turmeric

¼ cup fresh cilantro, chopped

Juice of 2 limes

1 lime, cut into wedges, for serving

1. In a large skillet, heat the coconut oil over medium heat. Add the garlic and cook for 1 minute.

2. Add in shrimp and sprinkle with the salt and turmeric.

3. When shrimp are starting to turn pink, add the cilantro and lime juice and cook until the shrimp are cooked through and the liquid has mostly cooked off.

4. Serve with the lime wedges.

PER SERVING (4 SERVINGS)

Cal: 271
Pro: 40g
Carb: 5g
Fat: 10g

Ginger Garlic Green Onion–Crusted Fish with Cream Sauce

Serves 4 · AIP WITH MODIFICATIONS AND WITHOUT SAUCE

This ginger garlic green onion crust is delicious on chicken, too. Serve warm, over cauliflower rice (page 254).

. . . .

2 to 3 tablespoons coarsely chopped fresh ginger

4 garlic cloves, coarsely chopped

½ cup coarsely chopped green onions

1 tablespoon olive oil

2 tablespoons coconut oil or olive oil

4 (6-ounce) skinless halibut or other firm white-fleshed fish fillets, patted dry and brought to room temperature

½ cup macadamia nuts, coarsely chopped (see Note)

Salt

1. Preheat the oven to 375°F.

2. Put the ginger, garlic, and green onions in a food processor and process until well combined. Add the olive oil and process until a smooth paste has formed. Set aside.

3. In a large ovenproof skillet, heat the coconut oil over medium-high heat until shimmering and just about to smoke. Add the fish, wiggling the pan as you place the pieces in the pan (this helps to prevent it from sticking). Sear for 3 to 5 minutes per side, or until the fish will easily release from the pan. Use a spatula to flip over each piece. Turn off the heat.

4. Coat the cooked side of the fish with the ginger-garlic paste. Sprinkle the nuts on top of the paste, pressing down lightly to help the nuts adhere to the paste. Place the pan in the oven and bake for 7 to 10 minutes, or until the fish is cooked through and the crust is slightly browned. Season with salt.

FOR THE CREAM SAUCE

- 1 shallot, minced
- 2 sprigs fresh thyme
- ¼ cup white wine (substitute with more white wine vinegar or chicken stock if desired)
- ¼ cup white wine vinegar
- ½ cup full-fat coconut milk or heavy cream
- ½ cup (1 stick) cold, unsalted butter, cut into 1-tablespoon pieces

5. To make the cream sauce, while the fish is in the oven, in a small saucepan, combine the shallot, thyme, wine, and vinegar and bring to a simmer. Cook until the liquid has almost completely reduced.

6. Add the coconut milk, stir, and bring the mixture to a boil. Use a slotted spoon to strain out and discard the shallots and thyme.

7. With the pan over medium heat, add the butter pieces one at a time, whisking after each addition until completely melted and incorporated.

8. Serve the fish with the sauce alongside.

Note: If AIP, instead of using the macadamia nuts, use ¾ to 1 cup crushed chicharrónes (pork rinds) for the "crunch" factor.

*To decrease the amount of fat, use less or no sauce (the sauce adds a total of about 30g of fat per serving).

Greek Kabobs with Tzatziki Sauce

Serves 6 to 8 · AIP

. . . .

FOR THE KABOBS

¼ cup olive oil, plus more for the grill grates

2 garlic cloves, minced

2 tablespoons fresh lemon juice

1 teaspoon red wine vinegar

1 teaspoon dried oregano

1 teaspoon dried basil

½ teaspoon salt

2 pounds boneless chicken breasts or thighs, cut into 1-inch cubes

2 bunches green onions, cut into 1-inch pieces

2 lemons, cut into slices

3 small zucchini, cut into ½-inch rounds

1. To make the kabobs, whisk together the olive oil, garlic, lemon juice, vinegar, oregano, basil, and salt in a large bowl.

2. Add the chicken and mix to coat well. Cover and marinate in the refrigerator for at least 30 minutes.

3. While the chicken is marinating, soak 8 to 12 large wooden skewers for at least 30 minutes to prevent burning.

4. Heat a grill to medium-high.

5. Thread the chicken, green onion, lemon, and zucchini pieces onto the skewers, alternating as you wish.

6. Lightly oil the grates and place the skewers on the grates. Cover and grill for 6 to 8 minutes per side, turning once.

FOR THE TZATZIKI

- 1 cup coconut milk yogurt or Greek yogurt
- 1 medium cucumber, peeled, seeded, and liquid squeezed out
- ½ teaspoon salt
- 1 garlic clove, mashed
- ¼ cup fresh lemon juice
- 1 tablespoon olive oil
- 2 tablespoons fresh flat-leaf parsley, roughly chopped
- ¼ cup fresh dill, roughly chopped

PER SERVING (8 SERVINGS)

Cal: 330
Pro: 37g
Carb: 5g
Fat: 17g

7. To make the tzatziki, combine all the tzatziki ingredients in a food processor and pulse to mix well. Serve alongside the skewers.

Grilled Strip Steaks

Serves 6 to 8 · AIP WITH MODIFICATIONS

- 2 pounds strip steak
- 1 teaspoon sea salt
- ¾ teaspoon garlic powder
- ¾ teaspoon ground fenugreek
- ¼ teaspoon onion powder
- ¾ teaspoon ground cinnamon
- ¾ teaspoon black pepper (omit if AIP)

1. Heat a grill to medium-high heat. Let the steaks come to room temperature and pat them dry with paper towels.

2. Combine the salt, garlic powder, fenugreek, onion powder, cinnamon, and pepper in a small bowl.

3. Liberally sprinkle both sides of the steaks with the seasoning mixture.

4. Grill the steaks for 4 to 5 minutes per side or to your desired doneness.

PER SERVING (8 SERVINGS)

Cal: 260
Pro: 25g
Carb: 0g
Fat: 18g

Guac-Stuffed Burgers (or Balls)

Serves 8 · AIP IF GUAC IS AIP-FRIENDLY

While these are stuffed with guacamole, you could just as easily stuff them with cheese or any filling of your choosing. The seasonings for the burger are kept simple, but you could spice up things by adding any flavors that suit your tastes.

2 pounds grass-fed ground beef

1 teaspoon garlic powder

1 teaspoon salt

1 cup Guacamole (page 334), with leftovers used for serving

1. Heat a grill to medium-high.

2. In a large bowl, mix together the beef, garlic powder, and salt. Do not overmix or the meat will be tough.

3. Divide the meat into 8 equal portions, then divide each individual portion in half and roll each piece into a ball.

4. Place a ball of meat on a flat surface (covered with foil or waxed paper is fine), cover with a piece of foil or waxed paper, and press down onto the patty with the bottom of a large mason jar or small skillet. You want the meat to be a uniform thickness, about ½ inch thick—not too thin, or it won't hold together. Repeat the flattening process with all the patties and place on a baking sheet.

(continued)

5. Spoon a tablespoon or so of the guacamole onto the center of one patty, cover with another patty, and carefully pinch together all the edges. Make sure it's totally sealed or your guacamole will ooze out. Repeat to make 8 stuffed burgers.

6. Grill for 6 to 8 minutes per side. Serve with additional guacamole.

Kitchen Sink Sauté

Serves 8 · AIP

This is a sample "kitchen sink" dish. Use what you have on hand or peruse your local grocery store or farmers' market for vegetables and seasonings that sound good to you. There are so many ways to change up this recipe. Use about 2 tablespoons curry paste and 2 cups coconut milk for a quick-and-easy curry, leaving out the herbs. Use a store-bought salsa (green or red) to make this more of a Mexican-inspired sauté. Use some canned artichokes, lemon juice, and olives instead of the other vegetables, along with extra oregano for an AIP-friendly sauté.

On your prep day, cook at least 2 pounds of ground beef (or any ground meat) to have on hand for the week. Then use it for this dish to make your life easier. Now you'll have dinner on the table in no time flat.

- 2 pounds ground grass-fed beef
- 1 tablespoon coconut oil or olive oil
- 1 onion, diced
- 2 garlic cloves, minced
- 1 12-ounce bag broccoli slaw, or 3 cups shredded broccoli stems
- 2 yellow squash, sliced into half-moons
- ¼ cup fresh parsley, minced
- 1 teaspoon dried oregano
- 1 cup beef stock or chicken stock
- ½ teaspoon salt
- ¼ cup ghee (optional)

1. Heat a large skillet over medium-high heat, and add the beef. Brown the beef, using a spoon to break apart the meat, stirring well. Remove the beef to a bowl.

2. In the same skillet, heat the coconut oil over medium heat. Add the onion and cook for 5 to 7 minutes, or until softened and translucent.

3. Add the beef, garlic, slaw, and squash to the skillet and cook for 3 to 5 minutes more, until heated through. Stir in the parsley, oregano, stock, and salt and cook for about 5 minutes more. Stir in the ghee at the end, if desired.

PER SERVING

Cal: 311
Pro: 36.6g
Carb: 3.8g
Fat: 15.5g

Lamb Chops

Serves 4 to 6 · AIP

- 2 tablespoons fresh rosemary
- 2 teaspoons fresh thyme
- 2 teaspoons sea salt
- 3 garlic cloves, minced
- ¼ cup olive oil
- 2 teaspoons orange zest
- 2 pounds lamb chops

PER SERVING (6 SERVINGS)

Cal: 301
Pro: 31g
Carb: 1g
Fat: 18g

1. Put the rosemary, thyme, salt, and garlic in a food processor and pulse to combine. Add the olive oil and orange zest and process until well combined.

2. Brush the herb paste on both side of the chops, set on a platter, cover, and marinate in refrigerator for 30 to 45 minutes or overnight.

3. When ready to cook, let the chops come to room temperature. Heat a grill to 450°F.

4. Grill the chops for 2 to 3 minutes per side, or until the desired doneness is reached.

Lemon-Herb Salmon

Serves 6 · AIP

. . . .

1   2-pound skin-on salmon fillet, cut evenly into 6 portions

1   tablespoon olive oil

2   garlic cloves, minced

½   teaspoon salt

2   tablespoons chopped fresh chives

¼   cup fresh dill, chopped

¼   cup fresh parsley, chopped

2   lemons, sliced

PER SERVING

Cal: 228
Pro: 30g
Carb: 2g
Fat: 12g

---

1. Preheat the oven to 450°F. Line a baking sheet with parchment paper.

2. Use paper towels to dry the salmon fillets and place them skin-side down on the prepared baking sheet.

3. Combine the olive oil with the garlic, then brush on top of each fillet.

4. Sprinkle the fillets with the salt and herbs, and top each one with a few lemon slices.

5. Bake for 8 to 12 minutes or until the salmon flakes easily.

Mashed Cauliflower

Serves 6 to 8 · AIP

. . . .

2   cups chicken stock

1   large head
    cauliflower, cored
    and chopped

1   garlic clove, minced

1   teaspoon fresh
    rosemary

    Salt

PER SERVING (8 SERVINGS)

Cal: 29
Pro: 2g
Carb: 3g
Fat: 0g

1. In a large pot or Dutch oven, bring the stock to a boil. Add the cauliflower, garlic, and rosemary. Cover and simmer for 15 to 20 minutes, or until most of the liquid has cooked off.

2. Puree the cauliflower using an immersion blender or, working in batches, transfer it to a food processor and puree. Season with salt.

VARIATIONS

Roasted Garlic Horseradish Mash

Preheat the oven to 400°F. Cut the top off a head of garlic and set the head in an 8-inch square of aluminum foil. Top the garlic with 1 teaspoon olive oil and enclose the head in the foil. Roast for 35 to 40 minutes. This can be done while you're preparing the cauliflower as directed. Omit the fresh garlic. Instead, after the cauliflower is done cooking, mix in 4 cloves roasted garlic and 1 table-spoon horseradish and puree as directed. Reserve the remaining garlic for other recipes.

Bacon Chive Mash

Prepare as above, mixing in a few slices of crumbled cooked bacon and 2 teaspoons minced fresh chives after pureeing the cauliflower.

Meatza

Serves 6 to 8 · AIP

Feel free to replace the Fauxmato Sauce with tomato sauce if you're not following AIP, and use other toppings as you like that fit your dietary needs (including peppers and pepperoni if you don't have to be on the AIP).

. . . .

2   pounds ground beef

2   teaspoons kosher salt

2   teaspoons garlic powder

1   teaspoon dried marjoram

1   teaspoon dried thyme

2   teaspoons dried oregano

2   cups Fauxmato Sauce (page 333)

½   cup sliced sweet onion

½   cup mushrooms, sliced

½   cup Kalamata olives, pitted and sliced

1. Preheat the oven to 350°F.

2. In a bowl, combine the beef, 1 teaspoon of the salt, the garlic powder, marjoram, thyme, and oregano and mix well.

3. Divide the meat mixture into 8 equal balls and press each into a disc about ½ inch thick. This will be the crust. Set the discs on a rimmed baking sheet and bake for 15 to 18 minutes. Remove from oven and drain off any liquid.

4. Sprinkle the remaining 1 teaspoon salt on the meat crusts and cover each with ¼ cup of the Fauxmato Sauce.

5. Top each pizza with some of the onion, mushrooms, and olives.

6. Return to the oven for 6 to 10 minutes to cook the vegetables.

PER SERVING (8 SERVINGS)

Cal: 259
Pro: 36g
Carb: 4g
Fat: 10g

Oven-Roasted Brisket

Serves 8 to 10 or more (depends on the fat cap and how much is not meat) · AIP

1 tablespoon kosher salt

2 teaspoons garlic powder

2 tablespoons prepared horseradish

2 teaspoons tamarind paste

1 (3-pound) beef brisket

2 tablespoons olive oil, coconut oil, or ghee

3 leeks, white part only, cleaned very well and sliced

1 cup beef stock, plus more if needed

¼ cup coconut aminos

¼ cup apple cider vinegar

PER SERVING (10 SERVINGS)

Cal: 301
Pro: 42g
Carb: 4g
Fat: 12g

1. Preheat the oven to 300°F.

2. Combine salt, garlic powder, horseradish, and tamarind paste in a bowl. Cover the brisket with the mixture and set aside.

3. While the brisket is marinating, in a large ovenproof roasting pan, heat the olive oil on the stovetop over medium-high heat (see Note). Add the leeks and cook until they begin to brown a bit. Add the stock and deglaze the pan, scraping up any browned bits. Add the coconut aminos and vinegar to the roasting pan and evenly distribute the leeks.

4. Place brisket fat-side up on top of the leeks and cover the pan tightly with aluminum foil. Roast in the oven for about 5 hours, checking after a few hours. If the leeks are looking too dried out, add a cup of water or beef stock.

5. Remove from oven and place the brisket on a cutting board to rest for 10 to 15 minutes. Slice the meat across the grain and serve with the pan sauce and leeks spooned on top of slices.

Note: If you don't have a roasting pan, use a large skillet to sauté the leeks. Once you deglaze the skillet, pour everything into a casserole dish for the oven and cover tightly.

Pork Chips

Makes 30 to 40 chips · AIP WITH MODIFICATIONS

These make a great snack or a wonderful chip for dips and guacamole.

. . . .

6 ounces thinly sliced prosciutto, cut into 2-inch pieces

1 teaspoon of your favorite spice blend (chipotle powder, chili powder, Cajun seasoning, Old Bay seasoning, etc.; see Note), optional

PER SERVING (4 CHIPS)

Cal: 41
Pro: 6g
Carb: 0g
Fat: 2g

1. Preheat the oven to 250°F. Line three or four baking sheets with wire racks.

2. Arrange the prosciutto pieces on the racks and sprinkle with any desired herbs or spices (do not use salt, as prosciutto is salty enough).

3. Bake for 20 to 25 minutes, or until crispy.

4. Remove from the oven, let cool completely, and store in an airtight container.

Note: If you are following the AIP, be cautious in your spice selection.

Pork Chops with Peach Chutney and Roasted Okra

Serves 4 to 6 · AIP WITH MODIFICATIONS

. . . .

FOR THE OKRA

- 1 pound okra, stem ends removed, halved lengthwise
- 1 tablespoon olive oil
- 1 teaspoon salt

FOR THE CHUTNEY

- 2 fresh peaches, pitted, peeled, and sliced
- 2 teaspoons apple cider vinegar
- ½ teaspoon ground ginger

FOR THE PORK

- 1½ pounds pork chops or cutlets
- 1 teaspoon salt
- ½ teaspoon white pepper (omit if AIP)
- 1 tablespoon coconut oil, lard, or other cooking fat

1. To make the okra, preheat the oven to 425°F.

2. In a large bowl, toss the okra with the olive oil and salt. Spread the okra on a large baking sheet and place in the oven. Roast for about 15 minutes, stirring every 5 to 7 minutes, until the okra is nicely browned.

3. To make the chutney, place the peaches and 2 tablespoons water in a small saucepan and bring to a simmer over medium-high heat, mushing down the peaches with a fork or spoon to break them apart. Add the vinegar and ginger and cook for 5 to 7 minutes; the longer you cook it, the thicker the chutney will be. (The chutney can be made up to a few days in advance and stored in an airtight container in the refrigerator.)

4. To make the pork, liberally season all sides of the pork with the salt and pepper.

PER SERVING (6 SERVINGS)

Cal: 447
Pro: 27g
Carb: 6g
Fat: 33g

5. In a large ovenproof skillet, heat the oil over medium-high heat, swirling to coat the pan. Add the pork chops and cook about 2 to 3 minutes per side, until a nice brown crust has formed. Turn over and repeat on the other side. You may need to work in batches if your chops are very thin.

6. Place all the chops in the skillet and cook for 10 to 12 minutes, or until the internal temperature of the pork reaches 140°F (once removed and resting, the pork will reach an internal temperature of 145°F).

7. Top each chop with some of the peach chutney and serve alongside the okra.

Pork Tenderloin and Roasted Asparagus with Hollandaise

Serves 6 to 8 · AIP WITHOUT HOLLANDAISE

. . . .

2   tablespoons olive oil, plus more for skillet

2   tablespoons fresh rosemary, or 2 teaspoons dried

3   garlic cloves, minced

2   teaspoons sea salt

2   pounds pork tenderloin (about 2 tenderloins), trimmed of silver skin

2   pounds asparagus, tough ends removed

2   recipes 5-Minute Hollandaise Sauce (page 325)

PER SERVING (8 SERVINGS WITHOUT HOLLANDAISE)

Cal: 219
Pro: 32g
Carb: 3g
Fat: 8g

PER SERVING (8 SERVINGS WITH 2 TABLESPOONS HOLLANDAISE EACH)

Cal: 436
Pro: 33g
Carb: 2g
Fat: 32g

1. Preheat the oven to 400°F.

2. In a small bowl, combine 1 tablespoon of the olive oil, the rosemary, garlic, and 1 teaspoon of the salt and mash to create a paste. Rub the paste all over the tenderloins and set aside.

3. In a large bowl, toss the asparagus with the remaining 1 tablespoon olive oil and remaining 1 teaspoon salt. Place on a large baking sheet.

4. Heat a large skillet over medium-high heat. Swirl a little bit of oil into the pan.

5. Place the tenderloins in the pan and brown on all sides, 5 to 7 minutes.

6. Put the tenderloins on the baking sheet, moving the asparagus so that no stalks are directly under the pork. Roast for 8 to 10 minutes, or until an instant-read thermometer inserted into the thickest part of the tenderloin registers 140 to 145°F. Remove from the oven and let rest for 5 to 10 minutes before slicing.

7. Serve the pork with the asparagus alongside. Top the asparagus with hollandaise.

Pork Cutlets or Chops with Cauliflower Medley

Serves 3 or 4 · AIP WITH MODIFICATIONS

- 1 tablespoon coconut oil, olive oil, or ghee
- 1 pound pork cutlets or pork chops, ½ inch thick or less

  Salt and black pepper (omit pepper if AIP)
- 1 yellow onion, sliced
- 2 garlic cloves, minced
- 1 tablespoon chopped fresh rosemary
- 1 cup sliced mushrooms
- ¼ cup sun-dried tomatoes, soaked in ½ cup boiling water (omit if AIP)
- 4 cups cauliflower florets
- 1 cup full-fat coconut milk

1. In a large skillet, heat the coconut oil over medium-high heat.

2. Liberally sprinkle the pork chops with salt and pepper. Add the chops to the skillet and brown for 3 to 4 minutes on each side to create a nice brown crust. Transfer the chops to a plate.

3. Reduce the heat to medium and add the onion to the pan, stirring to scrape up any of the browned bits from the chops. Stir in the garlic, rosemary, and mushrooms. Cook for 3 to 5 minutes more.

4. Add in the sun-dried tomatoes, cauliflower florets, and coconut milk. Place the pork chops on top of the cauliflower, cover, and simmer for 10 minutes, or until the cauliflower is softened and cooked through. Serve the pork chops alongside or on top of the cauliflower.

PER SERVING (4 SERVINGS)

Calories: 583
Pro: 30g
Carbs: 11g
Fat: 46.3g

Prime Rib

Serves 10 to 12

. . . .

1 (6-pound) standing rib roast

2 tablespoons kosher salt

¼ cup fresh rosemary, minced

1 tablespoon minced fresh oregano

4 tablespoons coconut oil, olive oil, or ghee

PER SERVING
(10 SERVINGS; ABOUT
6 OUNCES EACH)

Cal: 482
Pro: 39
Carb: 0g
Fat: 39

1. Let the roast come to room temperature. Use paper towels to pat the roast dry, then liberally season with 1 tablespoon of the salt.

2. In a small bowl, combine the rosemary, oregano, and 2 tablespoons of the coconut oil. Mix to combine.

3. Preheat the oven to 325°F.

4. In a large flameproof roasting pan, heat the remaining 2 tablespoons coconut oil over medium-high heat. Add the roast and sear on all sides until browned. Place the roast bone-side down in the roasting pan and coat the meat on all sides with the herb paste.

5. Bake for 90 to 120 minutes, or until the internal temperature reaches 120 to 130°F (longer if you prefer your meat more well done).

6. Let the meat rest for 10 to 15 minutes before slicing and serving.

Roasted Bok Choy

Serves 4 to 6 · AIP

If you cannot find baby bok choy, standard (larger) bok choy will work, too, but you will want to cut it into smaller pieces.

. . . .

4   heads baby bok choy, halved lengthwise

¼   cup olive oil

1   teaspoon kosher salt

½   teaspoon ground turmeric

2   tablespoons balsamic vinegar

1. Preheat the oven to 350°F.

2. Place the bok choy cut-side up on a baking sheet. Drizzle with the olive oil and sprinkle with the salt and turmeric.

3. Roast for 10 to 15 minutes, turning once.

4. Serve with a splash of the vinegar on each.

PER SERVING (6 SERVINGS)

Cal: 146
Pro: 8g
Carb: 7g
Fat: 4g

Roasted Broccoli and Cauliflower

Serves 6 to 8 · AIP WITH MODIFICATIONS

These veggies are delicious tossed in butter after cooking, or drizzled with some of the creamy dressings on pages 325–332. If not following AIP, sprinkle some cumin or smoked paprika on the vegetables to change up the flavor profile.

· ·

1 head cauliflower, cored and cut into florets (about 3 cups)

2 heads broccoli, cut into florets (about 4 cups)

¼ cup olive oil

5 garlic cloves, minced

1 teaspoon salt

½ teaspoon black pepper (omit if AIP)

1. Preheat the oven to 450°F.

2. Combine the cauliflower and broccoli in a large bowl and toss with the olive oil and garlic.

3. Spread out the vegetables on a large baking sheet and sprinkle with the salt and pepper.

4. Roast for 15 to 20 minutes, or until the vegetables are somewhat tender and slightly browned.

PER SERVING (6 SERVINGS)

Cal: 109
Pro: 3g
Carb: 5g
Fat: 9g

Rotisserie-Like Chicken

Serves 3 or 4

. . . .

1 (4- to 5-pound)
  whole chicken,
  giblets and neck
  (if yours came with
  them) removed
  from the cavity,
  patted dry

2 tablespoons butter
  or olive oil

  Seasoning blend of
  your choice (recipes
  follow)

  Salt

PER SERVING (4 SERVINGS)

Cal: 357
Pro: 41g
Carb: 0g
Fat: 20g

---

1. Rub the entire chicken with the butter and then rub with the seasonings/aromatics you choose and salt, always being sure to season inside the cavity, too.

2. Put some balled-up pieces of aluminum foil, a rack, or some large pieces of onion or lemon into the bottom of a large slow cooker. This will elevate the chicken.

3. Place the chicken breast-side down in the slow cooker on top of the foil/rack/vegetables and cook on Low for 6 to 8 hours or High for 4 to 6 hours, or until an instant-read thermometer inserted into the thickest part of the thigh without touching bone registers 155 to 160°F.

4. Remove the chicken from the slow cooker and place it breast-side up in a roasting pan. For crispy skin, place under a broiler set to high for about 5 minutes.

garlic herb seasoning

. . . .

3   garlic cloves, minced

2   teaspoons salt

1 to 2   teaspoons dried thyme, rosemary, poultry seasoning, or any other herbs

In a small bowl, mix all the ingredients together and set aside.

garlic paprika seasoning

. . . .

1   tablespoon smoked paprika

2   teaspoons salt

1   teaspoon garlic powder

In a small bowl, mix all the ingredients together and set aside.

lemon rosemary seasoning

. . . .

1   lemon, juiced and cut into pieces

3   sprigs fresh rosemary

In a small bowl, mix all the ingredients together and set aside.

Satay Skillet

Serves 6 to 8

Shrimp or beef would work well here in place of the chicken, though if using shrimp, marinate them for no more than 30 minutes. Yam noodles (*shirataki*) work great in this recipe, or if you want a cold salad to serve, you could use cold cucumber "noodles." Simply remove the chicken mixture from the heat after step 4, then mix with about 4 julienned/spiralized cucumbers, the green onions, and the sauce. Refrigerate until ready to serve.

1 tablespoon red curry paste

2 cups coconut milk

½ cup sunflower seed or almond butter (unsweetened)

2 teaspoons fish sauce

2 teaspoons lime juice

1 tablespoon honey (optional)

2 pounds chicken breasts or thighs, sliced into strips

1 tablespoon coconut or olive oil

2 red bell peppers, seeded and sliced (omit if AIP)

3 zucchini or squash, julienned or spiralized

4 green onions, white and green parts thinly sliced

1. In a medium bowl, combine the curry paste, coconut milk, sunflower seed butter, fish sauce, lime juice, and honey (if using). Stir to combine well (or use a food processor or blender to combine).

2. Place the chicken pieces into a zip-top bag or container with a lid and pour ½ cup of the sauce over the top. Stir to combine well. Seal the bag or cover the container, and marinate in the refrigerator for at least 30 minutes or overnight.

3. In a large skillet or wok, heat the oil over medium-high heat. When hot, add the chicken and stir. Cook for 5 to 7 minutes, or until the chicken is mostly cooked through.

4. Reduce the heat to medium and add the peppers (if using) and cook for a few minutes to slightly soften.

(continued)

PER SERVING (8 SERVINGS)

Cal: 480
Pro: 40g
Carb: 9.4
Fat: 29.7g

5. Stir in the zucchini, green onions, and reserved sauce. Stir to combine and cook for just a few minutes longer to slightly cook the zucchini (not too long—you don't want the zucchini to be mushy).

Sausage and Egg "Sandwiches"

Serves 4

If you prefer to keep the egg yolks intact, feel free, or for a more scrambled egg, whisk all the eggs in a spouted measuring cup first, then pour them into the egg molds to cook. If you want to get more veggies into your life, you could also use bell peppers as the "rings" to contain your eggs. Simply remove the top and bottom of any peppers, and remove the core and seeds. Slice into ½- to ¾-inch-thick slices and use as you would the egg rings.

2   tablespoons coconut or olive oil, plus more for greasing

¾   pound bulk sausage, formed into 4 patties

1   garlic clove, minced

2   cups fresh spinach, coarsely chopped

½   teaspoon salt

8   large eggs

1. Grease the inside of eight egg rings or eight Mason jar lids (about 3 inches in diameter). Set aside.

2. Heat a large cast-iron or other skillet over medium heat and add the sausage patties. Cook for 7 to 9 minutes on the first side, flip, and add about ½ cup water to the pan. Cover and cook for 5 minutes more, or until the sausage is cooked through.

3. Meanwhile, heat 1 tablespoon of the coconut oil in a large skillet over medium heat. When hot, add the garlic and the spinach and stir. Cook for 4 to 5 minutes, or until the spinach is softened. Transfer to a bowl and set aside.

(continued)

4. Wipe the skillet of any residue from the spinach and return it to the stovetop over medium heat. Add the remaining 1 tablespoon coconut oil and place the prepared egg rings or mason jar lids flat in the skillet. Crack one egg into each ring and use a fork to gently break up the egg yolk. Pour 1 to 2 cups water directly into the pan (not on top of the eggs), cover, and cook for 3 to 5 minutes, or until the eggs are cooked to your liking. Carefully remove the eggs from the molds (they will be hot), using a paring knife to loosen the egg from the edges of the mold.

5. To serve, place a sausage patty on each of 4 eggs, top with some of the spinach, and place another egg on top. Serve warm.

Sautéed Greens

Serves 6 to 8 · AIP WITH MODIFICATIONS

. . . .

½ pound bacon, diced (use AIP-friendly if AIP; see Note)

6 garlic cloves, sliced

4 cups coarsely chopped collards green leaves

2 cups coarsely chopped dandelion greens

4 cups coarsely chopped kale leaves

1 cup chicken stock

¼ cup olive oil

2 tablespoons balsamic vinegar

PER SERVING (8 SERVINGS)

Cal: 242
Pro: 13g
Carb: 5g
Fat: 19g

---

1. In a large pot, cook the bacon until crisp. Remove with a slotted spoon and set aside, keeping the bacon drippings in the pan.

2. Add garlic to the bacon drippings and cook for a minute, until fragrant.

3. Add the greens and stir until wilted. Pour in the stock and raise the heat to high. Cook, stirring frequently, until the liquid has cooked off.

4. Combine the olive oil and vinegar in a jar with a lid and shake well.

5. Sprinkle the oil and vinegar over the greens and garnish with the bacon bits.

Note: This dish can also be made without bacon. Just use ¼ cup olive oil instead of the bacon drippings to cook the garlic and greens.

Sautéed Mushrooms

Serves 4 to 6 · AIP

. . . .

3 tablespoons coconut oil, butter, or ghee

1 pound button mushrooms, sliced

2 garlic cloves, thinly sliced

½ cup beef stock

1 tablespoon coconut aminos

3 sprigs fresh thyme

Salt

1. In a large skillet, heat the coconut oil over medium heat. Add the mushrooms and cook for several minutes, until softened and lightly browned. Stir in the garlic and cook for 1 minute more.

2. Add the stock, coconut aminos, and thyme sprigs and cook for a few minutes more, until most of the liquid has cooked off. Season with salt. Discard the thyme sprigs before serving.

PER SERVING (4 SERVINGS)

Cal: 118
Pro: 4g
Carb: 3g
Fat: 10g

Savory Crispy Baked Chicken

Serves 4 to 8 · AIP

. . . .

3 pounds bone-in, skin-on chicken thighs and drumsticks

1 cup pickle juice (from a jar of pickles)

½ cup arrowroot powder

About 2 cups plain chicharrónes (pork rinds)

½ teaspoon garlic powder

½ teaspoon dried oregano

½ teaspoon dried thyme

¼ teaspoon dried rosemary

PER SERVING (4 SERVINGS)

Cal: 500
Pro: 40g
Carb: 0g
Fat: 35g

1. Put the chicken pieces in a large container or zip-top bag and pour over the pickle juice. Seal and marinate in the refrigerator for at least 30 minutes or overnight.

2. Preheat the oven to 375°F. Line a baking sheet with a wire rack.

3. Drain off the pickle juice and add the arrowroot powder to the bag or container with the chicken. Reseal the bag or container and massage the arrowroot powder onto/around the chicken.

4. In a food processor, pulse chicharrónes into a powder. Transfer to a bowl and stir in the garlic powder, oregano, thyme, and rosemary. Pour the mixture onto a large plate.

5. Working with one piece at a time, coat each chicken piece with the breading, being sure to press it firmly onto the chicken.

6. Place the chicken pieces on the prepared baking sheet and bake for 1 hour, or until the internal temperature of the chicken reaches 165°F and the juices run clear.

Seafood Chowder

Serves 6 to 8 · AIP WITH MODIFICATIONS

You want about 2 pounds total of seafood "meat" in this recipe. There may be bags of assorted fish/seafood at your local grocery store that would work well in this recipe. Just check to make sure they are wild caught or farmed responsibly.

. . . .

4   bacon (use AIP-friendly if AIP)

1   onion, minced

2   garlic cloves, minced

4   cups cauliflower florets

1½ cups chicken stock or fish stock

2   cups clam juice

2   cups coconut milk

1   teaspoon dried thyme

1   (10-ounce) can clams, drained

½   pound small sea scallops

1   pound wild-caught cod or other white-fleshed fish, cut into bite-size pieces

    Salt and black pepper (omit pepper if AIP)

PER SERVING (6 SERVINGS)
Cal: 361
Pro: 32g
Carb: 7.2g
Fat: 21g

1. In a large Dutch oven or soup pot, cook the bacon over medium-high heat until crispy, 6 to 8 minutes. Use a slotted spoon to transfer the bacon to a plate. Reserve the bacon drippings in the pan. Once the bacon has cooled, break into bite-size pieces.

2. Add the onion to the bacon drippings and cook over medium-high heat for 5 to 7 minutes, or until softened and translucent. Add the garlic, cauliflower, and stock, cover, and cook for 8 to 10 minutes more, or until the cauliflower is tender. Working in batches, transfer the contents of the pot to a blender. Cover the blender lid with a towel and while holding down the lid, puree (hot items in a blender can splatter all over your kitchen—use caution). Alternatively, puree the mixture directly in the pot using an immersion blender.

3. Return the puree to the pot (if necessary), set it over medium heat, and add the bacon pieces, clam juice, coconut milk, thyme, clams, scallops, and cod. Bring to a simmer and cook for 6 to 8 minutes, or until the cod is cooked through and flaky. Season with salt and pepper.

Seafood Stew

Serves 6 to 8 · AIP WITH MODIFICATIONS

. . . .

½ cup olive oil

1 pound monkfish, haddock, or sea bass, cut into bite-size pieces

2 leeks, cleaned well and coarsely chopped

3 garlic cloves, minced

1 cup white wine

4 cups fish, chicken, or vegetable stock

2 heads bok choy, leaves separated

2 tablespoons fresh tarragon leaves, chopped

1 to 2 tablespoons tomato paste (omit or use umeboshi paste if AIP)

½ pound crabmeat, picked over for shells

1 pound shrimp, peeled and deveined

Sea salt

1. In large heavy pot, heat ¼ cup of the olive oil over medium-high heat. Add the monkfish and sear on all sides, then transfer to a bowl and set aside.

2. Heat the remaining ¼ cup olive oil in the same pot. Add the leeks and garlic and cook for 3 to 5 minutes.

3. Pour the wine into the pot and stir, scraping up the browned bits from the bottom. When wine has nearly evaporated, add the stock, bok choy, tarragon, and tomato paste.

4. Bring to a boil, stirring frequently, then reduce the heat to maintain a simmer and cook for 10 to 15 minutes.

5. Return the monkfish to the pot, add the crabmeat and shrimp, and simmer until the shrimp are cooked through. Taste and season with salt as needed.

PER SERVING (6 SERVINGS)

Cal: 500
Pro: 40g
Carb: 0g
Fat: 35g

Shepherd's Pie

Serves 6 to 8 · AIP WITH MODIFICATIONS

. . . .

FOR THE CRUST

2 pounds parsnips, peeled and sliced

2 tablespoons olive oil

2 garlic cloves, mashed

1 teaspoon kosher salt

1 cup beef stock

FOR THE FILLING

2 tablespoons coconut oil

2 pounds ground lamb

1 onion, chopped

2 carrots, diced

3 garlic cloves, minced

1 cup button mushrooms, diced

2 zucchini, diced

2 tablespoons tomato paste (omit or use umeboshi paste if AIP)

½ cup beef stock

1 tablespoon minced fresh sage

2 teaspoons minced fresh rosemary

1 teaspoon dried oregano

1. Preheat the oven to 350°F.

2. To make the crust, on a large baking sheet, combine the parsnips with the olive oil. Roast for 20 to 25 minutes, turning once halfway.

3. Remove the pan from the oven and transfer the parsnips to a food processor. Add the garlic, salt, and half the stock. Process until smooth, adding more stock if needed to reach a mashed potato–like consistency. Set aside.

4. To make the filling, while the parsnips are cooking, in a large skillet, heat the coconut oil over medium heat. Add the lamb and cook, using a spoon to break it up, until cooked through and browned, about 8 minutes. Use a slotted spoon to transfer the lamb to a large bowl.

5. To the same skillet, add the onion and carrots and cook until the onion begins to soften.

6. Add the garlic, mushrooms, zucchini, and tomato paste and cook until the vegetables begin to brown and caramelize.

7. Pour in the stock, add the sage, rosemary, and oregano, and stir. Cook until very little liquid remains, 4 to 6 minutes.

8. Pour the vegetables into the bowl with the lamb and stir to combine.

9. Pour the filling into a 9 x 13-inch casserole dish, then top with the parsnip puree, using a spatula to evenly distribute it.

10. Bake for 15 to 20 minutes to incorporate the flavors.

Shrimp Kabobs

Serves 4 to 6 · AIP

. . . .

2 tablespoons coconut aminos

2 tablespoons olive oil

1 tablespoon honey

1 tablespoon fresh ginger, minced

2 garlic cloves, minced

½ teaspoon salt

1½ pounds shrimp, peeled (tails left on) and deveined

2 pounds pineapple, cut into 1-inch pieces

1 red onion, quartered

1 lemon, cut into wedges

1. Heat a grill to medium-high. Soak 8 to 12 bamboo skewers in water to prevent them from burning.

2. In a small bowl, stir together the coconut aminos, olive oil, honey, ginger, garlic, and salt.

3. Thread the shrimp, pineapple, and red onion pieces onto the skewers, alternating between them, and then liberally brush the marinade over all sides.

4. Grill for 2 to 4 minutes per side, until shrimp are pink and cooked through.

5. Serve with the lemon wedges.

PER SERVING (6 SERVINGS)

Cal: 235
Pro: 27g
Carb: 15g
Fat: 7g

Shrimp Stir-Fry

Serves 3 or 4

Serve over cauliflower rice (page 254).

. . . .

4 tablespoons coconut oil or ghee

1 pound shrimp, peeled and deveined

2 cups broccoli florets

2 cups button mushrooms, sliced

2 garlic cloves, minced

¼ cup chicken stock or fish stock

2 tablespoons coconut aminos

1 teaspoon Sriracha (omit if AIP)

2 tablespoons chopped fresh parsley

8 ounces sliced water chestnuts

Salt

1. In a wok or large skillet, heat 2 tablespoons of the coconut oil over medium-high heat. When hot, add the shrimp and cook for several minutes, until pink and cooked through. Remove from the pan and set aside.

2. Heat the remaining 2 tablespoons coconut oil in the same pan over medium-high heat. Add the broccoli and mushrooms and cook for 2 to 3 minutes. Stir in the garlic and cook for 1 minute more.

3. Pour in the stock and coconut aminos and stir. Cook for a few minutes, until the liquid has reduced and the broccoli is bright green and cooked to desired doneness. Stir in the Sriracha (if using), parsley, and water chestnuts. Return the cooked shrimp to the mixture, and stir to combine well. Season with salt.

PER SERVING (4 SERVINGS)

Cal: 368
Pro: 30g
Carb: 25g
Fat: 16g

Shrimp with Coconut-Lime Cauliflower Rice

Serves 6 to 8 · AIP WITH MODIFICATIONS

. . . .

2 tablespoons olive oil or melted ghee

Zest and juice of 2 limes

1 tablespoon fish sauce

3 garlic cloves, minced

4 tablespoons fresh cilantro, chopped

2 pounds wild-caught shrimp, peeled and deveined

1 head cauliflower, riced (see page 254; about 6 cups)

1½ cups coconut milk

½ cup chicken stock

3 green onions, green and white parts sliced

1 Thai chile, or ¼ teaspoon red pepper flakes (omit if AIP)

Salt and black pepper (omit pepper if AIP)

1. In a medium bowl, combine the olive oil, half the lime zest, half the lime juice, the fish sauce, garlic, and 2 tablespoons of the cilantro. Add the shrimp to the marinade and stir to coat. Marinate in the refrigerator for up to 30 minutes.

2. Heat a large skillet or wok over medium heat. Add the shrimp and cook until the shrimp are just starting to turn pink.

3. Stir in the cauliflower rice, coconut milk, stock, and the remaining lime zest, lime juice, and 2 tablespoons cilantro. Bring the mixture to a simmer and cook for 10 minutes, or until the liquid has mostly cooked off.

4. Stir in the green onions and chile. Season with salt and black pepper.

> **PER SERVING (8 SERVINGS)**
>
> Cal: 327
> Pro: 29g
> Carb: 7g
> Fat: 20g

Slow-Cooker Pork Butt

Serves 6 to 8 · AIP WITH MODIFICATIONS

It may sound crazy, but a pork butt will lose 40 to 50 percent of its weight in cooking and after removal of the bone. Since pulled pork is so delicious, it's always recommended to get a much bigger hunk of meat than you think you will need. Serve the pork in lettuce wraps, over a salad, or as a stand-alone protein.

. . . .

1 (4-pound) bone-in pork butt

Sea salt

2 teaspoons garlic powder

2 teaspoons juniper berries, crushed (omit if AIP)

Juice of 1 lime

PER SERVING (8 SERVINGS)

Cal: 230
Pro: 35g
Carb: 1g
Fat: 7g

1. Generously sprinkle the pork with salt and the garlic powder. Place in a slow cooker along with the crushed juniper berries.

2. Cover and cook on Low for 8 to 10 hours.

3. Once pork is fork-tender, transfer it to a cutting board. Remove the bone and use two forks to shred the pork (it's easiest to shred when it's still hot).

4. Squeeze the lime juice over pork and serve.

Slow-Cooker Pot Roast

Serves 6 to 8

Serve this pot roast over mashed cauliflower or potatoes.

. . . .

1   (3- to 4-pound) chuck roast

    Salt and black pepper

¼   cup coconut oil, lard, or other fat

1   large onion, chopped

4   celery stalks plus the heart, chopped into bite-size pieces

2   cups mushrooms, sliced

3   cups sliced parsnips

4   garlic cloves, mashed

2   cups diced tomatoes

2   cups beef stock

1   cup red wine

    Bouquet garni (a few sprigs each of fresh rosemary, oregano, and thyme, tied together with butcher twine)

1. Use paper towels to dry the chuck roast. Season it all over with salt and pepper.

2. In a large skillet, heat the coconut oil until almost smoking, then add the roast. Sear for a few minutes each side, until a nice brown crust has formed. Remove the meat from the skillet and set aside on a plate.

3. Add the chopped onion, celery, mushrooms, parsnips, and garlic to the skillet and cook for 3 to 5 minutes.

4. Transfer the vegetables to a slow cooker and set the meat on top.

5. Pour the tomatoes, stock, and wine into the slow cooker and add the bouquet garni.

6. Cook on Low for 6 to 8 hours, or until roast is fork-tender. Remove the bouquet garni before serving.

> **PER SERVING (8 SERVINGS)**
>
> Cal: 510
> Pro: 58g
> Carb: 9g
> Fat: 21g

Spaghetti Squash Pesto Casserole

Serves 4 to 6 · AIP WITH MODIFICATIONS

Instead of the pesto, use 1 to 2 cups of your favorite marinara sauce (not AIP), or try using a few tablespoons of buffalo sauce.

. . . .

1 spaghetti squash

½ cup olive oil, plus more for greasing

1 cup lightly packed fresh basil

¼ cup pine nuts, walnuts, or other nuts of your choosing (see Note)

Juice of ½ lemon

1 garlic clove, smashed

1½ pounds cooked turkey, chicken, steak, pork, or other protein of your choosing

5 eggs (see Note)

PER SERVING (6 SERVINGS)

Cal: 450
Pro: 39g
Carb: 6g
Fat: 30g

1. Preheat the oven to 350°F.

2. Cut off the ends of the spaghetti squash, then cut it crosswise into 3 or 4 pieces. Remove the seeds. Roast on a baking sheet for 20 minutes. (Alternatively, you can put it in the steamer basket of an InstantPot with 1 inch of water and cook at pressure for 7 minutes.)

3. Increase the oven temperature to 375°F. Grease a 9 x 13-inch baking dish with some olive oil.

4. In a food processor or blender, combine the basil, nuts, lemon juice, and garlic. Slowly add the olive oil to create the pesto.

5. Put the turkey, spaghetti squash, eggs, and pesto in a large bowl and mix to combine well. Pour the mixture into the prepared baking dish and bake for 30 to 40 minutes, or until the casserole has firmed up and the eggs have set and are cooked through.

Note: If AIP, you can create a basil pesto without the nuts, and instead of baking this together as a casserole serve almost like you would a pesto pasta with the protein on top (the eggs serve to bind everything together as a casserole, and flax eggs just don't work right in this recipe).

Spare Ribs

Serves 4 to 8

A general rule when cooking ribs is to plan for about 1 pound of ribs per person. Obviously, if the ribs are super meaty, you wouldn't need as many. There are some great no-sugar-added barbecue sauces on the market now, or you can make your own.

4 to 6 pounds pork spare ribs

2 tablespoons prepared mustard

1 tablespoon dried rosemary

1 teaspoon celery salt

1 teaspoon black pepper

2 teaspoons garlic powder

1 teaspoon dried thyme

½ cup barbecue sauce

PER SERVING (8 SERVINGS)

Cal: 451
Pro: 40g
Carb: 6g
Fat: 28g

1. Preheat the oven to 250°F. Line a baking sheet with aluminum foil and place a wire rack on top.

2. Place the ribs on the rack, meaty-side up, and coat with the mustard.

3. In a small bowl, combine the rosemary, celery salt, pepper, garlic powder, and thyme and sprinkle this seasoning mixture over the ribs, pressing it into the mustard lightly to adhere.

4. Cover the ribs with another sheet of foil and bake for 3 hours. Carefully remove the foil, brush the ribs with the barbecue sauce, then re-cover and bake for about 60 minutes more, until the ribs are very tender.

Squash Ribbon Salad

Serves 4 to 6 · AIP WITH MODIFICATIONS

If you tolerate dairy, try adding some freshly grated Parmesan cheese or some goat cheese to this salad.

- 2 pounds zucchini or yellow squash or a combination of both, ends trimmed

  Salt and black pepper (omit pepper if AIP)

- 2 tablespoons good-quality olive oil

- 1 tablespoon minced fresh chives

- 2 tablespoons finely chopped fresh flat-leaf parsley

- 1 tablespoon fresh mint, chopped

- 1 tablespoon fresh dill, chopped

  Juice of 2 lemons

1. Using a vegetable peeler or mandoline, shave the zucchini into "ribbons." Discard the center core of seeds. (If you don't have a peeler or mandoline, use a knife to slice the zucchini as thinly as possible.)

2. Place the zucchini in a colander and sprinkle with some salt to help extract some of the water. Set in the sink to drain for 5 to 10 minutes.

3. In a small bowl, whisk together the olive oil, chives, parsley, mint, dill, and lemon juice. Season with salt and pepper.

4. Place the zucchini in a medium bowl and toss with the dressing. Refrigerate for at least 30 minutes or until ready to serve (alternately, if the squash had been stored in your refrigerator, then you can serve immediately).

PER SERVING (4 SERVINGS)

Cal: 100
Pro: 3g
Carb: 5.5g
Fat: 7.5g

Stuffed Mushrooms

Serves 6 to 8 as an appetizer · AIP

If you have a good source for pork sausage, you can use that to stuff the mushrooms instead of making the pork mixture, to save time and measuring.

. . . .

24	large button mushrooms
1	pound ground pork
1½	teaspoons sea salt
1	teaspoon finely chopped fresh oregano
1	teaspoon finely chopped fresh rosemary
1	teaspoon finely chopped fresh sage
½	teaspoon garlic powder
½	teaspoon onion powder
2	teaspoons minced fresh thyme

1. Preheat the oven to 350°F.

2. Wipe clean all the mushrooms and remove and discard the stems. Place the mushrooms on a baking sheet top-side down.

3. In a bowl, stir together the pork, 1 teaspoon of salt, oregano, rosemary, sage, garlic powder, and onion powder. Scoop about a tablespoon of the pork mixture into each mushroom.

4. Bake the mushrooms for 15 to 18 minutes, or until pork is cooked through.

5. Remove from the oven and sprinkle the thyme and remaining ½ teaspoon of salt over the stuffed mushrooms.

PER SERVING (6 SERVINGS)

Cal: 131
Pro: 23g
Carb: 3g
Fat: 3g

Thai Coconut Soup

Serves 8 to 10 · AIP WITH MODIFICATIONS

- 3 cups chicken stock
- 3 kaffir lime leaves, or zest of 2 limes
- 3 (2-inch) pieces lemongrass, tough outer layer removed, inner core lightly smashed (to help release the flavor)
- 1 (2-inch) piece fresh ginger, peeled and cut in half
- 2 tablespoons fish sauce
- 2 tablespoons fresh lime juice
- 1 or 2 Thai chiles, finely chopped (omit if AIP)
- 1 cup sliced button mushrooms
- 3 cups full-fat coconut milk
- 2 pounds shrimp, peeled and deveined (or chicken breasts or thighs, thinly sliced)
- 2 to 3 tablespoons chopped fresh cilantro (optional)

1. In a large stockpot, combine the stock, lime leaves, lemongrass, ginger, fish sauce, lime juice, and chiles (if using) and bring to a boil. Reduce the heat to maintain a simmer and cook for at least 10 minutes and up to 1 hour—the longer the simmer, the deeper the flavor imparted to the stock.

2. Add in the mushrooms and coconut milk and bring to a simmer. Add the shrimp and cook for 5 minutes, or until the shrimp are pink and cooked through.

3. Garnish the soup with the cilantro, if desired, and serve hot.

PER SERVING (8 SERVINGS)

Cal: 349
Pro: 29g
Carb: 5g
Fat: 24g

Twice-Baked Sweet Potatoes

Serves 4 to 6 · AIP WITH MODIFICATIONS

- 3 sweet potatoes
- 1 cup coconut milk
- ½ yellow onion, minced
- ¼ cup chopped fresh chives
- 1 teaspoon ground cinnamon
- 1 teaspoon sea salt
- 1 teaspoon curry powder (see Note)

PER SERVING (6 SERVINGS)

Cal: 156
Pro: 2g
Carb: 14g
Fat: 10g

1. Preheat the oven to 375°F. Line a baking sheet with aluminum foil.

2. Using a fork, poke several holes in each potato and place them on the prepared baking sheet. Bake for 50 to 60 minutes, or until softened; keep the oven on.

3. Slice the cooked potatoes in half lengthwise and spoon the insides into a medium bowl. Be careful not to tear the potato skins. Set the potato skins cavity-side up on the baking sheet.

4. Add the coconut milk, onion, chives, cinnamon, salt, and curry powder to the potato flesh and mix thoroughly.

5. Spoon the potato mixture into the skins and bake for 10 minutes to finish.

Note: Replace the curry powder with ground turmeric if following AIP.

Ultimate Superfood Burgers

Serves 8 to 10 · AIP

. . . .

1 pound beef heart meat (from about a 1½ pound heart), trimmed of fat and sinew and cut into 1-inch chunks (see Note)

¼ pound beef liver

½ pound bacon

1 pound ground beef

2 teaspoons garlic salt

1 onion, finely chopped

1 cup button mushrooms, finely chopped

PER SERVING (8 SERVINGS)

Cal: 387
Pro: 48g
Carb: 2g
Fat: 19g

1. Heat a grill to 450 to 500°F. Make sure the grill grates are clean.

2. Put the heart, liver, and bacon in a food processor and pulse until well combined. Scoop into a large bowl.

3. Add the beef, garlic salt, onion, and mushrooms and use your hands to mix well. Form the meat mixture into 8 to 10 equal-size patties.

4. Use some paper towels to grease the grill grate. Cook the burgers over direct heat for 5 to 7 minutes per side, or until cooked through. Because of the bacon, liver, and heart, you will want to cook these burgers to more well-done.

Note: If you don't have heart or liver available, substitute another pound of ground beef.

Weeknight Chicken Breasts or Thighs

Serves 6 to 8 · AIP

. . . .

2 pounds boneless, skinless chicken breasts or thighs

Zest of 1 lemon

2 teaspoons fresh lemon juice

2 tablespoons minced fresh rosemary

4 garlic cloves, minced

¼ cup olive oil

1 teaspoon salt

1. Make sure your chicken pieces are at a uniform thickness, ½ to ¾ inch. If they are not, place them in a zip-top bag one at a time and use a meat mallet or heavy-bottomed skillet to pound them to a more even thickness.

2. In a covered dish or zip-top bag, combine the lemon zest, lemon juice, rosemary, garlic, olive oil, and salt. Add the chicken and marinate in the refrigerator for at least 30 minutes but preferably at least a few hours (overnight is great).

3. When ready to cook, heat a grill (outdoors) or grill pan (indoors) over medium-high heat, 375 to 400°F.

4. Grill the chicken for about 5 minutes on the first side, or until the chicken easily releases from the grill (or pan), then flip and cook for 5 minutes or so on the second side, until the juices run clear and an instant-read thermometer registers an internal temperature of 160°F—carryover cooking will bring this up to 165°F once the chicken has been removed from the oven.

5. Let sit for 5 to 10 minutes, then slice and eat as is or use in your favorite recipes.

Note: This marinade is delicious on grilled shrimp. Simply marinate the shrimp for no more than 30 minutes, thread onto skewers, then grill for a few minutes each side—until the shrimp are pink and cooked through.

Most of the fat comes from the oil used in the marinade, which is not consumed, so this calculation likely does not reflect an accurate fat content.

Whole Roast Chicken and Vegetables

Serves 4 to 6 · AIP WITH MODIFICATIONS

Drizzle some truffle oil over the chicken for a decadent take on things. If you'd like some gravy to go with your chicken, I've included a recipe here.

. . . .

1 (4- to 5-pound) chicken

Salt and black pepper (omit pepper if AIP)

2 shallots, sliced

2 or 3 carrots, cut into 1-inch pieces

1 pound radishes, halved

1 pound Brussels sprouts, halved

2 garlic cloves, gently smashed

1 teaspoon fresh thyme

1 teaspoon fresh rosemary

2 tablespoons olive oil

½ to 1 cup chicken stock

Pan gravy (optional, recipe follows)

1. Let the chicken come to room temperature (about 45 minutes) before cooking.

2. Preheat the oven to 450°F.

3. Dry chicken all over—including inside the cavity (making sure you have removed the giblets/chicken neck that may have been stored inside)—with paper towels. Liberally season the inside of the cavity and all over the outside of the bird with salt and pepper (if using). Truss together the legs and tuck the chicken wings under.

4. Put the vegetables, garlic, and herbs in a large roasting pan and toss with the olive oil. Sprinkle with salt.

5. Place the chicken breast-side up on top of the vegetables and place in the oven.

PER SERVING (6 SERVINGS, NOT INCLUDING PAN GRAVY)

Cal: 274
Pro: 30g
Carb: 7g
Fat: 12g

6. Bake for 40 to 50 minutes, checking after 15 minutes. If the vegetables are starting to get really brown, add some of the stock to prevent burning. As the chicken bakes its drippings will help to moisten the vegetables (while adding a great flavor).

7. When an instant-read thermometer inserted into the thickest part of the thigh registers 160°F, remove from the oven and let rest for at least 10 minutes. Carve and serve with the vegetables and, if using, the gravy.

pan gravy

Makes approximately 2½ cups

. . . .

Drippings and
browned bits from
roast chicken and
roasted garlic

Splash of white wine
(use chicken stock if
preferred)

2 onions, chopped

2 cups chicken stock

1 teaspoon fresh
thyme leaves,
chopped

¼ cup coconut milk
or heavy cream
(optional)

Salt and black
pepper

> NUTRITIONAL
> INFO VARIES

1. Remove the chicken and roasted vegetables (except the garlic) from the roasting pan. Place the roasting pan on the stovetop and heat over medium heat. Pour in a generous splash of wine to deglaze the pan. Use a wooden spoon to scrape up any of the browned bits from the bottom.

2. Add the onions and cook until translucent and softened.

3. Add the stock and thyme, stir, and bring to a simmer.

4. Pour the contents into a large heatproof measuring cup and use an immersion blender to puree. Or carefully transfer the mixture to a blender and puree (using caution as the hot liquid will cause the air inside to expand and can send hot liquid all over you). Add in the coconut milk (if using) and season with salt and pepper.

Dressings, Sauces, and More

5-Minute Hollandaise Sauce

Makes ½ cup

½ cup (1 stick) unsalted butter

1 egg yolk

1 teaspoon fresh lemon juice

¼ teaspoon sea salt

Pinch of cayenne pepper or tarragon (the latter for a closer to béarnaise sauce)

1. Melt the butter in a small saucepan, being careful not to brown or burn it.

2. In a Mason jar or small cup wide enough to fit the head of an immersion blender, place the egg yolk, lemon juice, salt, and 1 teaspoon water. Use an immersion blender to combine the ingredients. With the blender running, slowly pour in the melted butter until completely incorporated. Season with cayenne or tarragon, if desired. Serve warm.

PER SERVING
(2 TABLESPOONS)

Cal: 217
Pro: .9g
Carb: .2g
Fat: 24.2g

Asian Dressing

Makes about ¾ cup · AIP

- 2 tablespoons unseasoned rice vinegar
- 1 tablespoon fresh orange juice
- 1 tablespoon coconut aminos
- 1 teaspoon fish sauce
- 1 teaspoon minced fresh ginger
- 1 (1-inch) piece green onion, sliced
- 3 tablespoons MCT oil
- 3 tablespoons neutral oil (such as avocado oil or light olive oil)
- Salt

Put the vinegar, orange juice, coconut aminos, fish sauce, ginger, and green onion in a small food processor or blender and pulse to combine. Add in the oils and blend until well combined and emulsified. Taste and season with salt if needed.

PER SERVING
(2 TABLESPOONS)

Cal: 116
Pro: 0g
Carb: 1g
Fat: 14

Asian Marinade

Makes about ½ cup · AIP

. . . .

2   garlic cloves

2   tablespoons grated
    or minced fresh
    ginger

3   green onions, sliced

2   tablespoons coconut
    aminos

2   teaspoons fish sauce

¼   cup olive oil

Place all ingredients in a small food processor and blend to combine.

Caesar-Like Dressing

Makes ½ cup · AIP WITH MODIFICATIONS

½ avocado, pitted and peeled

3 tablespoons MCT oil

3 tablespoons olive oil

2 anchovy fillets, or 1 teaspoon anchovy paste

1 tablespoon fresh lemon juice

1 garlic clove, smashed

Salt and black pepper (omit pepper for AIP)

Put all the ingredients in a mini food processor or small blender. Process until no lumps of the avocado remain. Taste and season with salt and pepper. Thin with water to achieve your desired consistency (if you want a thicker dressing, use less water).

PER SERVING
(2 TABLESPOONS)

Cal: 215
Pro: 3g
Carb: 0g
Fat: 24g

Chimichurri

Makes about 1 cup · AIP

Serve this Argentinean sauce over or alongside chicken, fish, or steak or with your favorite vegetables.

. . . .

- 2 tablespoons fresh cilantro
- 1 tablespoon fresh oregano
- 1½ cups fresh flat-leaf parsley
- 2 garlic cloves, minced

  Juice of 1 lemon
- ½ cup olive oil or avocado oil
- 2 tablespoons red or white wine vinegar
- 1 teaspoon sea salt

Combine all the ingredients in a food processor or blender and blend.

PER SERVING
(2 TABLESPOONS)

Cal: 116
Pro: .5g
Carb: 1g
Fat: 13g

Cilantro-Lime Marinade

Makes about ½ cup · AIP WITH MODIFICATIONS

. . . .

¼ cup fresh cilantro, chopped

Zest and juice of 1 lime

¼ cup olive oil

1 teaspoon salt

1 jalapeño, minced (omit for AIP)

Place all the ingredients in a small food processor and blend to combine.

Compound Butter

Makes about 1¼ cups

. . . .

2 tablespoons minced fresh chives

1 tablespoon minced fresh parsley

2 garlic cloves, minced

¼ cup olive oil

1 cup (2 sticks) unsalted butter, at room temperature

1 teaspoon sea salt

PER SERVING
(1 TABLESPOON)

Cal: 104
Pro: 0g
Carb: 0g
Fat: 12g

1. Put the chives, parsley, garlic, and olive oil in a food processor and process to combine.

2. Put the butter and salt in a medium bowl and fold the herb mixture into the butter with spatula. Mix until well incorporated.

3. Spoon the mixture on a large piece of parchment paper and roll it into a round log, 1 to 2 inches in diameter.

4. Refrigerate for 1 to 2 hours before serving. Slice into discs, removing the parchment paper, when ready to use.

Creamy Dill Dressing

Makes ½ cup · AIP WITH MODIFICATIONS

. . . .

3 tablespoons MCT oil

¼ cup olive oil

½ avocado, pitted and peeled

2 tablespoons red wine vinegar or sherry vinegar

1 tablespoon fresh dill

1 teaspoon fresh lemon juice

Salt and black pepper (omit pepper if AIP)

Put all the ingredients in a mini food processor or small blender. Process until no lumps of the avocado remain. Taste and season with salt and pepper. Thin with water to achieve your desired consistency (if you want a thicker dressing, use less water).

> **PER SERVING (2 TABLESPOONS)**
>
> Cal: 194
> Pro: 0g
> Carb: 0g
> Fat: 23g

Fauxmato Sauce

Makes 5 to 6 cups · AIP

- 1 large beet, peeled and cut into 1-inch pieces
- 1 medium butternut squash, peeled, seeded, and cut into 1-inch pieces
- ½ cup olive oil
- 1 large leek, white and light green parts cleaned very well and chopped into small pieces
- 2 cups beef or chicken stock
- ¼ cup apple cider vinegar
- 1 tablespoon balsamic vinegar
- 2 tablespoons chopped fresh basil, or 1 tablespoon dried
- 1 teaspoon sea salt
- 2 teaspoons garlic powder
- 1 teaspoon dried oregano
- ½ teaspoon dried rosemary
- ½ teaspoon dried sage
- ¼ teaspoon dried thyme

1. Preheat the oven to 400°F.

2. Toss beets and butternut squash with ¼ cup of the olive oil and place on a baking sheet. Roast for 15 to 20 minutes, until softened, turning once during cooking.

3. Meanwhile, in a large saucepan or Dutch oven, heat the remaining ¼ cup olive oil over medium heat. Add the leeks and sauté until they begin to brown.

4. When beets and squash are done, remove the pan from oven and add them to the saucepan. Add the stock, vinegars, basil, sea salt, garlic powder, oregano, rosemary, sage, and thyme. Stir to combine and cook for a minute or two more.

5. Use an immersion blender to puree the sauce directly in the saucepan, then simmer for 10 to 15 minutes more. Thin with chicken stock or water if too thick.

> **PER SERVING (1 CUP)**
>
> Cal: 124
> Pro: 1.5g
> Carb: 10g
> Fat: 9g

Guacamole

Serves 6 to 8 · AIP WITH MODIFICATIONS

There's a long-standing debate about whether tomatoes have a place in guacamole. If you *do* want to add in tomatoes, seed and dice 2 Roma (plum) tomatoes, place them in a colander, and sprinkle with some salt. Let them stand for a bit to draw excess liquid out so your guac does not get too runny, then stir them in.

. . . .

3   ripe avocados, halved and pitted

½   yellow or red onion, finely diced (1/4 cup)

Juice of 1 lime

½   garlic clove, smashed and minced (optional)

1   serrano pepper or jalapeño, minced (omit if AIP)

¼   cup fresh cilantro, finely chopped

Salt

1. Scoop out the avocado flesh into a medium bowl (or a molcajete or mortar and pestle, if you have either of those). Add the onion, lime juice, garlic, serrano, and cilantro and stir to combine well. Season with salt. If you prefer a chunkier guacamole, use a fork and knife to break apart pieces of the avocado but still leave large chunks.

2. If not serving immediately, press a piece of plastic wrap directly against the surface of the guac, then cover the entire container with a lid or another piece of plastic wrap.

PER SERVING (6 SERVINGS)

Cal: 212
Pro: 2.1g
Carb: 3.3g
Fat: 19.6g

Pesto Sauce

Makes about 1¹/₂ cups

If you can't find water chestnuts and you are not on the autoimmune protocol, use any toasted nuts of your choosing.

. . . .

2 cups fresh basil

3 whole fresh water chestnuts, peeled, chopped, and toasted

2 garlic cloves

½ cup olive oil

Salt

½ cup grated Parmesan cheese (optional)

Put the basil, water chestnuts, garlic, and olive oil in a food processor and process until smooth. Season with salt, then stir in the Parmesan (if using) and serve.

PER SERVING (8 SERVINGS, WITHOUT CHEESE)

Cal: 126
Pro: .5g
Carb: 4g
Fat: 13g

Tangy Avocado Sauce

Makes about 2 cups · AIP

Use this as a dipping sauce, mayo substitute, or dressing—it's great with chicken, fish, or pork.

. . . .

2   ripe avocados, halved and pitted

Juice of 1 lime

1   tablespoon apple cider vinegar

3   garlic cloves, smashed

½   teaspoon kosher salt

¼   cup fresh flat-leaf parsley with stems

½   cup olive oil, plus more if needed

1. Scoop out the avocado flesh into a food processor. Add the lime juice, vinegar, garlic, salt, and parsley and process to combine.

2. With the motor running, slowly add the olive oil through the feed tube until the desired consistency is reached.

PER SERVING (¼ CUP)

Cal: 213
Pro: 1g
Carb: 2g
Fat: 22g

Tomato Meat Sauce

Serves 6 to 8

On your prep day, cook at least 2 pounds of ground beef to have on hand for the week. Then, take the cooked beef and use it for this sauce to make your life easier. You can make the tomato sauce ahead of time and refrigerate it for later—it cans and freezes well, too—then just add the ground beef when you're ready to eat. Serve the sauce over zucchini or squash noodles, cabbage noodles, or even cauliflower rice.

4 tablespoons olive oil

1 onion, diced

4 garlic cloves, smashed and minced

2 (28-ounce) cans San Marzano or other canned tomatoes

½ cup fresh basil, leaves torn

2 pounds cooked ground beef (or a mixture of cooked ground beef and Italian sausage, ground pork, etc.)

1. In a large Dutch oven, heat 1 tablespoon of the olive oil over medium heat. When hot, add the onion and cook, stirring, for 5 to 7 minutes, or until translucent and softened. Stir in the garlic and sauté for 1 minute more, being careful not to brown the garlic.

2. Pour in the tomatoes, basil, and remaining 3 tablespoons olive oil, stir, and bring to a boil.

3. Stir in the meat and simmer for at least 10 minutes; the longer it simmers, the more intense the flavors will be.

PER SERVING (8 SERVINGS)

Cal: 347
Pro: 25g
Carb: 12g
Fat: 22g

Afterword

We have come a long way together, and I have to offer you a sincere thank-you for sticking with me this far. We have looked at everything from the evolutionary biology of your appetite (how you are wired to eat) to your digestion and hormones to a fair amount of real-world psychology. My hope is that you now have the tools and the mental framework to live the life you want, unencumbered by the guilt normally associated with eating, to say nothing of extra pounds and health problems.

I love helping people and I hope that energy comes across in my writing. Part of helping people is hearing from them—I need to know what worked and what didn't. To that end, I hope this is not the end of our relationship, but rather just the beginning. Please reach out to me on social media, my podcast, and my blog, all of which you can find at robbwolf.com. I can't answer every question I receive, but you might be surprised by how many I *do* answer. This is not a popularity contest for me—this is my life's work. The way I succeed is by helping you to succeed, so please do contact me and let me know how *Wired to Eat* has affected you.

Yours in health,
Robb Wolf

Acknowledgments

I know books are written all the time, but in looking back on this project, I'm left wondering how the hell I got it done. The easy answer is lots of help and support. Lots. So much help in fact that I'd almost rather not put acknowledgments in the book, as I know I'm going to leave some folks out who really deserve credit for hard work. In an effort to not let too many people fall through the cracks I'll try to group folks a bit so I can keep things straight.

I'd had an idea for *Wired to Eat* for a long time, but it was not until I talked to my agent, Celeste Fine, that we actually decided to motor forward with the project. She managed to spiff me up and convince my editor and publisher, Diana Baroni, to take on this project. Thank you both. I know I'm not the easiest person to work with. Sometimes. A *huge* thank-you to my provisional editor, Cherise Fisher, who did an amazing job of asking great questions and helping to draw out my voice. I had significant help on the technical details of the book and I owe a huge debt to Matt Lalonde, PhD, for his suggestions on the organization of and veracity of the technical material, particularly on nutrient density. Bill Lagakos, PhD, was incredibly generous with his time and helped me understand the implications of the personalized nutrition research that is such a prominent feature of the book. A huge thank-you to both of these gentlemen, they helped make the book much better, but any technical errors are my own failings. A Big Foot–sized thank-you to my assistant, Chris "Squatchy" Williams. Chris helped me organize the references for the book, and if I had to do that on my own,

I would have hung myself with computer cables. The most practical part of this book (the recipes and meal plans) I owe to my dear friends Julie and Charles Mayfield. You guys outdid yourselves. My only complaint is we did not do this project from Eleuthera. Next time! A key feature of this book is the story about the Reno Risk Assessment program, which just might change the face of medicine if we can get the incentives of our health care system properly aligned. Thanks to the team who started and maintain that program: Jackie Cox, Dr. Jim Greenwald, Dr. Scott Hall, Shanti Wolfe, and Ethan Opdal.

I try to make a case in this book that community and activity are important for our health and happiness. For me that means Brazilian jiu-jitsu. There are a number of people who help me stay in the game with jits, but the following folks have played huge roles in my growth: Kelley Farrell, Ken Perotti, Patrick Johnston, Henry Akins, Jason Woodard, Marci Zavalla, Ray Price, Andrew Bowers, John Frankl, Matt Thornton, Scott Fitzinger, Sonny Bringas, Paul Hoch . . . this could spiral into a list of hundreds of names. Thank you to the folks mentioned and to all the folks I do not have space to thank right now.

A special thank-you to Coach Greg Glassman. Were it not for your interest and advice I'd not be doing what I'm doing.

Huge thanks goes out to the folks who have supported my work over the years. Blog readers, podcast listeners, folks who come out to live events—y'all are the reason any of this happens. We have changed the world for the better by tinkering with this ancestral health model . . . that feels pretty good.

Finally, thanks to my wife, Nicki. I'm still amazed you not only let me cook you dinner, but allowed me to share my life with you and our girls. Best. Gift. Ever.

Appendix
SHOPPING LISTS

ESSENTIALS

These are general kitchen essentials that are good to have on hand. You can make quick-and-easy meals with these when you need to, and you'll probably end up using these things somewhat regularly.

Meat

Ground beef

Whole chicken

Eggs*

Canned sardines or salmon (in olive oil or water)

Produce

Cauliflower

Green beans

Broccoli

Kale

Carrots

Onion

Mixed greens (for salad mix)

Avocado

Herbs/Spices

Salt

Black pepper*

Rosemary

Basil

Thyme

Oregano

Garlic powder

Ginger

Chili powder*

Cayenne pepper*

Turmeric

Oils/Cooking Fats

Coconut oil

Olive oil

Butter or ghee (optional)*

Other

Coconut aminos

Apple cider vinegar

Balsamic vinegar

= not AIP-friendly

These are the shopping lists for the ingredients to make the recipes as listed in the book for the various weeks and meal plans. Feel free to substitute or swap items and adjust quantities for your needs. This is definitely not something that is set in stone, and should be adjusted to the individual or family depending on preferences, health requirements, and how many servings you need.

EXAMPLE SHOPPING LIST FOR PALEO WEEK 1

This list corresponds with the meal plan on page 178.

Meat

1½ pounds chicken thighs or breasts

2 pounds flank steak

1 pound clams or mussels

½ pound baby scallops

½ pound shrimp

½ pound halibut

¾ pound bulk sausage (ground, not sausage links)*

12 large eggs*

1 (4- to 5-pound) whole chicken

Produce

3 yellow onions

1 pound okra

3 tomatoes

2 heads cauliflower

2 heads broccoli

3 sweet potatoes

1 fennel bulb

2 cups diced tomatoes (4 fresh tomatoes, or 1 [14.5-ounce] can of diced tomatoes)

2 cups fresh spinach

1 small head of cabbage (napa, green, or red—or any combination)

3 carrots

4 green onions

2 cups snow peas (about 10 ounces)

1 orange

1 lemon

1 smaller piece fresh ginger

Spices/Herbs

Garam masala

Ground ginger (or 1 tablespoon grated fresh ginger)

2 heads garlic

= not AIP-friendly

Ground turmeric

Red pepper flakes (optional)*

Fresh cilantro

Salt

Fresh parsley

Fresh oregano

Fresh rosemary

Black pepper*

Fresh chives

Cinnamon (Ceylon cinnamon is better than cassia)

Curry powder*

Dried oregano

Dried basil

Bay leaves

Garlic powder

Smoked paprika*

Oils/Cooking Fats

Ghee (optional)*

Olive oil

Coconut oil

MCT oil

Avocado oil (or light olive oil)

Other

Unsweetened coconut yogurt (or Greek yogurt, if you tolerate dairy, or coconut cream)

Tomato paste*

2 (13.5-ounce) cans coconut milk (Aroy-D is a great brand and also can be found in 8.5-ounce or 33.8-ounce boxes instead of a can)

Apple cider vinegar

1 (8-ounce) bottle clam juice

1 (750ml) bottle dry white wine (optional)*

6 cups fish stock or chicken stock

Bag of slivered almonds (or ½ cup)*

Coconut aminos

Fish sauce

Unseasoned rice vinegar*

EXAMPLE SHOPPING LIST FOR PALEO WEEK 2

This list corresponds with the meal plan on page 179.

Meat

4 pounds chicken (breast or thigh)

4 pounds grass-fed ground beef

12 bacon slices (use AIP-friendly for AIP)

2 pounds shrimp (or chicken breasts or thighs)

= not AIP-friendly

Produce

1 sweet onion

2 yellow or red onions

2 heads garlic

2 large heads cauliflower

6 limes

3 kaffir lime leaves (or 2 additional limes)

½ teaspoon capers

12 ounces button mushrooms

10 zucchini

3 yellow squash (or 3 additional zucchini)

3 ripe avocados

1 serrano pepper or jalapeño*

1 or 2 Thai chiles*

2 red bell peppers*

1 pound asparagus

1 (2-inch) piece fresh ginger

1 cup sliced button mushrooms

2 (28-ounce) cans San Marzano or other canned tomatoes*

4 green onions

Spices/Herbs

Sea salt

Garlic powder

Fresh rosemary

Fresh basil (½ cup)

Fresh cilantro (½ cup)

1 stalk of lemongrass

¼ cup fresh parsley

Oils/Cooking Fats

Coconut oil

Butter or ghee (optional)*

Olive oil

Other

6 cups chicken stock

4 (13.5-ounce) cans full-fat coconut milk

Balsamic vinegar

Fish sauce

Red curry paste

Almond butter (unsweetened)

Honey (optional)

= not AIP-friendly

EXAMPLE SHOPPING LIST FOR AIP WEEK 1

This list corresponds with the meal plan on page 180.

Meat

4 pounds boneless chicken breasts or thighs

½ pound bacon (make sure ingredients are AIP-friendly)

2 pounds ground lamb

4 (6-ounce) pieces cod or any other mild white-fleshed fish

Produce

6 lemons

2 limes

3 heads garlic

2 large heads cauliflower

4 cups collards greens

2 cups dandelion greens

4 cups kale

2 pounds parsnips

2 onions

2 carrots

7 zucchini

4 yellow squash

1 cucumber

1 cup button mushrooms

1 (12-ounce) bag broccoli slaw, or 3 cups broccoli stalks

2 small shallots

2 bunches green onions

Spices/Herbs

Salt

Fresh rosemary

Fresh sage

Fresh dill

Dried oregano

Fresh parsley

Fresh basil

Dried basil

Oils/Cooking Fats

Olive oil

Coconut oil

Butter or ghee (optional)

Other

5 cups chicken stock

Balsamic vinegar

2½ cups beef stock

Umeboshi paste (optional)

1 (13.5-ounce) can coconut milk

Red wine vinegar

1 cup unsweetened coconut milk yogurt

EXAMPLE SHOPPING LIST FOR AIP WEEK 2

This list corresponds with the meal plan on page 181.

Meat

2 pounds grass-fed ground beef

2 pounds chicken breast or thighs

1½ pounds pork chops or cutlets

1 pound shrimp

1 (6-pound) standing rib roast

Produce

2 medium and 1 large onions

3 ripe avocados

1 lime

2 heads garlic

1 large parsnip

2 carrots

4 celery stalks

1 pound okra

2 peaches

Broccoli florets (2 cups, or 1 bag)

1½ pounds button mushrooms

8 ounces fresh water chestnuts

1 head cauliflower

2 heads broccoli

Spices/Herbs

Salt

Kosher salt

Ground turmeric

Garlic powder

Onion powder

Dried oregano

Dried thyme

Fresh thyme

Dried parsley

Fresh parsley

Dried cilantro

Fresh cilantro

Dried chives

1 bay leaf

Ground ginger

Fresh rosemary

Fresh oregano

Oils/Cooking Fats

Coconut oil

Olive oil

Bacon fat (optional)

Other

4¼ cups chicken stock

½ cup beef stock

Apple cider vinegar

Fish sauce

Coconut aminos

EXAMPLE SHOPPING LIST FOR KETO TRANSITION WEEK 1

This list corresponds with the meal plan on page 235.

Meat

1½ pounds chicken (breast or thighs)

2 pounds strip steak

1 pound pork cutlets or pork chops (about ½ inch thick or less)

12 ounces bacon

1 (10-ounce) can clams

½ pound small sea scallops

1 pound wild-caught cod or other white-fleshed fish

1 (4- to 5-pound) whole chicken

Produce

1 onion

2 yellow onions

3 cups sliced mushrooms

1 pound button mushrooms

2 heads garlic

1 pound zucchini or yellow squash

2 cups fresh spinach

2 pounds Brussels sprouts

2 large heads cauliflower

4 cups collards greens

2 cups dandelion greens

4 cups kale

Spices/Herbs

Salt

Black pepper*

¼ cup fresh basil

Garlic powder

Ground fenugreek

Onion powder

Cinnamon (Ceylon cinnamon is better than cassia)

1 tablespoon fresh rosemary

Dried thyme

Fresh thyme

Smoked paprika

Oils/Cooking Fats

Olive oil

Coconut oil

Duck fat (optional)

Butter or Ghee (optional)

Other

3 (13.5-ounce) cans coconut milk

1½ cups chicken stock

½ cup beef stock

Balsamic vinegar

¼ cup sun-dried tomatoes

1½ cups chicken or fish stock

2 cups clam juice

Coconut aminos

EXAMPLE SHOPPING LIST FOR KETO TRANSITION WEEK 2

This list corresponds with the meal plan on page 238.

Meat

4 to 5 pounds beef short ribs

2 pounds skin-on salmon fillet, cut into 6 even portions

3 pounds bone-in, skin-on chicken thighs and drumsticks

1½ pounds cooked turkey, chicken, steak, pork, or any meat of your choosing

6 large eggs*

2 pounds wild-caught shrimp

Produce

2-inch piece fresh ginger

1 sweet yellow onion

2 oranges

3 lemons

= not AIP-friendly

2 limes

10 heads garlic

1 stalk lemongrass

1 bunch green onions

2 large heads cauliflower

Salt

2 tablespoons fresh chives

2 small heads green or red cabbage

3 carrots

2 cups snow peas

1 spaghetti squash

Spices/Herbs

1 cinnamon stick (Ceylon cinnamon is better than cassia)

Whole cloves*

¼ cup fresh dill

¼ cup fresh parsley

Garlic powder

Dried oregano

Dried thyme

Fresh rosemary

Dried rosemary

1 cup fresh basil

¼ cup fresh cilantro

1 Thai chile, or ¼ teaspoon red pepper flakes (optional)*

Oils/Cooking Fats

Coconut oil

Olive oil

Avocado oil or light olive oil

Butter or ghee (optional)

MCT oil

Other

Coconut aminos

2 cups beef stock

2½ cups chicken stock

Umeboshi paste (optional)

Unseasoned rice vinegar

1 cup pickle juice

1/2 cup arrowroot powder

2 cups plain chicharrónes (pork rinds)

½ cup slivered almonds*

Fish sauce

¼ cup pine nuts, walnuts, or other nuts of your choosing

1 (13.5-ounce) can coconut milk

= not AIP-friendly

EXAMPLE SHOPPING LIST FOR FULL-ON KETO WEEK 1

This list corresponds with the meal plan on page 239.

Meats

1 pound ground pork

1 (4-pound) bone-in pork butt

6 large eggs

1½ pounds skin-on wild-caught salmon fillets (4 to 6 fillets)

4 (6-ounce) halibut or other firm white-fleshed fish fillets

1½ pounds beef heart

¼ pound beef liver

½ pound bacon

1 pound ground beef

Produce

½ cup mushrooms, diced

1 cup button mushrooms

2 onions

2 heads garlic

1 (3-inch) piece fresh ginger

3½ ounces fresh shiitake mushrooms, sliced

7 heads baby bok choy

½ cup green onions

1 lime

1 head cauliflower

2 heads broccoli

Spices/Herbs

Kosher salt

Salt

Pepper*

Garlic powder

Garlic salt

Celery salt*

Dried rosemary

Dried basil

Juniper berries*

Ground turmeric

Oils/Cooking Fats

Coconut oil

Olive oil

Butter or ghee (optional)

Sesame oil*

Other

Coconut aminos

Rice vinegar

Fish sauce

½ cup macadamia nuts

Balsamic vinegar

* = not AIP-friendly

EXAMPLE SHOPPING LIST FOR FULL-ON KETO WEEK 2

This list corresponds with the meal plan beginning on page 239.

Meats

2 pounds lamb chops

2 pounds pork tenderloin (about 2 tenderloins)

1 (3-pound) beef brisket

1 (4- to 5-pound) whole chicken

1½ pounds tail-on shrimp

1 pound beef sirloin or top round steak

Produce

2 heads garlic

1 orange

3 lemons

3 limes

1 avocado

1 pound mixed greens

2 pounds asparagus

3 leeks

2 shallots

2 pounds zucchini or yellow squash (or a combination)

5 or 6 large carrots (about 1½ pounds)

1 pound radishes

1 pound Brussels sprouts

2 heads cauliflower

2 cups mushrooms, sliced

2 heads baby bok choy

1 (1-inch) piece fresh ginger

4 green onions

Spices/Herbs

Salt

Kosher salt

Black pepper*

Garlic powder

Fresh cilantro

Fresh rosemary

Fresh dill

Fresh chives

Fresh parsley

Fresh thyme

Horseradish

Fresh mint

Ground turmeric

= not AIP-friendly

Oils

Olive oil

Coconut oil

Butter or ghee (optional)

MCT oil

Other

Red wine vinegar or sherry vinegar

Tamarind paste

1¼ cups beef stock

2½ to 3 cups chicken stock

Coconut aminos

Apple cider vinegar

Arrowroot powder

References

Chapter 2: It's Not Your Fault

Egger G, Dixon J. "Should Obesity Be the Main Game? or Do We Need an Environmental Makeover to Combat the Inflammatory and Chronic Disease Epidemics?" *Obes Rev*. 2009 Mar; 10(2): 237–49.

Larsen CS. "The Agricultural Revolution as Environmental Catastrophe: Implications for Health and Lifestyle in the Holocene." *Quaternary International*. 2006 May; 150(1): 12–20.

Lloyd E, Wilson DS, Sober E. "Evolutionary Mismatch and What to Do About It: A Basic Tutorial." Wesley Chapel: Evolution Institute, 2014.

Heitmann BL, Westerterp KR, Loos RJ, Sørensen TI, O'Dea K, Mclean P, Jensen TK, Eisenmann J, Speakman JR, Simpson, et al. "Obesity: Lessons from Evolution and the Environment." *Obes Rev*. 2012 Oct; 13(10): 910–22.

Pijl H. "Obesity: Evolution of a Symptom of Affluence." *Neth J Med*. 2011 Apr; 69(4): 159–66.

Ruiz-Núñez B, Pruimboom L, Dijck-Brouwer DAJ, Muskiet FAJ. "Lifestyle and Nutritional Imbalances Associated with Western Diseases: Causes and Consequences of Chronic Systemic Low-Grade Inflammation in an Evolutionary Context." *Journal of Nutritional Biochemistry*. 2013 Jul 1; 24(7): 1183–201.

Koren D, Levitt Katz LE, Brar PC, Gallagher PR, Berkowitz RI, Brooks LJ. "Sleep Architecture and Glucose and Insulin Homeostasis in Obese Adolescents." *Diabetes Care*. 2011 Nov; 34(11): 2442–7.

Burger O, Baudisch A, Vaupel JW. "Human Mortality Improvement in Evolutionary Context." *PNAS*. 2012 Oct 30; 109(44): 18210–4.

Carrera-Bastos P, Fontes, O'Keefe, Lindeberg, Cordain. "The Western Diet and Lifestyle and Diseases of Civilization." *Research Reports in Clinical Cardiology*. 2011 Mar; 15.

Ekirch AR. "Sleep We Have Lost: Pre-Industrial Slumber in the British Isles." *Am Hist Rev*. 2001; 106(2): 343–86.

Aubrey A. "Many Americans Say Doing Taxes Is Easier Than Eating Right." NPR.Org. May 23, 2012. www.npr.org/sections/thesalt/2012/05/23/153416865/many-americans-saying-doing-taxes-is-easier-than-eating-right.

Chapter 3: Mosquitos, Appetite, and Hyperpalatable Food

Spreadbury IA and Samis AJW. "Evolutionary Aspects of Obesity, Insulin Resistance, and Cardiovascular Risk." *Curr Cardiovasc Risk Rep.* 2013; 7:136–46.

Karnani MM, Apergis-Schoute J, Adamantidis A, Jensen LT, De Lecea L, Fugger L, Burdakov D. "Activation of Central Orexin/Hypocretin Neurons by Dietary Amino Acids." *Neuron.* 2011 Nov 17; 72(4): 616–29.

Dunn JP, Kessler RM, Feurer ID, Volkow ND, Patterson BW, Ansari MS, Li R, Marks-Shulman P, Abumrad NN. "Relationship of Dopamine Type 2 Receptor Binding Potential with Fasting Neuroendocrine Hormones and Insulin Sensitivity in Human Obesity." *Diabetes Care.* 2012 May; 35(5): 1105–11.

Bray GA. "Is Sugar Addictive?" *Diabetes.* 2016; 65:1797–99.

Richards MP. "A Brief Review of the Archaeological Evidence for Paleolithic and Neolithic Subsistence." *Eur J Clin Nutr.* 2002 Dec; 56(12): 1262–78.

Brooking LA, Williams SM, Mann JI. "Effects of Macronutrient Composition of the Diet on Body Fat in Indigenous People at High Risk of Type 2 Diabetes." *Diabetes Res Clin Pract.* 2012 Apr; 96(1): 40–6.

Schwartz M, Cohen IR. "Autoimmunity Can Benefit Self-Maintenance." *Immunol Today.* 2000 Jun; 21(6): 265–8.

Myers MG Jr, Olson DP. "Central Nervous System Control of Metabolism." *Nature.* 2012 Nov 15; 491(7424): 357–63.

Zhernakova A, Elbers CC, Ferwerda B, Romanos J, Trynka G, Dubois PC, De Kovel CG, Franke L, Oosting M, Barisani D et al. "Evolutionary and Functional Analysis of Celiac Risk Loci Reveals SH2B3 as a Protective Factor Against Bacterial Infection." *Am J Hum Genet.* 2010 Jun 11; 86(6): 970–7.

Laland KN, Sterelny K, Odling-Smee J, Hoppitt W, Uller T. "Cause and Effect in Biology Revisited: Is Mayr's Proximate-Ultimate Dichotomy Still Useful?" *Science.* 2011 Dec 16; 334(6062): 1512–6.

Sajantila A. "Major Historical Dietary Changes Are Reflected in the Dental Microbiome of Ancient Skeletons." *Investig Genet.* 2013; 4:10.

Muskiet F.A.J. "Adaptation to the Conditions of Existence." *Ned Tijdschr Klin Chem Labgeneesk.* 2006; 31:187–93.

Leonti M. "The Co-Evolutionary Perspective of the Food-Medicine Continuum and Wild Gathered and Cultivated Vegetables." *Genet Resour Crop Evol.* 2012; 59:1295–1302.

Armelagos GJ. "Brain Evolution, the Determinates of Food Choice, and the Omnivore's Dilemma." *Critical Reviews in Food Science and Nutrition.* 2014; 54:1330–41.

Pennisi E. "Evolution. Darwinian Medicine's Drawn-Out Dawn." *Science.* 2011 Dec 16; 334(6062): 1486–7.

Lucock MD, Martin CE, Yates ZR, Veysey M. "Diet and Our Genetic Legacy in the Recent Anthropocene: A Darwinian Perspective to Nutritional Health." *J Evid Based Complementary Altern Med.* 2014 Jan; 19(1): 68–83.

Tattersall I. "Diet as Driver and Constraint in Human Evolution." *J Hum Evol.* 2014 Dec; 77:141–2.

Eisenstein M. "Evolution: The First Supper." *Nature.* 2010 Dec 23; 468:S8–S9.

Brüne M and Hochberg Z. "Evolutionary Medicine—The Quest for a Better Understanding of Health, Disease and Prevention." *BMC Medicine.* 2013; 11:116.

Knight C. " 'Most People Are Simply Not Designed to Eat Pasta': Evolutionary Explanations for Obesity in the Low-Carbohydrate Diet Movement." *Public Underst Sci.* 2011 Sep; 20(5): 706–19.

Rangel A. "Regulation of Dietary Choice by the Decision-Making Circuitry." *Nat Neurosci.* 2013 Dec; 16(12): 1717–24.

Spreadbury I and Samis AJW. "Evolutionary Aspects of Obesity, Insulin Resistance, and Cardiovascular Risk." *Curr Cardiovasc Risk Rep.* 2013; 7:136.

Simpson SJ and Raubenheimer D. "The Nature of Nutrition: A Unifying Framework." *Aus J Zoology.* 2011; 59:350–68.

Cordain L, Hickey MS, Kim K. "Malaria and Rickets Represent Selective Forces for the Convergent Evolution of Adult Lactase Persistence." In *Biodiversity in Agriculture: Domestication, Evolution and Sustainability* (Cambridge, UK: Cambridge University Press).

Wynne-Edwards, KE. "Evolutionary Biology of Plant Defenses Against Herbivory and Their Predictive Implications for Endocrine Disruptor Susceptibility in Vertebrates." *Environ Health Perspect.* 2001 May; 109(5): 443–48.

Li Z, Henning SM, Zhang Y, Zerlin A, Li L, Gao K et al. "Antioxidant-Rich Spice Added to Hamburger Meat During Cooking Results in Reduced Meat, Plasma, and Urine Malondialdehyde Concentrations 1234." *Am J Clin Nutr.* 2010 May; 91(5): 1180–4.

Bengmark S. "Gut Microbiota, Immune Development and Function." *Pharmacol Res.* 2013 Mar; 69(1): 87–113.

De Vadder F, Kovatcheva-Datchary P, Goncalves D, Vinera J, Zitoun C, Duchampt et al. "Microbiota-Generated Metabolites Promote Metabolic Benefits Via Gut-Brain Neural Circuits." *Cell.* 2014 Jan 16; 156(1–2): 84–96.

Straub R. *The Origin of Chronic Inflammatory Systemic Diseases and Their Sequelae* (Academic Press; 2015).

Gurven M, Kaplan H, Winking J, Eid Rodriguez D, Vasunilashorn S, Kim JK et al. "Inflammation and Infection Do Not Promote Arterial Aging and Cardiovascular Disease Risk Factors Among Lean Horticulturalists." *PLoS One.* 2009; 4(8): e6590.

Ege MJ, Bieli C, Frei R, Van Strien RT, Riedler J, Ublagger E et al. "Prenatal Farm Exposure Is Related to the Expression of Receptors of the Innate Immunity and to Atopic Sensitization in School-Age Children." *J Allergy Clin Immunol.* 2006 Apr; 117(4): 817–23.

Aiello LC. "Brains and Guts in Human Evolution: The Expensive Tissue Hypothesis." *Braz. J. Genet. Ribeirão Preto.* 1997 Mar; 20(1).

Ruvolo J. "How Much of the Internet Is Actually for Porn?" *Forbes.* September 7, 2011. www .forbes.com/sites/julieruvolo/2011/09/07/how-much-of-the-internet-is-actually-for-porn.

Hamblin J. "Science Compared Every Diet, and the Winner Is Real Food." *The Atlantic.* March 24, 2014. www.theatlantic.com/health/archive/2014/03/science-compared-every -diet-and-the-winner-is-real-food/284595.

"Why Do Some People Put on Weight and Not Others—And Can We Change It?" *Trust Me, I'm a Doctor* [BBC Two]. Episode 4, Series 4. www.bbc.co.uk/programmes/articles /2lw8qkp7nff7n7mhbxmsy34/why-do-some-people-put-on-weight-and-not-others-and -can-we-change-it.

Chapter 4: On Digestion and Obesity

Bray GA, Smith SR, De Jonge L, Xie H, Rood J, Martin CK, Most M, Brock C, Mancuso S, Redman LM. "Effect of Dietary Protein Content on Weight Gain, Energy Expenditure, and Body Composition During Overeating: A Randomized Controlled Trial." *JAMA.* 2012 Jan 4; 307(1): 47–55.

Goran MI, Ball GD, Cruz ML. "Obesity and Risk of Type 2 Diabetes and Cardiovascular Disease in Children and Adolescents." *J Clin Endocrinol Metab.* 2003 Apr; 88(4): 1417–27.

Halatchev IG, Ellacott KL, Fan W, Cone RD. "Peptide YY3–36 Inhibits Food Intake in Mice Through a Melanocortin-4 Receptor-Independent Mechanism." *Endocrinology.* 2004 Jun; 145(6): 2585–90.

Smith RG. "From GH to Billy Ghrelin." *Cell Metab.* 2009 Aug; 10(2): 82–3.

Kirchner H, Gutierrez JA, Solenberg PJ, Pfluger PT, Czyzyk TA, Willency JA, Schürmann A, Joost HG, Jandacek RJ, Hale JE et al. "GOAT Links Dietary Lipids with the Endocrine Control of Energy Balance." *Nat Med.* 2009 Jul; 15(7): 741–5.

Colagiuri S, Brand Miller J. "The 'Carnivore Connection'—Evolutionary Aspects of Insulin Resistance." *Eur J Clin Nutr.* 2002 Mar; 56(Suppl 1): S30–5.

Esteve E, Ricart W, Fernández-Real JM. "Dyslipidemia and Inflammation: An Evolutionary Conserved Mechanism." *Clin Nutr.* 2005 Feb; 24(1): 16–31.

Alcock J, Franklin ML, Kuzawa CW. "Nutrient Signaling: Evolutionary Origins of the Immune-Modulating Effects of Dietary Fat." *Q Rev Biol.* 2012 Sep; 87(3): 187–223.

McKnight SL. "On Getting There from Here." *Science.* 2010 Dec 3; 330(6009): 1338–9.

Ruiz-Núñez, Begoña et al. "Lifestyle and Nutritional Imbalances Associated with Western Diseases: Causes and Consequences of Chronic Systemic Low-Grade Inflammation in an Evolutionary Context." *J Nutr Biochem.* 24(7): 1183–1201.

Dowling JK. "Unravelling the Anti-Inflammatory Mechanisms of Dietary Fatty Acids [Doctoral]." Dublin City University. School of Biotechnology; 2009 [Cited 2016 Aug 4].

Sun S, Ji Y, Kersten S, Qi L. "Mechanisms of Inflammatory Responses in Obese Adipose Tissue." *Annu Rev Nutr*. 2012 Aug 21; 32:261–86.

Minihane AM, Vinoy S, Russell WR, Baka A, Roche HM, Tuohy KM et al. "Low-Grade Inflammation, Diet Composition and Health: Current Research Evidence and Its Translation." *Br J Nutr*. 2015 Oct 14; 114(7): 999–1012.

Frayn KN. "Adipose Tissue and the Insulin Resistance Syndrome." *Proc Nutr Soc*. 2001 Aug; 60(3): 375–80.

Tönjes A, Fasshauer M, Kratzsch J, Stumvoll M, Blüher M. "Adipokine Pattern in Subjects with Impaired Fasting Glucose and Impaired Glucose Tolerance in Comparison to Normal Glucose Tolerance and Diabetes." *PLoS One*. 2010; 5(11): e13911.

Cao H, Sekiya M, Ertunc ME, Burak MF, Mayers JR, White et al. "Adipocyte Lipid Chaperone AP2 Is a Secreted Adipokine Regulating Hepatic Glucose Production." *Cell Metab*. 2013 May 7; 17(5): 768–78.

Berglund ED, Vianna CR, Donato J, Kim MH, Chuang J-C, Lee CE et al. "Direct Leptin Action on POMC Neurons Regulates Glucose Homeostasis and Hepatic Insulin Sensitivity in Mice." *J Clin Invest*. 2012 Mar; 122(3): 1000–9.

Hauner H, Bechthold A, Boeing H, Brönstrup A, Buyken A, Leschik-Bonnet E et al. "Evidence-Based Guideline of the German Nutrition Society: Carbohydrate Intake and Prevention of Nutrition-Related Diseases." *Ann Nutr Metab*. 2012; 60(Suppl 1): 1–58.

Cholerton B, Baker LD, Craft S. "Insulin Resistance and Pathological Brain Ageing." *Diabet Med*. 2011 Dec; 28(12): 1463–75.

Ohtsubo K, Chen MZ, Olefsky JM, Marth JD. "Pathway to Diabetes Through Attenuation of Pancreatic Beta Cell Glycosylation and Glucose Transport." *Nat Med*. 2011 Sep; 17(9): 1067–75.

Unger RH, Cherrington AD. "Glucagonocentric Restructuring of Diabetes: A Pathophysiologic and Therapeutic Makeover." *J Clin Invest*. 2012 Jan; 122(1): 4–12.

Hoehn KL, Salmon AB, Hohnen-Behrens C, Turner N, Hoy AJ, Maghzal GJ et al. "Insulin Resistance Is a Cellular Antioxidant Defense Mechanism." *Proc Natl Acad Sci USA*. 2009 Oct 20; 106(42): 17787–92.

Johnson AMF, Olefsky JM. "The Origins and Drivers of Insulin Resistance." *Cell*. 2013 Feb 14; 152(4): 673–84.

Williams KJ, Wu X. "Imbalanced Insulin Action in Chronic Over Nutrition: Clinical Harm, Molecular Mechanisms, and a Way Forward." *Atherosclerosis*. 2016 Apr; 247:225–82.

Badman MK, Flier JS. "The Adipocyte as an Active Participant in Energy Balance and Metabolism." *Gastroenterology*. 2007 May; 132(6): 2103–15.

Storlien L, Oakes ND, Kelley DE. "Metabolic Flexibility." *Proc Nutr Soc*. 2004 May; 63(2): 363–8.

Rodin J. "Insulin Levels, Hunger, and Food Intake: An Example of Feedback Loops in Body Weight Regulation." *Health Psychol*. 1985; 4(1): 1–24.

Ahrén B. "Glucagon Secretion in Relation to Insulin Sensitivity in Healthy Subjects." *Diabetologia*. 2006 Jan; 49(1): 117–22.

Berthoud H-R. "The Vagus Nerve, Food Intake and Obesity." *Regul Pept*. 2008 Aug 7; 149(1–3): 15–25.

Ventral Tegmental Area. In: Wikipedia, the Free Encyclopedia [Internet]. 2016. Available from: https://en.wikipedia.org/w/index.php?title=ventral_tegmental_area&oldid =730026894.

Nucleus Accumbens. In: Wikipedia, the Free Encyclopedia [Internet]. 2016. Available from: https://en.wikipedia.org/w/index.php?title ucleus_accumbens&oldid=731923053.

Reward System. In: Wikipedia, the Free Encyclopedia [Internet]. 2016. Available from: https://en.wikipedia.org/w/index.php?title=reward_system&oldid=732386280.

Reinforcement. In: Wikipedia, the Free Encyclopedia [Internet]. 2016. Available from: https://en.wikipedia.org/w/index.php?title=reinforcement&oldid=731653112.

Colocalize. In: Wiktionary [Internet]. Available from: https://en.wiktionary.org/wiki /colocalize.

Acetylcholine. In: Wikipedia, the Free Encyclopedia [Internet]. 2016. Available from: https:// en.wikipedia.org/w/index.php?title=acetylcholine&oldid=732618822.

Yeung EH, Appel LJ, Miller ER, Kao WHL. "The Effects of Macronutrient Intake on Total and High Molecular Weight Adiponectin: Results from the OMNI-Heart Trial." *Obesity (Silver Spring)*. 2010 Aug; 18(8): 1632–7.

Chavan R, Feillet C, Costa SSF, Delorme JE, Okabe T, Ripperger JA et al. "Liver-Derived Ketone Bodies Are Necessary for Food Anticipation." *Nat Commun*. 2016 Feb 3; 7:10580.

Mobbs CV, Mastaitis JW, Zhang M, Isoda F, Cheng H, Yen K. "Secrets of the Lac Operon. Glucose Hysteresis as a Mechanism in Dietary Restriction, Aging and Disease." *Interdiscip Top Gerontol*. 2007; 35:39–68.

Mesolimbic Pathway. In: Wikipedia, the Free Encyclopedia [Internet]. 2016. Available from: https://en.wikipedia.org/w/index.php?title esolimbic_pathway&oldid=732399434.

Chapter 5: Glucose, Guts, and Genes

Dekking EHA, Van Veelen PA, De Ru A, Kooy-Winkelaar EMC, Gröneveld T, Nieuwenhuizen WF, Koning F. "Microbial Transglutaminases Generate T Cell Stimulatory Epitopes Involved in Celiac Disease." *Journal of Cereal Science*. 47(2008): 339–46.

Parodi A, Paolino S, Greco A, Drago F, Mansi C, Rebora A, Parodi A, Savarino V. "Small Intestinal Bacterial Overgrowth in Rosacea: Clinical Effectiveness of Its Eradication." *Clin Gastroenterol Hepatol*. 2008 Jul; 6(7): 759–64.

Figura N, Palazzuoli A, Vaira D, Campagna M, Moretti E, Iacoponi F, Giordano N, Clemente S, Nuti R, Ponzetto A. "Cross-Sectional Study: Caga-Positive Helicobacter Pylori Infection, Acute Coronary Artery Disease and Systemic Levels of B-Type Natriuretic Peptide." *J Clin Pathol*. 2014 Mar; 67(3): 251–7.

Al Khalidi H1, Kandel G, Streutker CJ. "Enteropathy with Loss of Enteroendocrine and Paneth Cells in a Patient with Immune Dysregulation: A Case of Adult Autoimmune Enteropathy." *Hum Pathol*. 2006 Mar; 37(3): 373–6.

Ketelhuth DF, Hansson GK. "Modulation of Autoimmunity and Atherosclerosis—Common Targets and Promising Translational Approaches Against Disease." *Circ J*. 2015; 79(5): 924–33.

Doria A, Zen M, Bettio S, Gatto M, Bassi N, Nalotto L, Ghirardello A, Iaccarino L, Punzi L. "Autoinflammation and Autoimmunity: Bridging the Divide." *Autoimmun Rev*. 2012 Nov; 12(1): 22–30.

Zen M, Gatto M, Domeneghetti M, Palma L, Borella E, Iaccarino L, Punzi L, Doria A. "Clinical Guidelines and Definitions of Autoinflammatory Diseases: Contrasts and Comparisons with Autoimmunity-A Comprehensive Review." *Clin Rev Allergy Immunol*. 2013 Oct; 45(2): 227–35.

Humbert P, Bidet A, Treffel P, Drobacheff C, Agache P. "Intestinal Permeability in Patients with Psoriasis." *J Dermatol Sci*. 1991 Jul; 2(4): 324–6.

Fasano A. "Leaky Gut and Autoimmune Diseases." *Clin Rev Allergy Immunol*. 2012 Feb; 42(1): 71–8.

Sildorf SM, Fredheim S, Svensson J, Buschard K. "Remission without Insulin Therapy on Gluten-Free Diet in a 6-Year Old Boy with Type 1 Diabetes Mellitus." *BMJ Case Rep*. 2012 Jun 21; Pii: Bcr0220125878.

Waterhouse JC, Perez TH, Albert PJ. "Reversing Bacteria-Induced Vitamin D Receptor Dysfunction Is Key to Autoimmune Disease." *Ann N Y Acad Sci*. 2009 Sep; 1173:757–65.

Blasi C. "The Autoimmune Origin of Atherosclerosis." *Atherosclerosis*. 2008 Nov; 201(1): 17–32.

Sollid LM, Jabri B. "Triggers and Drivers of Autoimmunity: Lessons from Coeliac Disease." *Nat Rev Immunol*. 2013 Apr; 13(4): 294–302.

Sapone A, Bai JC, Ciacci C, Dolinsek J, Green PH, Hadjivassiliou M, Kaukinen K, Rostami K, Sanders DS, Fasano a et al. "Spectrum of Gluten-Related Disorders: Consensus on New Nomenclature and Classification." *BMC Med*. 2012 Feb 7; 10:13.

Nijeboer P, Bontkes HJ, Mulder CJ, Bouma G. "Non-Celiac Gluten Sensitivity. Is It in the Gluten or the Grain?" *J Gastrointestin Liver Dis*. 2013 Dec; 22(4): 435–40.

Hadjivassiliou M, Sanders DS, Grünewald RA, Woodroofe N, Boscolo S, Aeschlimann D. "Gluten Sensitivity: From Gut to Brain." *Lancet Neurol*. 2010 Mar; 9(3): 318–30.

Meresse B, Malamut G, Cerf-Bensussan N. "Celiac Disease: An Immunological Jigsaw." *Immunity*. 2012 Jun 29; 36(6): 907–19.

Rieder F, Cheng L, Harnett KM, Chak A, Cooper GS, Isenberg G, Ray M, Katz JA, Catanzaro A, O'Shea R et al. "Gastroesophageal Reflux Disease-Associated Esophagitis Induces Endogenous Cytokine Production Leading to Motor Abnormalities." *Gastroenterology*. 2007 Jan; 132(1): 154–65.

Vojdani A and Tarash I. "Cross-Reaction Between Gliadin and Different Food and Tissue Antigens." *Food Nutr Sci.* 2013; 44:20–32.

Drago S, El Asmar R, Di Pierro M, Grazia Clemente M, Tripathi A, Sapone A, Thakar M, Iacono G, Carroccio A, D'Agate C et al. "Gliadin, Zonulin and Gut Permeability: Effects on Celiac and Non-Celiac Intestinal Mucosa and Intestinal Cell Lines." *Scand J Gastroenterol.* 2006 Apr; 41(4): 408–19.

Carlo Catassi, Julio C. Bai, Bruno Bonaz, Gerd Bouma, Antonio Calabrò, Antonio Carroccio, Gemma Castillejo, Carolina Ciacci, Fernanda Cristofori, Jernej Dolinsek et al. "Non-Celiac Gluten Sensitivity: The New Frontier of Gluten Related Disorders." *Nutrients.* 2013 Oct; 5(10): 3839–53.

Papista C, Gerakopoulos V, Kourelis A, Sounidaki M, Kontana A, Berthelot L, Moura IC, Monteiro RC, Yiangou M. "Gluten Induces Coeliac-Like Disease in Sensitised Mice Involving Iga, CD71 and Transglutaminase 2 Interactions That Are Prevented by Probiotics." *Lab Invest.* 2012 Apr; 92(4): 625–35.

Zhernakova A, Elbers CC, Ferwerda B, Romanos J, Trynka G, Dubois PC, De Kovel CG, Franke L, Oosting M, Barisani D et al. "Evolutionary and Functional Analysis of Celiac Risk Loci Reveals SH2B3 as a Protective Factor Against Bacterial Infection." *Am J Hum Genet.* 2010 Jun 11; 86(6): 970–7.

Spreadbury I. "Comparison with Ancestral Diets Suggests Dense Acellular Carbohydrates Promote an Inflammatory Microbiota, and May Be the Primary Dietary Cause of Leptin Resistance and Obesity." *Diabetes Metab Syndr Obes.* 2012; 5:175–89.

Guandalini S, Polanco I. "Nonceliac Gluten Sensitivity or Wheat Intolerance Syndrome?" *J Pediatr.* 2015 Apr; 166(4): 805–11.

Hollon J, Puppa EL, Greenwald B, Goldberg E, Guerrerio A, Fasano A. "Effect of Gliadin on Permeability of Intestinal Biopsy Explants from Celiac Disease Patients and Patients with Non-Celiac Gluten Sensitivity." *Nutrients.* 2015 Mar; 7(3): 1565–76.

Jobin C. "GPR109a: The Missing Link Between Microbiome and Good Health?" *Immunity.* 2014 Jan 16; 40(1): 8–10.

Nakamura YK, Omaye ST. "Metabolic Diseases and Pro- and Prebiotics: Mechanistic Insights." *Nutrition & Metabolism.* 2012; 9:60.

Feingold KR, Funk JL, Moser AH, Shigenaga JK, Rapp JH, Grunfeld C. "Role for Circulating Lipoproteins in Protection from Endotoxin toxicity." *Infect Immun.* 1995 May; 63(5): 2041–6.

Kootte RS, Vrieze A, Holleman F, Dallinga-Thie GM, Zoetendal EG, De Vos WM et al. "The Therapeutic Potential of Manipulating Gut Microbiota in Obesity and Type 2 Diabetes Mellitus." *Diabetes Obes Metab.* 2012 Feb; 14(2): 112–20.

Bowe WP, Logan AC. "Acne Vulgaris, Probiotics and the Gut-Brain-Skin Axis—Back to the Future?" *Gut Pathog.* 2011; 3(1): 1.

Grześkowiak Ł, Collado MC, Mangani C, Maleta K, Laitinen K, Ashorn P et al. "Distinct Gut Microbiota in Southeastern African and Northern European Infants." *J Pediatr Gastroenterol Nutr.* 2012 Jun; 54(6): 812–6.

Garn H, Neves JF, Blumberg RS, Renz H. "Effect of Barrier Microbes on Organ-Based Inflammation." *J Allergy Clin Immunol.* 2013 Jun; 131(6): 1465–78.

Assimakopoulos SF, Papageorgiou I, Charonis A. "Enterocytes' Tight Junctions: from Molecules to Diseases." *World J Gastrointest Pathophysiol.* 2011 Dec 15; 2(6): 123–37.

Kussmann M, Van Bladeren PJ. "The Extended Nutrigenomics—Understanding the Interplay Between the Genomes of Food, Gut Microbes, and Human Host." *Front Genet.* 2011; 2:21.

Zupancic ML, Cantarel BL, Liu Z, Drabek EF, Ryan KA, Cirimotich S et al. "Analysis of the Gut Microbiota in the Old Order Amish and Its Relation to the Metabolic Syndrome." *PLoS One.* 2012; 7(8): e43052.

Delzenne NM, Cani PD. "Gut Microbiota and the Pathogenesis of Insulin Resistance." *Curr Diab Rep.* 2011 Jun; 11(3): 154–9.

Rook GAW, Lowry CA, Raison CL. "Hygiene and Other Early Childhood Influences on the Subsequent Function of the Immune System." *Brain Res.* 2015 Aug 18; 1617:47–62.

Jayashree B, Bibin YS, Prabhu D, Shanthirani CS, Gokulakrishnan K, Lakshmi BS et al. "Increased Circulatory Levels of Lipopolysaccharide (LPS) and Zonulin Signify Novel Biomarkers of Proinflammation in Patients with Type 2 Diabetes." *Mol Cell Biochem.* 2014 Mar; 388(1–2): 203–10.

Reid G. "Neuroactive Probiotics." *Bioessays.* 2011 Aug; 33(8): 562.

Kelly CJ, Colgan SP, Frank DN. "Of Microbes and Meals: The Health Consequences of Dietary Endotoxemia." *Nutr Clin Pract.* 2012 Apr; 27(2): 215–25.

Pearson JP, Brownlee IA, Pearson JP, Brownlee IA. "The Interaction of Large Bowel Microflora with the Colonic Mucus Barrier." *International Journal of Inflammation.* 2010 Oct 3: e321426.

Pastorelli L, De Salvo C, Mercado JR, Vecchi M, Pizarro TT. "Central Role of the Gut Epithelial Barrier in the Pathogenesis of Chronic Intestinal Inflammation: Lessons Learned from Animal Models and Human Genetics." *Front Immunol.* 2013; 4:280.

Teixeira TFS, Collado MC, Ferreira CLLF, Bressan J, Peluzio M Do CG. "Potential Mechanisms for the Emerging Link Between Obesity and Increased Intestinal Permeability." *Nutr Res.* 2012 Sep; 32(9): 637–47.

Blaser M. "Antibiotic Overuse: Stop the Killing of Beneficial Bacteria." *Nature.* 2011 Aug 25; 476(7361): 393–4.

Koloski NA, Jones M, Kalantar J, Weltman M, Zaguirre J, Talley NJ. "The Brain-Gut Pathway in Functional Gastrointestinal Disorders Is Bidirectional: A 12-Year Prospective Population-Based Study." *Gut.* 2012 Sep; 61(9): 1284–90.

Peterson LW, Artis D. "Intestinal Epithelial Cells: Regulators of Barrier Function and Immune Homeostasis." *Nat Rev Immunol.* 2014 Mar; 14(3): 141–53.

Teixeira TFS, Souza NCS, Chiarello PG, Franceschini SCC, Bressan J, Ferreira CLLF et al. "Intestinal Permeability Parameters in Obese Patients Are Correlated with Metabolic Syndrome Risk Factors." *Clin Nutr.* 2012 Oct; 31(5): 735–40.

Murch O, Collin M, Hinds CJ, Thiemermann C. "Lipoproteins in Inflammation and Sepsis. I. Basic Science." *Intensive Care Med.* 2007 Jan; 33(1): 13–24.

Wendel M, Paul R, Heller AR. "Lipoproteins in Inflammation and Sepsis. II. Clinical Aspects." *Intensive Care Med.* 2007 Jan; 33(1): 25–35.

Amin F, Gilani AH. "Fiber-Free White Flour with Fructose Offers a Better Model of Metabolic Syndrome." *Lipids Health Dis.* 2013; 12:44.

Dandona P, Ghanim H, Bandyopadhyay A, Korzeniewski K, Ling Sia C, Dhindsa S et al. "Insulin Suppresses Endotoxin-Induced Oxidative, Nitrosative, and Inflammatory Stress in Humans." *Diabetes Care.* 2010 Nov; 33(11): 2416–23.

Beck J. "Taking Antibiotics Can Change the Gut Microbiome for Up to a Year." *The Atlantic.* November 16, 2015. www.theatlantic.com/health/archive/2015/11/taking-antibiotics-can -change-the-gut-microbiome-for-up-to-a-year/415875.

"Western Diets Damage Gut Microbiota Over Generations, in Ways Hard to Reverse." *Los Angeles Times.* January 13, 2016. www.latimes.com/science/la-sci-sn-low-fiber-diet-gut -microbiota-generation-20160112-story.html.

Moeller AH, Foerster S, Wilson ML, Pusey AE, Hahn BH, Ochman H. "Social Behavior Shapes the Chimpanzee Pan-Microbiome." *Science Advances.* 2016 Jan 15; 2(1): e1500997 –e1500997.

Lagakos W. "Impact of a Low-Carbohydrate, High-Fat Diet on Gut Microbiota." Calories Proper. December 2013. http://caloriesproper.com/impact-of-a-low-carbohydrate-high-fat -diet-on-gut-microbiota.

Deans E. "The Gut-Brain Connection, Mental Illness, and Disease: Psychobiotics, Immunology, and the Theory of All Chronic Disease." *Psychology Today.* April 6, 2014. www .psychologytoday.com/blog/evolutionary-psychiatry/201404/the-gut-brain-connection -mental-illness-and-disease.

Onuora S. "Rheumatoid Arthritis: Could Glucose Metabolism Be a Sweet Target for RA Therapy?" *Nat Rev Rheumatol.* 2016 Mar; 12(3): 131.

Li X, Atkinson MA. "The Role for Gut Permeability in the Pathogenesis of Type 1 Diabetes—A Solid or Leaky Concept?" *Pediatr Diabetes.* 2015 Nov; 16(7): 485–92.

Shirai T, Nazarewicz RR, Wallis BB, Yanes RE, Watanabe R, Hilhorst M et al. "The Glycolytic Enzyme PKM2 Bridges Metabolic and Inflammatory Dysfunction in Coronary Artery Disease." *Journal of Experimental Medicine.* 2016 Mar 7; 213(3): 337–54.

"Glucose-Guzzling Immune Cells May Drive Coronary Artery Disease, Study Finds." Sciencedaily. February 29, 2016. www.sciencedaily.com/releases/2016/02/160229095432 .htm.

Chapter 6: Personalized Nutrition: The Future Is Now

David Zeevi, Tal Korem, Niv Zmora, David Israeli, Daphna Rothschild, Adina Weinberger, Orly Ben-Yacov, Dar Lador, Tali Avnit-Sagi, Maya Lotan-Pompan, Jotham Suez, Jemal Ali Mahdi, Elad Matot, Gal Malka, Noa Kosower, Michal Rein, Gili Zilberman-Schapira, Lenka Dohnalová, Meirav Pevsner-Fischer, Rony Bikovsky, Zamir Halpern. "Personalized Nutrition by Prediction of Glycemic Responses." *Cell.* 2015 Nov 19; 163(5): 1079–94. DOI: 10.1016/J .Cell.2015.11.001.

Chapter 7: Is There a Case for the Paleo Diet?

Cordain L and Campbell TC. "The Protein Debate. The Performance Menu." www .catalystathletics.com/articles/downloads/proteindebate.pdf.

Richards MP. "A Brief Review of the Archaeological Evidence for Paleolithic and Neolithic Subsistence." *Eur J Clin Nutr*. 2002 Dec; 56(12): 1262–78.

Brooking LA, Williams SM, Mann JI. "Effects of Macronutrient Composition of the Diet on Body Fat in Indigenous People at High Risk of Type 2 Diabetes." *Diabetes Res Clin Pract*. 2012 Apr; 96(1): 40–6.

Ströhle A, Hahn A. "Diets of Modern Hunter-Gatherers Vary Substantially in their Carbohydrate Content Depending on Ecoenvironments: Results from an Ethnographic Analysis." *Nutr Res*. 2011 Jun; 31(6): 429–35.

Mellberg C, Sandberg S, Ryberg M, Eriksson M, Brage S, Larsson C, Olsson T, Lindahl B. "Long-Term Effects of a Paleolithic-Type Diet in Obese Postmenopausal Women: A 2-Year Randomized Trial." *Eur J Clin Nutr*. 2014 Mar; 68(3): 350–7.

Muskiet FAJ. "Adaptation to the Conditions of Existence." *Ned Tijdschr Klin Chem Labgeneesk*. 2006; 31:187–93.

Coyne JA, Hoekstra HE. "Evolution of Protein Expression: New Genes for a New Diet." *Curr Biol*. 2007 Dec 4; 17(23): R1014–6.

Kuipers RS, Joordens JC, Muskiet FA. "A Multidisciplinary Reconstruction of Palaeolithic Nutrition That Holds Promise for the Prevention and Treatment of Diseases of Civilisation." *Nutr Res Rev*. 2012 Jun; 25(1): 96–129.

Shanks N and Pyles RA. "Evolution and Medicine: The Long Reach of 'Dr. Darwin.' " *Philos Ethics Humanit Med*. 2007; 2:4.

Kaplan H, Hill K, Lancaster J, and Hurtado AM. "A Theory of Human Life History Evolution: Diet, Intelligence, and Longevity." *Evol Anthropol*. 2000; 9:156–85.

Raichlen DA, Alexander GE. "Exercise, APOE Genotype, and the Evolution of the Human Lifespan." *Trends Neurosci*. 2014 May; 37(5): 247–55.

Lindeberg S, Cordain L, Eaton SB. "Biological and Clinical Potential of a Palaeolithic Diet." *Journal of Nutritional & Environmental Medicine*. 2003 Sep 1; 13(3): 149–60.

Brand-Miller JC, Griffin HJ, Colagiuri S. "The Carnivore Connection Hypothesis: Revisited." *Journal of Obesity*. 2011 Dec 22; 2012:E258624.

Domínguez-Rodrigo M, Pickering TR, Diez-Martín F, Mabulla A, Musiba C, Trancho G et al. "Earliest Porotic Hyperostosis on a 1.5-Million-Year-Old Hominin, Olduvai Gorge, Tanzania." *PLoS One*. 2012; 7(10): E46414.

Osterdahl M, Kocturk T, Koochek A, Wändell PE. "Effects of a Short-Term Intervention with a Paleolithic Diet in Healthy Volunteers." *Eur J Clin Nutr*. 2008 May; 62(5): 682–5.

Frassetto LA, Schloetter M, Mietus-Synder M, Morris RC, Sebastian A. "Metabolic and Physiologic Improvements from Consuming a Paleolithic, Hunter-Gatherer Type Diet." *Eur J Clin Nutr*. 2009 Aug; 63(8): 947–55.

Jönsson T, Granfeldt Y, Lindeberg S, Hallberg A-C. "Subjective Satiety and Other Experiences of a Paleolithic Diet Compared to a Diabetes Diet in Patients with Type 2 Diabetes." *Nutr J*. 2013; 12:105.

Kuipers RS, Joordens JCA, Muskiet FAJ. "A Multidisciplinary Reconstruction of Palaeolithic Nutrition That Holds Promise for the Prevention and Treatment of Diseases of Civilisation." *Nutr Res Rev*. 2012 Jun; 25(1): 96–129.

Lindeberg S. "Paleolithic Diets as a Model for Prevention and Treatment of Western Disease." *Am J Hum Biol*. 2012 Apr; 24(2): 110–5.

Eaton SB, Konner M. "Paleolithic Nutrition. A Consideration of Its Nature and Current Implications." *N Engl J Med*. 1985 Jan 31; 312(5): 283–9.

Boers I, Muskiet FA, Berkelaar E, Schut E, Penders R, Hoenderdos K et al. "Favourable Effects of Consuming a Palaeolithic-Type Diet on Characteristics of the Metabolic Syndrome: A Randomized Controlled Pilot-Study." *Lipids Health Dis*. 2014; 13:160.

Metzgar M, Rideout TC, Fontes-Villalba M, Kuipers RS. "The Feasibility of a Paleolithic Diet for Low-Income Consumers." *Nutr Res*. 2011 Jun; 31(6): 444–51.

Bligh HFJ, Godsland IF, Frost G, Hunter KJ, Murray P, Macaulay K et al. "Plant-Rich Mixed Meals Based on Palaeolithic Diet Principles Have a Dramatic Impact on Incretin, Peptide YY and Satiety Response, but Show Little Effect on Glucose and Insulin Homeostasis: aAnn Acute-Effects Randomised Study." *Br J Nutr*. 2015 Feb 28; 113(4): 574–84.

Pontzer H, Raichlen DA, Wood BM, Mabulla AZP, Racette SB, Marlowe FW. "Hunter-Gatherer Energetics and Human Obesity." *PLoS One*. 2012; 7(7): E40503.

Bettinger RL. "Prehistoric Hunter–Gatherer Population Growth Rates Rival Those of Agriculturalists." *Proc Natl Acad Sci USA*. 2016 Jan 26; 113(4): 812–14.

Calvez J, Poupin N, Chesneau C, Lassale C, Tomé D. "Protein Intake, Calcium Balance and Health Consequences." *Eur J Clin Nutr*. 2012 Mar; 66(3): 281–95.

Carrera-Bastos P, Fontes, O'Keefe, Lindeberg, Cordain. "The Western Diet and Lifestyle and Diseases of Civilization." *Research Reports in Clinical Cardiology*. 2011 Mar; 15.

Eaton SB, Konner M. "Paleolithic Nutrition." *New England Journal of Medicine*. 1985 Jan 31; 312(5): 283–9.

Lindeberg S, Jönsson T, Granfeldt Y, Borgstrand E, Soffman J, Sjöström K et al. "A Palaeolithic Diet Improves Glucose Tolerance More Than a Mediterranean-Like Diet in Individuals with Ischaemic Heart Disease." *Diabetologia*. 2007 Sep; 50(9): 1795–807.

Jönsson T, Granfeldt Y, Ahrén B, Branell U-C, Pålsson G, Hansson A et al. "Beneficial Effects of a Paleolithic Diet on Cardiovascular Risk Factors in Type 2 Diabetes: A Randomized Cross-Over Pilot Study." *Cardiovasc Diabetol*. 2009 Jul 16; 8:35.

Frassetto LA, Schloetter M, Mietus-Synder M, Morris RC, Sebastian A. "Metabolic and Physiologic Improvements from Consuming a Paleolithic, Hunter-Gatherer Type Diet." *Eur J Clin Nutr*. 2009 Aug; 63(8): 947–55.

Bisht B, Darling WG, Grossmann RE, Shivapour ET, Lutgendorf SK, Snetselaar LG et al. "A Multimodal Intervention for Patients with Secondary Progressive Multiple Sclerosis: Feasibility and Effect on Fatigue." *J Altern Complement Med*. 2014 May; 20(5): 347–55.

Cordain, L. "The Nutritional Characteristics of a Contemporary Diet Based Upon Paleolithic Food Groups." *JANA*. Summer 2002; 5(3): 15–24.

Misner B. "Food Alone May Not Provide Sufficient Micronutrients for Preventing Deficiency." *J Int Soc Sports Nutr*. 2006 Jun 5; 3(1): 51–5.

Novella S. "Vitamins and Cancer Risk « Science-Based Medicine." May 6, 2015. www .sciencebasedmedicine.org/vitamins-and-cancer-risk.

Violanti JM, Fekedulegn D, Hartley TA, Andrew ME, Gu JK, Burchfiel CM. "Life Expectancy in Police Officers: A Comparison with the U.S. General Population." *Int J Emerg Ment Health*. 2013; 15(4): 217–28.

Chapter 8: Rebalancing the Pillars of Sleep, Community, and Movement

Di Rosa M, Malaguarnera M, Nicoletti F, Malaguarnera L. "Vitamin D_3: A Helpful Immuno-Modulator." *Immunology*. 2011 Oct; 134(2): 123–39.

Rosenkranz MA, Davidson RJ, Maccoon DG, Sheridan JF, Kalin NH, Lutz A. "A Comparison of Mindfulness-Based Stress Reduction and an Active Control in Modulation of Neurogenic Inflammation." *Brain Behav Immun*. 2013 Jan; 27(1): 174–84.

Ritterhouse LL, Crowe SR, Niewold TB et al. "Vitamin D Deficiency Is Associated with an Increased Autoimmune Response in Healthy Individuals and in Patients with Systemic Lupus Erythematosus." *Annals of the Rheumatic Diseases*. 2011; 70(9): 1569–74.

Caini S, Boniol M, Tosti G, Magi S, Medri M, Stanganelli I, Palli D, Assedi M, Marmol VD, Gandini S. "Vitamin D and Melanoma and Non-Melanoma Skin Cancer Risk and Prognosis: A Comprehensive Review and Meta-Analysis." *Eur J Cancer*. 2014 Oct; 50(15): 2649–58.

Seyfried TN and Mukherjee P. "Targeting Energy Metabolism in Brain Cancer: Review and Hypothesis." *Nutr Metab* (Lond). 2005; 2:30.

Andersen ML, Alvarenga TF, Mazaro-Costa R, Hachul HC, Tufik S. "The Association of Testosterone, Sleep, and Sexual Function in Men and Women." *Brain Res*. 2011 Oct 6; 1416:80–104.

Cohen C, Janicki-Deverts D, Doyle WJ et al. "Chronic Stress, Glucocorticoid Receptor Resistance, Inflammation, and Disease Risk." *Proc Natl Acad Sci USA*. 2012 Apr 17; 109(16): 5995–99.

Hamer M, Steptoe A. "Cortisol Responses to Mental Stress and Incident Hypertension in Healthy Men and Women." *J Clin Endocrinol Metab*. 2012 Jan; 97(1): e29–34.

Loucks AB, Callister R. "Induction and Prevention of Low-T3 Syndrome in Exercising Women." *Am J Physiol*. 1993 May; 264(5 Pt. 2): R924–30.

Schulkin J, ed. *Allostasis, Homeostasis, and the Costs of Physiological Adaptation* (New York: Cambridge University Press, 2004).

Hawley JA, et al. "Integrative Biology of Exercise." *Cell*. 2014 Nov 6; 159(4): 738–49.

Noakes T, Spedding M. "Olympics: Run for Your Life." *Nature*. 2012 Jul 19; 487(7407): 295–6.

Kilpeläinen TO, Qi L, Brage S, Sharp SJ, Sonestedt E, Demerath E et al. "Physical Activity Attenuates the Influence of FTO Variants on Obesity Risk: A Meta-Analysis of 218,166 Adults and 19,268 Children." *PLoS Med*. 2011 Nov; 8(11): E1001116.

Soskin DP, Cassiello C, Isacoff O, Fava M. "The Inflammatory Hypothesis of Depression." *FOC*. 2012 Oct 1; 10(4): 413–21.

Koren D, Levitt Katz LE, Brar PC, Gallagher PR, Berkowitz RI, Brooks LJ. "Sleep Architecture and Glucose and Insulin Homeostasis in Obese Adolescents." *Diabetes Care*. 2011 Nov; 34(11): 2442–7.

Siervo M, Wells JCK, Cizza G. "The Contribution of Psychosocial Stress to the Obesity Epidemic: An Evolutionary Approach." *Horm Metab Res*. 2009 Apr; 41(4): 261–70.

Gouin J-P. "Chronic Stress, Immune Dysregulation, and Health." *Am J Lifestyle Med*. 2011 Nov 1; 5(6): 476–85.

Gremeaux V, Gayda M, Lepers R, Sosner P, Juneau M, Nigam A. "Exercise and Longevity." *Maturitas*. 2012 Dec; 73(4): 312–7.

Guerra B, Olmedillas H, Guadalupe-Grau A, Ponce-González JG, Morales-Alamo D, Fuentes T et al. "Is Sprint Exercise a Leptin Signaling Mimetic in Human Skeletal Muscle?" *J Appl Physiol*. 2011 Sep; 111(3): 715–25.

Tetley M. "Instinctive Sleeping and Resting Postures: An Anthropological and Zoological Approach to Treatment of Low Back and Joint Pain." *BMJ*. 2000 Dec 23; 321(7276): 1616–8.

Donga E, Van Dijk M, Van Dijk JG, Biermasz NR, Lammers G-J, Van Kralingen KW et al. "A Single Night of Partial Sleep Deprivation Induces Insulin Resistance in Multiple Metabolic Pathways in Healthy Subjects." *J Clin Endocrinol Metab*. 2010 Jun; 95(6): 2963–8.

Knutson KL. "Does Inadequate Sleep Play a Role in Vulnerability to Obesity?" *Am J Hum Biol*. 2012 Jun; 24(3): 361–71.

Leproult R, Van Cauter E. "Effect of 1 Week of Sleep Restriction on Testosterone Levels in Young Healthy Men." *JAMA*. 2011 Jun 1; 305(21): 2173–4.

Ohkuma T, Fujii H, Iwase M, Kikuchi Y, Ogata S, Idewaki Y et al. "Impact of Sleep Duration on Obesity and the Glycemic Level in Patients with Type 2 Diabetes: The Fukuoka Diabetes Registry." *Diabetes Care*. 2013 Mar; 36(3): 611–7.

Broussard JL, Ehrmann DA, Van Cauter E, Tasali E, Brady MJ. "Impaired Insulin Signaling in Human Adipocytes After Experimental Sleep Restriction: A Randomized, Crossover Study." *Ann Intern Med*. 2012 Oct 16; 157(8): 549–57.

Spiegel K, Knutson K, Leproult R, Tasali E, Van Cauter E. "Sleep Loss: A Novel Risk Factor for Insulin Resistance and Type 2 Diabetes." *J Appl Physiol*. 2005 Nov; 99(5): 2008–19.

Gu JK, Charles LE, Burchfiel CM, Fekedulegn D, Sarkisian K, Andrew ME et al. "Long Work Hours and Adiposity Among Police Officers in a US Northeast City." *J Occup Environ Med*. 2012 Nov; 54(11): 1374–81.

Pan A, Schernhammer ES, Sun Q, Hu FB. "Rotating Night Shift Work and Risk of Type 2 Diabetes: Two Prospective Cohort Studies in Women." *PLoS Med.* 2011 Dec; 8(12): e1001141.

St-Onge M-P, O'Keeffe M, Roberts AL, Roychoudhury A, Laferrère B. "Short Sleep Duration, Glucose Dysregulation and Hormonal Regulation of Appetite in Men and Women." *Sleep.* 2012 Nov; 35(11): 1503–10.

Ekirch AR. "Sleep We Have Lost: Pre-Industrial Slumber in the British Isles." *Am Hist Rev.* 2001; 106(2): 343–86.

Watson NF, Harden KP, Buchwald D, Vitiello MV, Pack AI, Weigle DS et al. "Sleep Duration and Body Mass Index in Twins: A Gene-Environment Interaction." *Sleep.* 2012 May; 35(5): 597–603.

Santhi N, Thorne HC, Van Der Veen DR, Johnsen S, Mills SL, Hommes V et al. "The Spectral Composition of Evening Light and Individual Differences in the Suppression of Melatonin and Delay of Sleep in Humans." *J Pineal Res.* 2012 Aug; 53(1): 47–59.

Wang J, Yang D, Yu Y, Shao G, Wang Q. "Vitamin D and Sunlight Exposure in Newly-Diagnosed Parkinson's Disease." *Nutrients.* 2016 Mar; 8(3): 142.

Lindqvist PG, Epstein E, Landin-Olsson M, Ingvar C, Nielsen K, Stenbeck M et al. "Avoidance of Sun Exposure Is a Risk Factor for All-Cause Mortality: Results from the Melanoma in Southern Sweden Cohort." *J Intern Med.* 2014 Jul; 276(1): 77–86.

Holick MF. "Go Ahead, Soak Up Some Sun." *Washington Post.* July 24, 2015. www.washingtonpost.com/opinions/go-ahead-soak-up-some-sun/2015/07/24/00ea8a84–3189 –11e5–97ae-30a30cca95d7_story.html.

Egan KM, Sosman JA, Blot WJ. "Sunlight and Reduced Risk of Cancer: Is the Real Story Vitamin D?" *J Natl Cancer Inst.* 2005 Feb 2; 97(3): 161–3.

Gangwisch JE, Babiss LA, Malaspina D, Turner JB, Zammit GK, Posner K. "Earlier Parental Set Bedtimes as a Protective Factor Against Depression and Suicidal Ideation." *Sleep.* 2010 Jan; 33(1): 97–106.

McGonigal K. "How to Make Stress Your Friend." TED Talks. 2013. www.ted.com/talks /kelly_mcgonigal_how_to_make_stress_your_friend.

Derbyshire D. "Loneliness Is a Killer: It's as Bad for Your Health as Alcoholism, Smoking and Over-Eating, Say Scientists." *Daily Mail.* 2010. www.dailymail.co.uk/health/article-1298225/ loneliness-killer-its-bad-health-alcoholism-smoking-eating-say-scientists.html.

Cheung IN, Zee PC, Shalman D, Malkani RG, Kang J, Reid KJ. "Morning and Evening Blue-Enriched Light Exposure Alters Metabolic Function in Normal Weight Adults." *PLoS One.* 2016 May 18; 11(5): E0155601.

Johnston JD, Ebling FJP, Hazlerigg DG. "Photoperiod Regulates Multiple Gene Expression in the Suprachiasmatic Nuclei and Pars Tuberalis of the Siberian Hamster (*Phodopus sungorus*)." *Eur J Neurosci.* 2005 Jun; 21(11): 2967–74.

Tournier BB, Menet JS, Dardente H, Poirel VJ, Malan A, Masson-Pévet M, et al. "Photoperiod Differentially Regulates Clock Genes' Expression in the Suprachiasmatic Nucleus of Syrian Hamster." *Neuroscience.* 2003; 118(2): 317–22.

Weller RB. "Sunlight Has Cardiovascular Benefits Independently of Vitamin D." *Blood Purif.* 2016; 41(1–3): 130–4.

Zhou H. "Evolutionary Anthropologists Tout Benefits of Human Sleep." *The Chronicle.* January 20, 2016. www.dukechronicle.com/article/2016/01/evolutionary-anthropologists -tout-benefits-of-human-sleep.

Bernstein A. *The Myth of Stress: Where Stress Really Comes from and How to Live a Happier and Healthier Life* (New York: Simon & Schuster, 2010).

Chapter 10: Get Testy! The Plan for Success

Mallappa RH, Rokana N, Duary RK, Panwar H, Batish VK, Grover S. "Management of Metabolic Syndrome Through Probiotic and Prebiotic Interventions." *Indian J Endocrinol Metab.* 2012 Jan; 16(1): 20–7.

Calder PC, Ahluwalia N, Albers R, Bosco N, Bourdet-Sicard R, Haller D et al. "A Consideration of Biomarkers to Be Used for Evaluation of Inflammation in Human Nutritional Studies." *Br J Nutr.* 2013 Jan; 109(Suppl 1): S1–34.

Shah NR, Braverman ER. "Measuring Adiposity in Patients: The Utility of Body Mass Index (BMI), Percent Body Fat, and Leptin." *PLoS One.* April 2, 2012 [Cited August 4, 2016]; 7(4). www.ncbi.nlm.nih.gov/pmc/articles/pmc3317663.

Coelho M, Oliveira T, Fernandes R. "Biochemistry of Adipose Tissue: An Endocrine Organ." *Arch Med Sci.* 2013 Apr 20; 9(2): 191–200.

Ames B. "The 'Triage Theory': Micronutrient Deficiencies Cause Insidious Damage That Accelerates Age-Associated Chronic Disease." www.bruceames.org/triage.pdf.

"Are You Carrying Dangerous Fat Around Your Midsection?" Mercola.com. http://articles .mercola.com/sites/articles/archive/2012/11/14/waist-size-matters.aspx.

Wood LE. "Obesity, Waist-Hip Ratio and Hunter-Gatherers." *BJOG.* 2006 Oct; 113(10): 1110–6.

Virtue MA, Furne JK, Nuttall FQ, Levitt MD. "Relationship Between GHB Concentration and Erythrocyte Survival Determined from Breath Carbon Monoxide Concentration." *Diabetes Care.* 2004 Apr 1; 27(4): 931–5.

Kresser C. "How to Prevent Diabetes and Heart Disease for $16." Chriskresser.com. November 26, 2010. http://chriskresser.com/how-to-prevent-diabetes-and-heart-disease -for-16.

"Fructosamine: Reference Range, Interpretation, Collection and Panels." April 10, 2016. http://emedicine.medscape.com/article/2089070-overview.

Kresser C. "When Your 'Normal' Blood Sugar Isn't Normal (Part 1)." Chriskresser.Com. 2010. http://chriskresser.com/when-your-normal-blood-sugar-isnt-normal-part-1.

Kresser C. "Why Your 'Normal' Blood Sugar Isn't Normal (Part 2)." Chriskresser.Com. 2010. http://chriskresser.com/when-your-%e2%80%9cnormal%e2%80%9d-blood-sugar -isn%e2%80%99t-normal-part-2.

Guyenet S. "Whole Health Source: Glucose Tolerance in Non-Industrial Cultures." Whole Health Source. 2010. http://wholehealthsource.blogspot.com/2010/11/glucose-tolerance-in-non-industrial.html.

Lagakos W. "Insulin Resistance Is a Spectrum." Calories Proper. April 25, 2016. http://caloriesproper.com/insulin-resistance-is-a-spectrum.

Chapter 11: Phase One—The 30-Day Reset

Ströhle A, Hahn A. "Diets of Modern Hunter-Gatherers Vary Substantially in Their Carbohydrate Content Depending on Ecoenvironments: Results from an Ethnographic Analysis." *Nutr Res*. 2011 Jun; 31(6): 429–35.

Kaur B, Chin RQY, Camps S, Henry CJ. "The Impact of a Low Glycaemic Index (GI) Diet on Simultaneous Measurements of Blood Glucose and Fat Oxidation: A Whole Body Calorimetric Study." *Journal of Clinical & Translational Endocrinology*. 2016 Jun 1; 4:45–52.

Chapter 12: Phase Two—The 7-Day Carb Test Plan

David Zeevi, Tal Korem, Niv Zmora, David Israeli, Daphna Rothschild, Adina Weinberger, Orly Ben-Yacov, Dar Lador, Tali Avnit-Sagi, Maya Lotan-Pompan, Jotham Suez, Jemal Ali Mahdi, Elad Matot, Gal Malka, Noa Kosower, Michal Rein, Gili Zilberman-Schapira, Lenka Dohnalová, Meirav Pevsner-Fischer, Rony Bikovsky, Zamir Halpern, "Personalized Nutrition by Prediction of Glycemic Responses." *Cell*. 2015 Nov 19; 163(5): 1079–94. DOI: 10.1016/j.cell.2015.11.001.

Chapter 14: Hammers, Drills, and Ketosis

IOM (Institute of Medicine). 2011. "Nutrition and Traumatic Brain Injury: Improving Acute and Subacute Health Outcomes in Military Personnel." (Washington, DC: The National Academies Press).

Cox P et al. "Nutritional Ketosis Alters Fuel Preference and Thereby Endurance Performance in Athletes." *Cell Metabolism*. 2016; 24(2): 256–68.

Cox and Clarke. "Acute Nutritional Ketosis: Implications for Exercise Performance and Metabolism." *Extreme Physiology & Medicine*. 2014; 3:17.

The Defense Science Board Report On: Technology and Innovation Enablers for Superiority in 2030. The Defense Science Board (DSB). October 2013.

Paoli et al. "Effect of Ketogenic Mediterranean Diet with Phytoextracts and Low Carbohydrates/High-Protein Meals on Weight, Cardiovascular Risk Factors, Body Composition and Diet Compliance in Italian Council Employees." *Nutrition Journal*. 2011; 10:112.

Jordy AB and Kiens B. "Regulation of Exercise-Induced Lipid Metabolism in Skeletal Muscle." *Exp Physiol*. 2014 Dec 1; 99(12): 1586–92.

Gonzalez-Lima F, Barksdale BR, Rojas JC. "Mitochondrial Respiration as a Target for Neuroprotection and Cognitive Enhancement." *Biol Pharmacol*. 2014 Apr 15; 88(4): 584–93.

Prins M. "Diet, Ketones, and Neurotrauma." *Epilepsia*. 2008; 49(Suppl 8): 111–13.

Zou X, Meng J, Li L, Wanhong Han et al. "Acetoacetate Accelerates Muscle Regeneration and Ameliorates Muscular Dystrophy in Mice." *J Biol Chem*. December 8, 2015.

Katz DL and Meller S. "Can We Say What Diet Is Best for Health?" *Annu Rev Public Health*. 2014; 35:83–103.

Cotter DG, Schugar RC, Crawford PA. "Ketone Body Metabolism and Cardiovascular Disease." *Am J Physiol Heart Circ Physiol*. 2013; 304(8): h1060–h1076.

Ford K, Raj A, D'Agostino D. "Ketones and Astronaut Safety, Performance, and Resilience." *IHMC*. 2014 May.

Ford K, Attia P, Clark K, Crook S, Eisenstadt E, Johnson E, Raj A, Rappaport A, Veech R, Volek J. "Enhancing Human Performance: Ketones." *IHMC*. 2012 Oct.

Rich J. "Ketone Bodies as Substrates." *Proceedings of the Nutrition Society*. 1990; 49:361–73.

Shimazu T, Hirschey MD, Newman J et al. "Suppression of Oxidative Stress by β-Hydroxybutyrate, an Endogenous Histone Deacetylase Inhibitor." *Science*. 2013 Jan 11; 339(6116): 211–4. DOI: 10.1126/science.1227166.

Pérez-Guisado J, Muñoz-Serrano A, and Alonso-Moraga A. "Spanish Ketogenic Mediterranean Diet: a Healthy Cardiovascular Diet for Weight Loss." *Nutrition Journal*. 2008; 7:30.

Prins ML and Matsumoto J. "The Collective Therapeutic Potential of Cerebral Ketone Metabolism in Traumatic Brain Injury." *J Lipid Res*. 2014 Dec; 55(12): 2450–7.

Ford K. "Warfighter Performance and Resilience (Ver. 8.2)." *IHMC*. 2012 Dec.

Ford K and Glymour C. "The Enhanced Warfighter." *Bulletin of the Atomic Scientists*. 2014; 70:43.

Schmidt M, Pfetzer N, Schwab M, Strauss I, Kämmerer U. "Effects of a Ketogenic Diet on the Quality of Life in 16 Patients with Advanced Cancer: A Pilot Trial." *Nutr Metab* (Lond). 2011 Jul 27; 8(1): 54.

Priolo C, Henske EP. "Metabolic Reprogramming in Polycystic Kidney Disease." *Nat Med*. 2013 Apr; 19(4): 407–9.

Seyfried TN, Sanderson TM, El-Abbadi MM, McGowan R, Mukherjee P. "Role of Glucose and Ketone Bodies in the Metabolic Control of Experimental Brain Cancer." *Br J Cancer*. 2003 Oct 6; 89(7): 1375–82.

Nishi Y, Hiejima H, Hosoda H, Kaiya H, Mori K, Fukue Y, Yanase T, Nawata H, Kangawa K, Kojima M. "Ingested Medium-Chain Fatty Acids Are Directly Utilized for the Acyl Modification of Ghrelin." *Endocrinology*. 2005 May; 146(5): 2255–64.

Morley WA, Seneff S. "Diminished Brain Resilience Syndrome: A Modern Day Neurological Pathology of Increased Susceptibility to Mild Brain Trauma, Concussion, and Downstream Neurodegeneration." *Surg Neurol Int*. 2014 Jun 18; 5:97.

Cronise RJ, Sinclair DA, Bremer AA. "The 'Metabolic Winter' Hypothesis: A Cause of the Current Epidemics of Obesity and Cardiometabolic Disease." *Metab Syndr Relat Disord*. 2014 Sep; 12(7): 355–61.

Wallace DC. "A Mitochondrial Paradigm of Metabolic and Degenerative Diseases, Aging, and Cancer: A Dawn for Evolutionary Medicine." *Annu Rev Genet*. 2005; 39:359.

Paoli A, Grimaldi K, D'Agostino D, Cenci L, Moro T, Bianco A et al. "Ketogenic Diet Does Not Affect Strength Performance in Elite Artistic Gymnasts." *J Int Soc Sports Nutr*. 2012; 9(1): 34.

Forsythe CE, Phinney SD, Fernandez ML, Quann EE, Wood RJ, Bibus DM et al. "Comparison of Low Fat and Low Carbohydrate Diets on Circulating Fatty Acid Composition and Markers of Inflammation." *Lipids*. 2008 Jan; 43(1): 65–77.

Swerdlow RH, Burns JM, Khan SM. "The Alzheimer's Disease Mitochondrial Cascade Hypothesis: Progress and Perspectives." *Biochim Biophys Acta*. 2014 Aug; 1842(8): 1219–31.

Mattson MP. "Lifelong Brain Health Is a Lifelong Challenge: from Evolutionary Principles to Empirical Evidence." *Ageing Res Rev*. 2015 Mar; 20: 37–45.

Shanley DP, Kirkwood TBL. "Caloric Restriction Does Not Enhance Longevity in All Species and Is Unlikely to Do So in Humans." *Biogerontology*. 2006 Jun; 7(3): 165–8.

Phelan JP, Rose MR. "Caloric Restriction Increases Longevity Substantially Only When the Reaction Norm Is Steep." *Biogerontology*. 2006 Jun; 7(3): 161–4.

Kerti L, Witte AV, Winkler A, Grittner U, Rujescu D, Flöel A. "Higher Glucose Levels Associated with Lower Memory and Reduced Hippocampal Microstructure." *Neurology*. 2013 Nov 12; 81(20): 1746–52.

Varady KA. "Intermittent Versus Daily Calorie Restriction: Which Diet Regimen Is More Effective for Weight Loss?" *Obes Rev*. 2011 Jul; 12(7): e593–601.

Mattson MP, Allison DB, Fontana L, Harvie M, Longo VD, Malaisse WJ et al. "Meal Frequency and Timing in Health and Disease." *Proc Natl Acad Sci USA*. 2014 Nov 25; 111(47): 16647–53.

Rothschild J, Hoddy KK, Jambazian P, Varady KA. "Time-Restricted Feeding and Risk of Metabolic Disease: A Review of Human and Animal Studies." *Nutr Rev*. 2014 May; 72(5): 308–18.

Rothschild J, Lagakos W. "Implications of Enteral and Parenteral Feeding Times: Considering a Circadian Picture." *J Parenter Enteral Nutr*. 2015 Mar; 39(3): 266–70.

Schaumberg K, Anderson DA, Reilly EE, Anderson LM. "Does Short-Term Fasting Promote Pathological Eating Patterns?" *Eat Behav*. 2015 Dec; 19:168–72.

Tóth C, Clemens Z. "A Child with Type 1 Diabetes Mellitus (T1DM) Successfully Treated with the Paleolithic Ketogenic Diet: A 19-Month Insulin-Freedom." *International Journal of Case Reports and Images*. 2015; 6(12): 752.

Wheless JW. "History of the Ketogenic Diet." *Epilepsia*. 2008 Nov; 49(Suppl 8): 3–5.

Keller U, Schnell H, Sonnenberg GE, Gerber PPG, Stauffacher W. "Role of Glucagon in Enhancing Ketone Body Production in Ketotic Diabetic Man." *Diabetes*. 1983 May 1; 32(5): 387–91.

Mobbs CV, Mastaitis J, Isoda F, Poplawski M. "Treatment of Diabetes and Diabetic Complications with a Ketogenic Diet." *J Child Neurol*. 2013 Aug; 28(8): 1009–14.

Aylward NM, Shah N, Sellers EA. "The Ketogenic Diet for the Treatment of Myoclonic Astatic Epilepsy in a Child with Type 1 Diabetes Mellitus." *Can J Diabetes*. 2014 Aug; 38(4): 223–4.

Poff A M, Ari C, Arnold P, Seyfried T N, D'Agostino D P. "Ketone Supplementation Decreases Tumor Cell Viability and Prolongs Survival of Mice with Metastatic Cancer." *Int J Cancer*. 2014 Oct 1; 135(7): 1711–20.

Shen R, Wang B, Giribaldi MG, Ayres J, Thomas JB, Montminy M. "Neuronal Energy-Sensing Pathway Promotes Energy Balance by Modulating Disease Tolerance." *Proceedings of the National Academy of Sciences*. 2016 Jun 7; 113(23): e3307–14.

Dashti HM, Mathew TC, Hussein T, Asfar SK, Behbahani A, Khoursheed MA et al. "Long-Term Effects of a Ketogenic Diet in Obese Patients." *Exp Clin Cardiol*. 2004; 9(3): 200–5.

General Index

References to footnotes are indicated by *n* following page reference.

blood lipids, 52
blood pressure, elevated. *See* hypertension
blood pressure readings, 154–55
"blue blocker" sunglasses, 119–20
blue light, 117
body fat
    effect on appetite control, 49–50
    as fuel source, 221
    visceral, 52, 152–53
body mass index (BMI), 150
body temperature, and sleep, 120, 122
bone density, 132
bone wasting, 53
brain-gut connection, 49–55
breakfast
    carb testing at, 205
    foods for, 171–72, 175
breast milk, 71–72

C

caffeine, 186, 235
calcium, 101, 102
calorie restriction. *See* fasting
calories, 22–23, 131, 166, 224
cancer
    high insulin levels and, 54
    ketogenic diet and, 174, 227–28, 234
    metabolic theory of, 227
    receiving diagnosis of, 86
    reducing risk of, 82, 223
    senescent cells leading to, 51
    from sun exposure, 118
    treating as genetic disease, 227–28
capsaicin, 65
carbohydrates. *See also* low-carb diets; 7-Day
    Carb Test plan
    in 30-Day Reset, 165
    adding variety in, 206
    "bad," permitting, 210
    body's response to, 40–41
    daily amounts, in Paleo diet, 211
    digestion of, 43, 62
    effect on insulin release, 46
    fiber-rich, satiating effects of, 27
    forms of, 40
    as fuel source, 54
    intake, adjusting, 5
    net carb counts, 176
    pro-inflammatory, 63
    refined, digestion of, 62

refined, effect on gut bacteria, 6, 44, 70
volume and weight measurements, 202–4
cardiovascular disease
    cholesterol as predictor of, 160–61
    epidemic of, 12
    high insulin levels and, 53–54
    inflammation and, 51, 63
    Paleo diet for, 94, 95, 96
    role of gut in, 17–18, 57
    sun exposure and, 118
    waist-to-hip ratios and (WHR), 153–54
celiac disease, 40, 68, 69, 73, 74
cell membranes, 59
cells, DNA expression in, 45
change
    resistance to, 84–87, 88–89
    tracking progress, 182
cheating, mind-set of, 8, 137–45
chewing food, 42
chocolate, 185
cholesterol, 98, 160–61, 236
Christofferson, Travis, 228
chronic inflammation. *See* systemic
    inflammation
coconut oil, 229
coffee, 66, 186
cognitive impairment, 114, 221, 222
colon, 44, 62
community, 9, 18, 129–31
The Complete Guide to Fasting (Fung), 229
computers, 116, 120
cooking at home, 193
Cordain, Loren, 74, 100, 101
cortisol, 47, 51, 122
cravings, 114
C-reactive protein, 113
Crohn's disease, 44
cytokines, 68

D

dairy (cow), 72, 73
Deans, Emily, 57
degenerative diseases. *See also specific types*
    anthropological observations of, 92
    mitochondrial dysfunction and, 6–7, 69
    root causes of, 6–7, 94
    systemic inflammation and, 113
    Western, increasing rates in, 14, 32, 69
dementia, 228
dessert effect, 34

fullness. *See* satiety
Fung, Jason, 51n, 229, 231

G
gallbladder, 43
gastrointestinal (GI) tract, 44, 58
General Adaptation Syndrome (GAS) model
    of stress, 124
Glassman, Greg, 182
glucagon, 46, 48, 51
gluconeogenesis, 46, 221
glucose, 40. *See also* blood glucose
gluten
    avoiding, on 30-Day Reset, 193, 202,
      210
    digestibility of, 68
    -free food options, 145, 193
    inflammatory response from, 67, 125
    problems, symptoms of, 145
glycogen, 52
goals, choosing, 188–89
grains
    and celiac disease, 64
    chemical defense substances in, 66–67
    eating in moderation, 64
    effect on gut lining, 71
    volume and weight measurements,
      202
Greenwald, Jim, 104
gut bacteria. *See also* small intestine
    bacterial overgrowth (SIBO)
    altered, link with insulin resistance, 64
    altered, link with type 2 diabetes, 64
    beneficial, 58
    effect on health and disease, 44
    growing in wrong places, 44
    harmful, 44, 58
    of non-Westernized populations, 60
    overgrowth and/or change in, 61, 70
    pathogenic shift in, 63
    properly feeding, importance of, 44
    of urban vs. rural children, 60
    of Westernized populations, 60
    whole grains and beans and, 64
gut health
    damage to gut lining, 58, 61, 71
    food irritants to, 65–67
    immunogenic foods and, 71
    of infants, 71–72
    link with disease, 56–58

gut microbiome. *See also* gut bacteria; gut
    health
    and ancestral diet, 64
    changes throughout history, 17–18
    influence on blood glucose response,
      78, 81

H
hand sanitizers, 17, 60
"hangry"
    as sign of insulin resistance, 152, 183,
      184–85
    what it means, 46
HDL cholesterol, 98, 160, 161
health issues. *See also* diseases
    getting accurate picture of, 149
    lab work for, 149
    major types of, 148
    overlap in, 148–49
    tracking progress in, 149
    treating, importance of, 162
hedonic centers of the brain, 36
herbs, 170
heterozygous individuals, 30–31
high-fructose corn syrup, 40
homozygous individuals, 30–31
hormesis, 223
hormones. *See also specific hormones*
    anabolic, 114
    bonding to receptor sites, 45
    defined, 45
    digestive, primary types, 45
    effect on appetite, 23
    influences on, 6
    released in anticipation of
      food, 41
    sensitivity to receptor sites, 47
hot peppers, 65–66
human cultural evolution
    agriculturalist life, 28–30
    food scarcity in, 220–21
    four pillars in, 15–19
    genetic adaptation, 30–32
    Neolithic foods in, 73–74
hunger. *See also* "hangry"
    becoming comfortable with,
      184
    blunting, with ketones, 223
    glucagon released by, 46
    how we think about, 23–24

hunter-gatherers
anthropological observations of, 92
daily miles walked by, 18
food scarcity of, 221
lifestyle of, 15–16
transition to agricultural life, 29, 74
hydrochloric acid, 42
Hygiene Hypothesis, 60–61
hyperpalatability of food, 17
hypertension, 154–55
hypochondria, 56–57

I
immune system
Hygiene Hypotheses and, 60–61
immunogenic foods and, 71, 125, 201
inadequate sleep and, 114
stress and, 124
immunogenic foods
avoiding, during 30-Day Reset, 201
effect on gut lining, 71
and systemic inflammation, 125
infants, 71–72
infectious diseases, in history, 59–60
inflammation. *See also* systemic
inflammation
effect of fiber on, 62
in gut, 67
markers, 63
and mitochondrial function, 71
prednisone shots for, 47
from sepsis, 63
from stress, 124
insulin. *See also* insulin resistance
low, from underfeeding, 51
receptors, 47–48
released by sight or smell of food, 41–42
role of, 45–46
-sensitive individuals, 47–48, 70, 113,
153
insulin resistance
detecting, 5, 7
fat storage and, 152–53
how it develops, 46, 48, 53
hypertension and, 154
influence on appetite, 184–85
link with gut bacteria, 64
low-carb diets for, 46n, 190
Paleo-type diet for, 231
in police and fire personnel, 104–5

predisposition to, 6
from stress, 124
subjective signs of, 151–52
waist-to-hip ratios and, 153–54
intact gut lining, 43
Internet, 35–37, 116
interval training, 134–35
intestinal permeability, 68–71, 113
intestines. *See* large intestine; small
intestine
iron, 101
irritable bowel syndrome (IBS), 44

J
jerky, 185, 194
journal writing, 120–21
junk food, discarding, 166–67

K
Kendall, Marty, 232
ketoacidosis, 51, 225–26
ketogenic state, 51n
ketone bodies, 222
ketones, 51, 221–23, 225
ketone salts, 229
ketosis (ketogenic diet). *See also* nutritional
ketosis
about, 9
benefits of, 227
cancer and, 174, 227–28, 234
description of, 220–26
downsides of, 236–37
insulin resistance and, 184, 185
keto transition meal plans, 235–39
neurodegeneration and, 228–30
repairing mitochondria with, 70, 133
starvation, state of, 51–52
suggested guidelines, 234–35
therapeutic uses for, 219–40
Transitional Ketosis plan, 174
type 1 diabetes and, 232–33
type 2 diabetes and, 9, 51n, 230–31
weight loss and, 233
kidneys, 53, 54, 154, 155
Konner, Melvin, 93

L
lab tests, 147–48
lactase persistence, 32
Lalonde, Mat, 102

large intestine, 44, 62
LDL cholesterol, 98, 160, 161
LDL-P, 160, 161, 236
leaky gut, 68–71, 113
lectins, 67
legumes, 66–67, 71, 73, 203
lentils, 200–201
leptin resistance, 53, 70
Letter on Corpulence (Banting), 233
lifestyle changes, resistance to, 84–87, 88–89
light, artificial
    blue light, 117, 119–20
    effect on human innovation, 16–17
    effect on sleep, 115, 116
    impact on metabolism, 117
Lindeberg, Staffan, 94
lipids. *See* blood lipids; fats
lipopolysaccharide (LPS), 63
lipoproteins, 161
liver
    damage, from refined carbs, 70
    in digestive process, 43
    excess glucose in, 52
    glucose released by, 47, 51
loneliness, 129–31
low-carb diets
    controversy over, 197–98
    criticisms of, 155
    for insulin-resistant individuals, 46n, 190
    Paleo diet viewed as, 102–3
    police and fire personnel study, 105
    for small intestine bacterial overgrowth (SIBO), 64, 237
    well-known types of, 91–92
lower-fat diets, 190
lunch foods, 173
lupus, 68, 71, 73

M

macronutrients. *See also* carbohydrates; fats; protein
    in ancestral diets, 63
    satiety from, 27–28, 164–65
magnesium, 101, 102, 123
malaria, 29–32
Man v. Food (tv show), 33–34
mattresses, 121
McGonigal, Kelly, 125–26

MCT oil, 174, 229, 230
MCTs, 228–29
meal delivery services, 195
meal plans
    keto transition, 235–39
    nutritional ketosis, 239–40
    30-Day Reset, 174–77
meal trackers, 199
meat, grass-fed, 177
Mediterranean diet, 94–95
medium-chain triglycerides. *See* MCTs
melatonin, 117, 123
mental illness, 57
metabolic syndrome, 150
metabolic ward conditions, 77, 95
metabolism, 54, 223, 224
microbiota. *See* gut microbiome
microvilli, 43
mitochondria
    aging process and, 223
    density, 132–33, 135, 224
    function of, 54
    repairing, 70, 71, 133, 228
mobility, 132
moderators, 191–92
molecular mimicry, 71
monounsaturated fats, 41
morality, and food choices, 37–38, 138–45
mosquitos, malaria-carrying, 29
movement. *See* exercise
multiple sclerosis (MS), 68, 69, 70
muscle glycogen, 52
muscle mass, 53, 132, 134
The Myth of Stress (Bernstein), 126

N

Neolithic culture and foods, 73, 74
neurodegenerative diseases
    Alzheimer's, 4, 6, 14, 40, 57, 227, 228
    ketosis and fasting for, 228–30
    MCT oil supplements for, 229–30
    Parkinson's, 4, 6, 14, 40, 57, 227, 228
    triggers for, 228
neurotransmitters, 23. *See also specific neurotransmitters*
nighttime social life, 116
normal fed state, 54–55
nutrients and nutrition, 26–27, 43–44, 101–2, 176

nutritional ketosis
  following, guidelines for, 174, 234
  increasing information about, 226
  ketone production during, 225
  meal plans, 239–40
  for serious health conditions, 174
  treating epilepsy with, 226
nuts, 167, 185, 194

O
obesity, 12, 14, 17, 46n, 150. *See also*
    overweight individuals
The Obesity Code (Fung), 231
optimum foraging strategy (OFS), 25–27
oral glucose tolerance test (OGTT), 157,
    158–59
organic produce, 177
outcome-based medicine, 77
overfeeding. *See also* overweight individuals
  body's response to, 52–54, 224
  feeling of fullness from, 23–24
  health consequences from, 55
overweight individuals
  aesthetic considerations, 150
  BMI measures, 150
  body fat and, 49–50, 52, 152–53, 221
  correlation with health issues, 149–50
  documenting weight loss in, 151
  obese, 14, 46n, 150
  research on, 149–50

P
palatability of food, 17
palate fatigue, 26–27, 34
Paleo diet
  Autoimmune Paleo (AIP) plan, 70, 174
  carbohydrate sources in, 211
  for cardiovascular disease, 94, 95, 96
  clinical research on, 93–99, 100
  criticisms of, 97, 100–103
  discovery of, 74
  effect on author's health, 74
  foods excluded from, 89
  foods included on, 89, 100–101
  global sustainability of, 103
  highlights of, 89–90
  for insulin resistance, 231
  misconceptions around, 7, 100–103
  nutrients provided by, 101–2
  origins of, 92

overly simplistic view of, 2
real-world example, 211–16
trying foods outside of, 90–91
for type 2 diabetes, 231
using as "rough" tool, 3
viewed as another "low-carb diet,"
    102–3
pancreas, 43, 53, 232
parents, sleep-deprived, 123
Parkinson's, 4, 6, 14, 40, 57, 227, 228
Parsley, Kirk, 109–12, 115, 123
pepsin, 42
Personalized Nutrition. *See also* 7-Day Carb
    Test plan; 30-Day Reset
  detecting problematic foods with, 79
  introduction to, 3–5
  long-term motivation for, 216–17
  Phase One, 5, 87
  Phase Two, 5
  Phase Three, 207–17
  scientific research project on,
    76–82
Phase One, 5, 87
Phase Three, 207–17
  avoiding backsliding, 208
  having "bad carbs" during, 210
  seasonal resets, 207–8
Phase Two, 5
phosphorus, 101
Pillars of Health, 15–20. *See also*
    community; exercise; food; sleep
plants, selective breeding of, 66
police officers, 104–5, 123, 160–61
polyphenolics, 27
polyunsaturated fats, 41
pornography and sex, 35–37
portion sizes, 176
prediabetes, 157–59
prednisone, 47
processed foods, 17, 114, 186
protein
  in 30-Day Reset, 164, 165, 167, 176
  in calorie restricted state, 51
  conversion to glucose, 46
  digestion of, 40, 42, 43
  effect on insulin release, 46
  satiating effects of, 27, 164
  stocking up on, 167
Prozac, 36
Puritan Work Ethic, 115

R

receptor sites, 45, 47
recipe nutritional estimates, 176
registered dietitians, 192
resilience, 126, 127
resistance training, 134
resistant starches, 44
rheumatoid arthritis, 68, 70, 71, 73, 106
rice, 200–201
Richman, Adam, 33–34
Rubin, Gretchen, 191–92
running, 134

S

sardines, 167
satiety
    academic research on, 27–28
    from different macronutrients, 27–28,
        164–65
    how people think about, 23–24
    signals of, 53
saturated fats, 41
school and work, 193–94
seizures, 226
Selye, Hans, 124
senescence, 51
sepsis, 62–63, 70
serotonin, 36
7-Day Carb Test plan, 197–206
    about, 5, 7–8
    blood glucose testing in, 198–99, 205
    information gained from, 204–6
    noting subjective responses to food, 201
    testing carbs in, 200–204
    tracking foods eaten, 199
sex and pornography, 35–37
short-chain fatty acids, 44, 62
showers, 121
SIBO. See small intestine bacterial
        overgrowth
sickle cell anemia, 30–32
skin cancer, 118
skin conditions, 211, 213–14, 215
slash-and-burn process, 29
sleep
    alcohol and, 112, 123, 187
    importance of, 112–13, 196
    improving, strategies for, 119–22
    inadequate, effects of, 8, 109–11, 113–14
    inadequate, reasons for, 115–16, 123

nonprescription aids for, 112
operational definition of, 112
patterns, influences on, 116–19
prescription aids for, 112
prioritizing, 123, 190
statistics on, 17, 115
supplements for, 123
Sleep Number mattresses, 121
Sleep Remedy supplement, 123
small intestine, 42–44
small intestine bacterial overgrowth (SIBO)
    effect on inflammation, 82
    low-carb diets for, 64, 237
    LPS molecules and, 63
    refined carbohydrates effect on, 62, 70
smartphones, 116, 120
snacks, 183–85
social isolation, 9, 18, 129–31
social life, nighttime, 116
sodium, 154, 155
spices, 65–66, 170
sprint interval training, 134–35
starches, resistant, 44
step goals, 133
stomach, acid in, 42, 44
stomach distension, 24
strep throat, 72
stress
    body's response to, 114
    changing our perception of, 8
    from finances, 128–29
    General Adaptation Syndrome (GAS)
        model of, 124
    hormone (cortisol), 47
    recognizing and reframing, 125–28
    from social isolation, 18
    sources of, 125
stretching, 135
sugar, 187
sunblock, 118, 119
sunburns, 118
sun exposure, 116–17, 118–19
sunglasses, "blue blocker," 119–20
supernormal stimuli (SNS), 35–36
sweetened beverages, 186, 187
sweeteners, artificial, 187
systemic inflammation
    AIP protocol for, 174
    from high levels of LPS, 63
    in police and fire personnel, 104–5

systemic inflammation (*cont.*)
  from poor sleep, 113
  from stress, 125
systolic blood pressure number, 154, 155

T
tea, 186
technology, and sleep, 116, 120
television, and sleep, 116, 120
tetracycline, 72
30-Day Reset, 163–96
  about, 5, 7, 164–66
  artificial sweeteners and sugar in, 187
  autoimmune plan—week 1, 180–81
  autoimmune plan—week 2, 181
  benefits of, 87
  beverages, 186–87
  eating out during, 192–93
  evaluating results from, 144, 182, 188–89
  features of, 87
  following guidelines of, after 7-Day Carb
    Test, 206
  Food Matrix, 168–73
  food quantities, 176, 181–83
  ingredient notes, 177
  insufficient progress from, 189–90
  meal delivery services, 195
  meal plans, 174–77
  motivation for starting, 87
  phase one—week 1, 178–79
  phase one—week 2, 179–80
  portion sizes, 176
  "program minimum," 196
  recipe nutritional estimates, 176
  shopping for ingredients, 168
  snacks and, 183–85
  strategies for success, 191–92
  tips and tricks for, 166–68
  work and school considerations, 193–94
time-restricted feeding (TRF), 234–35
toxins, in plants, 26
Transitional Ketosis, 174, 229, 234
trigger foods, 4, 167, 187, 192
triglycerides, 98, 160
triglycerides, medium-chain. *See* MCTs
Tripping Over the Truth (Christofferson), 228
type 1 diabetes, 14, 70, 232–33
type 2 diabetes, 156–62
  causes of, 53, 70
  diagnosis of, 157–59, 230

dietary studies on, 96
elevated ketones and, 51
fasting for, 9, 51n
increase in rates of, 12, 14
ketogenic diet for, 9, 51n, 230–31
link with gut bacteria, 57, 64
muscle and bone wasting from, 53
Paleo-type diet for, 231
symptoms of, 63

U
ulcerative colitis, 44, 72
underfeeding, and metabolism, 50–52, 221
urban life, 16

V
vaginal delivery, 71
vegetables, 167, 177, 203
villi, 43
"virtual" communities, 130
visceral fat, 52, 152–53
vitamin D, 102, 118, 123
vitamins, 44, 101
vitiligo, 211, 213–14

W
Wahls, Terry, 69
waist-to-hip ratios (WHR), 153–54
walking, 134
Warburg, Otto, 227
water intake, 186
water retention, 154, 155
weight lifting, 134
weight loss. *See also* Personalized Nutrition
  environmental challenges to, 5–7
  failed attempts at, 11–19, 21–22
  ketogenic diet for, 233
Western degenerative diseases, 14, 32, 69
wheat, 64, 68
Wilson, Gary, 35–36
wine, 187
work and school, 193–94
Wunderlist app, 175

Y
yoga, 135
Your Brain on Porn (Wilson), 35–36

Z
zinc, 101

Recipe Index